BURN FAT FOR FUEL

FAT TO FABULOUS IN ONLY 28 DAYS

USING MY

REVOLUTIONARY

LIVE IT OR DIET

SYSTEM™

DONNA MICHAELS-SURFACE

WITH

DR. GARY S. SNYDER

Published by the Magni Group, P.O. Box 849, McKinney, Texas 75070

www.magnico.com

Printed in the U.S.A.

ISBN 1-882330-58-7

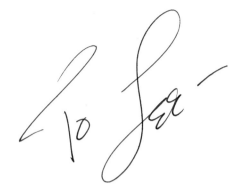

To Lee —

Understanding is the fountain of life to those who have it.
PROVERBS 16:22

Awesome to
meet you,
Hope you
are empowered by
my book. God Bless —
Donna

Recipes by Judith Lynne

Illustrations (Featuring "Minnie Pauz") by Dee Adams
(Minnie Pauz Trademark—Dee Adams/Dream Studio—All Rights Reserved)

Photography by Paul Greco

Design: Paul Perlow Design

This book is not intended to supply a "program." As you will see, we
do not subscribe to a "one size fits all" philosophy.
We recommend that you consult your health care practitioner
before beginning any new regimen.

American College of Sports Medicine recommends
a stress test for individuals over the age of 45 before
beginning an exercise program.

TABLE OF CONTENTS

Please Do Not Skip This Part

(Usually Called "Acknowledgments")

Why do we put this section in a book? It's just more stuff for you to read before you get to the stuff you are looking for, right? Oh, my friend, it is so much more than that. It tells you that an effort like a book just doesn't happen without a team. Even if an author is isolated in some little remote beach shack banging away at an antique Remington, someone still has to recognize the value of the work before it can get to you.

And so, meet my team. This book could not have happened without:

God—my Divine Inspiration. He blessed me with incredible gifts and taught me how to share them.

Ann and Mike—my Mom and Dad. All my life they have been a source of support, comfort, encouragement, boundless enthusiasm for my efforts, and a perpetual example of unconditional love.

Pat—my husband. His gentle nature, beautiful music, patience and understanding, and wonderful humor permeate my life and my work.

Dr. Gary Snyder—my partner. His brilliant direction and constant reminders to "Let go and let God" keep me going.

Judith Lynne—my natural foods expert. Her generosity of spirit, knowledge, and experience has impacted my work (and this book) in countless ways.

Paul Greco—my photographer and oldest friend (not in age, he'll want me to tell you, but in time shared on this planet with me). Paul has been taking my pictures for over 25 years! He is a gifted and special person.

Dee Adams—illustrator and creator of "Minnie Pauz" Dee has a wonderful sense of irony, and "Minnie" keeps the text of this book light and fun. I am very grateful to Dee for allowing "Minnie" to participate in this project.

Marilyn Murray Willison—my editor. Marilyn edited the very first "incarnation" of this book. She taught me style, structure, and appropriate literary license.

Tom Byrne and Jeff Burton—my advisors. Their guidance and council protects Dr. Gary and I in the world of business—a place completely alien to us!

Evan Reynolds—my publisher. He saw in my manuscript something that needed to be shared, and took a chance on an unknown.

Colin Furness—my International Marketing Consultant, and a great friend to Doc Gary and myself. He has elevated the world's perception of this project through his elegant and articulate demeanor. (Always get someone with a British accent on your side. Everything they say is pretty!)

And my circle of clients, colleagues, and friends. This process could not have happened without their commitment and input.

Special love and thanks to: JoJo, Francine, Bobby, Andrea, Cori, Wesley, Chelsea, Austin, and Trevor.

Dr. Gary wishes to acknowledge his family: Jane, Garret, Alexa, Sean, Danny, and his Mom, Dad, and sister, Barbara. Their unconditional love has enriched his life in countless ways. The many years of education, the long hours required in clinical practice, and the commitment required to complete this project would have been impossible without their support.

This book has been a collaboration of experiences, knowledge, and passion. My team and I hope you enjoy it, and grow from it.

Donna

A Note from the Doctor

I t pleases me greatly that you have chosen this book. It has been a constant frustration to me that most of what is contained on these pages has not yet been revealed to you in a comprehensive and organized manner. The mind is like an umbrella—it works best when it is opened. So, open your mind and be prepared to learn, become exasperated, even infuriated, and through this process, hopefully enlightened!

When Donna first came to me over three years ago, she had a variety of symptoms and complaints. Identifying and dealing with Donna's issues was like peeling an artichoke—there were many layers to the heart of it all. With each layer, symptoms abated and relief was found, only to uncover another problem. This is often the case in my clinical practice. Every day I see people who have been failed by conventional methods that only address the symptom, not the "heart" of the matter—the cause. Symptoms are the body's way of talking to us—"Hey, there's a problem here!" Why do we want to silence that communication, that very link to our inner selves But, how often we do that in life—stick a Band-Aid on it and hope for the best.

I've been intending to get a book out there for years, but my research and my practice have kept me so busy it has never happened—until now. Donna was so excited about the work we did together on her problems, she wanted to combine our knowledge and experience in Live It Or Diet. This collaboration is the perfect solution to my dilemma. By directing Donna, I am finally able to get this vital information to you. I am blessed to have at my disposal (and now yours) not only the benefits of my own years of clinical encounters, but the vast world of research and knowledge available to me through many distinguished colleagues and friends. I am equally blessed to be working with Donna and her; passion, honesty, boundless energy, and special gift of communicating often complex information, simply and eloquently.

So, what you will find in this book is Donna's personal journey, along with her exploration of both my 25 years of clinical experience, and the exciting work of doctors I know and admire. Among this long list of brilliant and dedicated colleagues who have enlightened and inspired me (many of whom you will find in this book) are: Dr. John Teale, Dr. C. T. Smith, Dr. Earl Lankau, Dr. Gary Douglas, Dr. Sam Walters, Dr. Ken Brockman, Dr. Steve Bittiker, Dr. David Beaulieu, Dr. Dwight McKee, Dr. Emanuel Revici, Dr. Jeffrey Bland, Dr. Jonathan Wright, Dr. Broda Barnes, Dr. John Lee, Dr. Sydney Baker, Dr. James Braly, Dr. Theodore Baroody, Dr. Devi Nambudripad, Dr. Rob Greenberg, Dr. Harold J. Kristal, Dr. William Kelley, Dr. George Watson, and especially Dr. Dan Clark and Dr. Jack Hinze.

Author Eric Hoffer once wrote: "In times of change, learners inherit the earth while the learned find themselves beautifully equipped to deal with a world that no longer exists." This book is written by learners—for learners.

I applaud you for reaching for this book instead of another Band-Aid.

—Dr. Gary S. Snyder

WELCOME TO MY BOOK

Hi.

I'd like to begin by asking you a question.

If you lost 10 pounds of fat and bloat, how do you think you'd feel?

Lighter? Happier? More confident? More energetic?

More comfortable in your skin?

And wouldn't that be *fabulous?*

Wouldn't you enjoy waking up in the morning...not cowering from your reflection in the mirror? Not having to painfully hold your stomach in...(squeeze-oof-youch-pop)? Not avoiding the scale like it was a serpent coiled up in the corner waiting to strike?

Wouldn't you love to feel loose in your clothes (and need to shop for a smaller size!)? Put on something you haven't been able to wear for years? Demurely respond to the inevitable observations of others with...*Why yes...about 10 pounds, I guess...*

Well???

Mmmmmm...yeah. Sweet satisfaction.

Try this.

Pick up a gallon of milk and a pound of spaghetti.

Now walk around.

Imagine that they are with you when you are doing your housework...walking through a mall...hurrying across the street...strapped to your butt.

Now set them down (heck, throw them out).

Wouldn't that put a spring in your step!

What a difference 10 pounds makes...on anyone!

28 Days.

You could safely lose 8 to 10 pounds of fat and bloat in 28 days.

Now, you could just turn to *PHASE I: Starting The Process-Your First 28 Days* and bypass hundreds of pages of valuable information and nearly 6 years of work to cut to *The Plan, The Program, The Solution, The Chase...*

But I ask you to *not* do that so you can <u>understand</u> what the concept is all about...and become empowered with *knowing*.

Listen. One of the hardest things I have ever learned to do is to focus on the moment—the *journey*—and not the *destination*. I used to look down the road to the result without enjoying the *process*. And, that's really a waste of time, (especially in this endeavor) because becoming fit is not a single event—it is an *evolution*.

I have a lot to share with you.

I have been striving for perfection for 20 years! Am I there yet? Heck no! Perfection is an illusive prize—an ever-changing concept—a subjective paragon that transforms with age, experience, and a taste of reality. And so, we must experience the *experience*—learn and grow and feel satisfaction at the end of the day that we did what we could to become the best we can be. Otherwise, it will be another frustrating obsession that we have willed ourselves to endure. Been there. Done that. Let's try something a little less nerve-wracking, shall we?

Come, take this journey with me.

INTRODUCTION

South Beach. Land of the beautiful people.

If you haven't already witnessed the parade down Ocean Drive where each female is more stunning than the last...let me share this little reality check with you. Either you are a spectator (seated at an outdoor cafe turning three shades of green and wondering whatever in this world possessed you to come to this place with your significant other) or you are a beautiful, skinny participant, slithering down the sidewalk, feeling the admiring gaze of the crowd.

This is the place where models from all over the world come to work. This is the place where the rich and famous frolic in their finery. This is the place where you feel like Gulliver wearing what you thought was a pretty frock (back when you triumphantly purchased it on sale in a department store) until you see designer ads come to life as they sashay before you on a balmy Miami evening.

This is the place where I chose to put my office.

Was I nuts?

As a fitness professional, I have worked with many models. And I've discovered that, in spite of being envied and admired by we "ordinary"mortals, many of them are the most insecure people on the planet. Think about it. Way too much emphasis is put on their looks; all of the attention, the fuss, the attraction is because they are beautiful on the *outside*. It is their job to look "perfect." And when they stop looking that way, they are replaced.

I know, I know...you'd take it if you could. But remember, this is the way

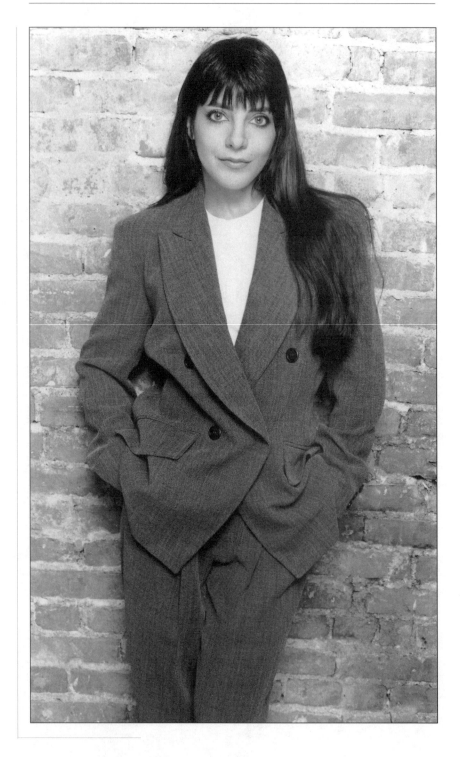

society has set up the world for all women. We are all constantly afraid of being replaced; even when we know we have other compelling attributes. We may be talented, clever, funny, nurturing, compassionate...but, you just can't parade all that stuff down Ocean Drive on South Beach, can you?

My work has evolved to address the women's issues that go beyond the pull of gravity, the deception of the diet industry, and the obsession to compete. We know that we are being victimized by cultural stereotypes, but we still do what we can to fit in—to be acknowledged and desired—to "hang in there" one more year. We buy promises of youth and beauty in the form of diets, pills, surgery, and "fashion" because we somehow got the message that this is our job. Women are supposed to be sexy, stay young, and stay *thin*. A man doesn't get older—he becomes distinguished. His face develops *character*, not wrinkles. His fat is called "love handles."

Cute.

Sorry, guys—but you know this is true. What part of our fat have you given cute names to? *Saddlebags??*

Thank you.

As a woman who has been fat, I know what it is like to live in a body that you are ashamed of. Having conquered that, I know what it is like to feel pride, confidence, and yes, what it's like to strut. And, now that I am 50, I understand how one could struggle with the feeling that life is like Christmas afternoon—when the best stuff is over. How do we come to terms with aging and learn to appreciate what else of value there is to us beyond our looks? How do we give this obsession up, and gracefully, elegantly glide into another phase of life with dignity and purpose? Youth is such a short event in the game of life. Why can't we go into overtime? It is, after all, wasted on the young, isn't it?

When I first began writing this book, the title was, *How To Get A Little Behind In A Big Hurry*, and my focus was primarily superficial, external concerns. This was also how I functioned in life—"Hi, this is my body." But, my journey has profoundly impacted my perception, and my message. I have learned that we must nurture all of the other aspects of ourselves that are truly valuable, and that without building a body on a solid foundation of health and well-being, all you really have is a facade—empty on the inside and doomed to crumble with time and stress.

My story is not just of a woman who transformed her physical body, but it is also about a woman who obsessed over this physical body to the point of believing it was the only thing of value she possessed. So, what happens when you need to look behind you to see fifty? Better get a new perspective or you'll wind up directing traffic in Times Square— pushing all of your possessions around in a shopping cart muttering, "I'm ready for my close-up, Mr. DeMille." This book is no longer just about how to get a "little behind" and keep it through menopause, but it explores the means to obtain optimum health and wellness. It also examines the psychological and emotional aspects of dealing with the aging process, the signposts that signal the absence of self-love, the profound value of spiritual growth, and how to mature without getting *old*.

Mature. I've always hated that word. As Webster defines it, to mature is to: Age, mellow, harden, ripen (yuck). But it also means to unfold, progress, and evolve. Although this book has been written for both women and men, there are sections that speak directly to women who are entering and *leaving* the fourth decade of life. Some people call the fourth decade "The Passage Decade," but does this have to mean that these years are where we are passing from a gloriously unbridled time of youth to a dismally restricted time of old age?

We are the baby-boomers—78 million strong! Nearly every second one of us is turning fifty. Imagine. Wasn't it just yesterday when we were all dancing ecstatically in the rain to the sounds of Jimmy Hendrix in an obscure little town in upstate New York? How did we get here? Where is the manual for this time of life? How are we supposed to act? How are we supposed to feel? And, dang it...*how are we supposed to look??* What is the best we can hope for? When there is no schematic to work from...well you just can't seem to construct the thing, can you? How do I function without instructions? What tool do I use? Hold it...who took my tools?? The search for these tools has been the most formidable challenge of my life.

I have spent the past six years researching and writing this book, which is a vivid journey through the minefields in the diet industry terrain. It explores all of the conventional and opposing philosophies and asks the question: "When are 'they' going to stop treating us like laboratory rats!" I've read over 200 books, studies, and articles on nutrition, exercise, and aging, and I discuss the many paradigms out there. You will read verbal tennis matches between doctors—with baby-boomers being the "ball." Back and forth—back and forth—where is the truth? The extraordinary opposition between experts in their respective fields leads to one conclusion: We must each discover our own uniqueness, and build a nutrition/exercise/anti-aging/lifestyle game plan on this foundation of knowledge. Certain concepts, however, *do* keep making appearances throughout the following chapters. Pay very close attention to them. They are some of the few things my sources agree on.

This book is intended to amuse you as well as educate you. I have punched the text with cartoon illustrations to underscore the irony in the baby-boomer's unique time of life...with all of its challenges and confusion.

"Minnie Pauz," a creation by Dee Adams, makes an appearance here and there to depict our determination...and frustration. I've been on my own "Roller-coaster Ride From Hell," and have suffered like countless other females, but in that is humor. There has to be. Research shows that a happy person gets sick less frequently than an unhappy person. *The surly bird gets the germ,* my friend. Laugh...and learn.

As we age, maintaining a youthful physique does become more challenging for both sexes. But, we mature women are not only dealing with the already confounding and complex matter of unwanted fat, we also have to cope with the depressing domino effect caused by the interactive dance of our fickle, sputtering hormones. It is not our imagination that our bodies bloat by five pounds in a single day. It is not our lack of discipline that makes it more difficult to lose fat now. Our bodies seem to betray us. Sometimes we believe they're downright alien! Certain foods attack us. Our hormones decline and then surge, thus manipulating our responses to food, stress, and life in general.

The aging process comes with lots of little free "gifts;" increased body fat, decreased muscle mass, hormonal changes, free radical damage, cellular death, and many more goodies that are not on your wish list. How many of these consequences can we control? Depending on which book or scientific journal you read, the answer is either: All, some, or none of the above. The problem with citing just one of these findings is that it does not give us the whole picture, and if I have learned one thing during this quest, it is that all of these principles and arguments relate back to one another in an intricately directed play perpetually performed by the mechanisms of our bodies. One actress forgets her lines...and the play falters! (I just love metaphors, as you will see throughout this book.)

I believe that we have been tragically misled in the arenas of health, fitness and nutrition. My work takes me to cities all over the country, and some of the most rewarding moments of my life happen at the seminars that I give in all of these different places to people with common issues. There are so many of us out there...so many confused and frustrated people who simply do not know which direction to turn in anymore. And, as my story unfolds, they lean forward and listen harder as they realize I'm one of them...and I might have something new to say. My lecture is not just another "sharing" of a personal battle with high body fat and low self-esteem. I am presenting alternatives to the standard guidance that has disillusioned us all. The application of this tailored knowledge to my daily life has been greatly responsible for the woman who stands before her audience, and I do not know who has more urgency...they, to learn...or I, to teach.

Let me put it to you this way (look out, here comes another metaphor).

Did you ever buy one of those jigsaw puzzles that come in a big box? On the cover of that box was a beautiful picture that promised to be the outcome of the persistence and discipline required to piece together the hundreds of complex little configurations that you eagerly dumped on the table. Then, didn't you find that it was a more challenging and frustrating event than you imagined when you first decided to purchase it? Consider that the puzzle in that box is *you*, and all of the tiny pieces within that box must precisely fit together to create the complete and beautiful you pictured on the cover. You cannot cheat, or leave any piece out, or it will not complete your picture. Each piece represents a separate issue or component that must be present for optimum health and fitness. But, remember that we are all unique, so the puzzle pieces within each of our boxes will vary in size and shape from individual to individual. Some issues may be of more concern to you than others, so those particular pieces of your puzzle will be larger, and require a more predominant position in your picture. My intention is to acquaint you with many of the components it will take to help successfully complete your puzzle. What should you do???" Well, the answer my friends *is different for everyone*. I am an enigma. Aren't *you*? Ultimately, I have learned that the most rewarding approach is a combination of many distinguished individuals' works. With the direction of Dr. Gary Snyder, I have synthesized and incorporated these works in this book.

I will also introduce to you *Live It Or Diet Lifestyle Systems*, our schematic for constructing individualized weight-management systems. "Dr. Gary," (as he is referred to throughout the text) guided me through the incredibly confusing, (treacherous) and constantly colliding worlds of conventional and alternative medicine and nutrition. Together we developed several applications of *Live It Or Diet Lifestyle Systems*: Clinical (for pharmacies and different types of medical practices), health club industry, and our virtual *Live It Or Diet Lifestyle Center*, LiveItOrDiet.com.

So, don't look for a "program" in this book. That would conflict with our philosophy of one *size does not fit all*. Instead, we offer a "Phase One" plan that will help you begin on your own discovery cruise. *A Live It Or Diet Lifestyle System* can be built for you at one of our many locations, and not taken "off the rack." After all, my friend, haven't you finally had it with blindly following the program du jour? When you bang into the concrete wall that ultimately awaits you at the dead end of one of these programs and open your eyes—the sign that you see clearly reads FAILURE, doesn't it?

Enough of that nonsense!

CHAPTER 1

THE ROLLER-COASTER RIDE FROM HELL

When I tell people I wasn't born this way, I mean that literally—*genetically* speaking, I wasn't born this way. My siblings were slender, athletic, fearless wildcats. I came out a chunky, unathletic scaredy-cat. And back when I was a kid, President Kennedy was enthusiastically enforcing his "Council on Physical Fitness," which meant we had to go to the gym. So, there I was, in my olive-drab gym-suit (remember how flattering *those* things were?), humiliated, mortified, and tearful as I attempted to participate in the mandatory program under the militant direction of our frustrated drill sergeant/gym teacher. I was hopeless, and neither she nor my classmates were patient with my lack of athletic prowess. I was always the last to be picked for any team. The gymnastic horse loomed before me like a giant monolith, I couldn't connect a bat with a ball if it were the size of a bean bag chair, jump hurdles...you want a real laugh? Tumbling, running, you name the event, I was the clumsiest, the slowest, and the least confident.

Thankfully all that has changed, and I'm now strong, secure, and fit. The point is that you do not have to be a *born* athlete. I would give anything to reconnect with the genetic wonders of my youth—the competitive, spunky, aggressive little dynamos, the adorable, agile, ever-popular cheerleaders, the girls who won the hearts of the captains of the school athletic teams; the pretty, perky, fit little prom queens from 30 years ago. I do not know what's become of them, but I know that *I* conquered my genetics and my fears—as I learned to replace my resignation and failure with fierce determination and success.

1

WHO AM I?

I have spent most of my life trying not to answer that question. Although in the 60's it was fashionable to exclaim to anyone who would listen that "I am finding myself," it seemed that I looked everywhere but where *I* was. If the 60's were about "finding yourself," then the 70's were about "throwing yourself away." Of course, the 90's are about "learning to love yourself." What will the new millennium bring us..."get over yourself, already?"

This brings me to why I am compelled to write. I want to share my quest for an enduring positive self-image with others who are also in search of this elusive prize. And, as I reflect on my journey through life thus far, I am at once horrified and amused. At times, my only comment can be "what lunacy."

Well, I guess you do not survive as much "lunacy" as I have without purpose. Yes, I feel that I've learned and grown and evolved, in part by applying my lessons in the positive, enlightened manner that befits a 90's inhabitant of the "New Age." But, at the risk of appearing obsolete, I must admit to you that I really do not subscribe to the overtly celestial attitudes of the day. The past few decades have provided me with a fool-proof approach to growth— if you slam into something hard enough and it doesn't move, eventually you'll need to go around it or over it or *under* it to get anywhere. And as I've propelled my bruised and battered soul through these fifty years, I have been (and still am) strengthened by my obstacles. This book is a presentation of my obstacle course, and I offer this volume of personal discovery to you as a beacon in the distance, signaling a refuge from confusion. For, if you are like me, your journey has left you in deep, uncharted waters, too—halfway between a place that was cruel, but familiar—and a promising, but alien shore. Well, land ho, my friends. You already know it's futile to go back, and I know you can reach the other side. If I did (even if it was with controlled drowning), anyone can.

THE THIN WORLD

My odyssey into this uncharted territory began in my senior year of high school when I was preparing to go to college. I desperately wanted to be thin. Thin was in—Twiggy set the standard—and "Future Homemakers of America" was replaced by "Future Anorexics of America." Genetically short, round females like me were definitely not in vogue. I had to do <u>something</u> so I would be popular in college. So, I went on my first DIET.

Graham crackers. I loved them. So, <u>they</u>, I decided, would be my diet. Graham crackers for breakfast, lunch, and dinner. It worked. Nutritionally and metabolically speaking, of course, it was a catastrophe. But the scale said 87 pounds, and I was ecstatic. Bring on the fraternities, the beer blasts...

THE DORM FOOD.

And so began *"The Roller-coaster Ride From Hell."* Dorm food, of course, included the four major food groups: Starch, sugar, fat, and macaroni and cheese. So, with a metabolism in the dumper, by Thanksgiving vacation I was 135 pounds! (Since I'm only five feet tall, you've got to figure that's probably not an appropriate weight for me.) I was unrecognizable to my family. My father wanted to know what I had done with his little girl... "eaten her?" I wore a ton of makeup and streaked my dark hair blonde in a vain attempt to call the attention away from my body. I was probably the only virgin on campus, but I looked like "The Whore of Babylon." What happened to my precious graham-cracker-starved dream of popularity? It went into the dumper along with my metabolism.

Enter DIET #2. In Third World countries it's called starvation. In America in the late 60's it was called *fasting*. Very trendy, and very effective. I dropped 35 pounds— along with my eyelashes, clumps of my hair, and a couple of teeth—not to mention that most of what I lost was muscle, and, viola, I was once again a "skinny fat person." But who knew? And who cared? Certainly not me. The scale said 100, and I was on my way down. Really down.

Time to return to school. The dead of winter in Potsdam, New York, where the average temperature was 30 below zero and the most popular activity was staying indoors. And ordering pizzas and heroes. All night. You could *hear* your body grow. In two months I was up to 150 pounds. I couldn't stand with my feet together; my thighs were in the way. I was <u>fat</u>. I hated me. I used to back out of rooms so people wouldn't see how wide my butt was. I wore muumuus. I couldn't have run a half a block if Godzilla were chasing me. I started smoking because someone said it cut down your appetite. I got up to two packs a day, and found that a cigarette was just the thing after a large meal. Or with a drink. It worked with gluttony. I heard it was good after sex as well, but I still hadn't experienced *that*. Expose my fat butt to a man? *No one* saw me naked, let alone a man. *I* wouldn't even look at me in the nude.

Summer vacation. Time to wear next to nothing, go to the beach, play volleyball, parade on the boardwalk. Who's kidding whom? I might as well have been in Siberia. I was taking this act *nowhere*.

Then, I discovered speed—diet pills, crystal methadrine, amphetamines— WOW! Guess what happened? Again, I got down to 87 pounds. Almost immediately. Of course I didn't want to develop a habit so I only "used" on the weekends. I would literally be up from Friday to Monday, eating absolutely nothing and jabbering nonstop. Monday it was back to old behavior, and by Thursday I was invariably 20 to 30 pounds heavier. But that's okay. The next day was Friday and it would all be gone by Saturday. I carried on like this for a whole year. Guess what happened to my thyroid? And I did sacrifice a few more teeth. Well, there's always bridgework. Anyway, none of that mattered. For three days out of every week I was <u>skinny</u>! It's funny though, when I look at pictures of myself from back then, my basic shape was the same as when I was fat—hips wider than my shoulders, tube arms, flabby legs. I looked like death. I felt even worse. But the alternative—no way.

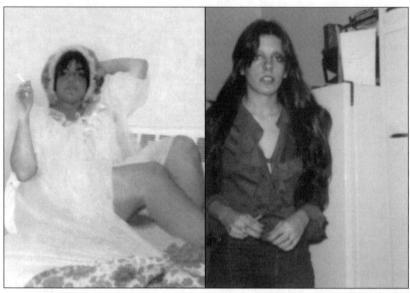

FROM ONE EXTREME...
A butt "the size of New Jersey"...weighing in
somewhere between 135 and 140 pounds.
(The outfit was a joke..but the cigarette, and the
thighs were not!)

...TO THE OTHER
The "speed freak" look...
No sleep (or food) for three days,
But the scale said 87 pounds!

THE SUMMER OF LOVE

It was 1969, and I was 19 years old. Woodstock—drugs, sex, rock and roll—free love. I wanted to start having sex, so I went on the pill. But, nothing's free, babe, and the price I paid for this bright idea was that my fat got fatter. Oops. Not acceptable. So my doctor informed me of a handy little device he could insert and my troubles would be over. He neglected to say *permanently.*

4

The IUD—Intra-Uterine Device—was my ticket to intimacy without the embarrassment of an even fatter butt. It was also my ticket to the emergency room at Bellevue Hospital in New York City. That is where I was rushed when I was found on the floor, passed out, with a raging fever and an abdomen distended as if I were nine months pregnant. I had Pelvic Inflammatory Disease—PID from an IUD. And a few other complications as well; peritonitis, endometriosis, possible sterility. Also, I had a fever that was as high as a human's could go without "checking out." In a hospital where the state picks up the tab, there aren't too many amenities, so I was in a ward with twenty other women. They came and went one way or the other. I stayed, hooked up to IVs, for a month.

Do you know what happens when the only nourishment you have for a month is intravenous glucose and Jell-O? You get skinny. You waste away to nothing. I left Bellvue weighing 80 pounds. I had lost so much muscle and strength that I couldn't move on my own. I was so wasted that even I didn't like the way I looked. And almost every pound I gained back during recovery was fat. Purchase your tickets here, ladies, to *"The Roller-coaster Ride From Hell."*

IN SEARCH OF ANOTHER DIET.

If it was published, I bought it. "The Fruit Only Diet," "The Carbohydrate Only Diet," "The Protein Only Diet," "The Liquid Only Diet," "The Air Only Diet," you name it, I tried it. I lost 50 pounds—twelve times. By the time I turned 30, I practically had only fat hanging from my bones. I lived in high heels to raise my "wide load" up farther from the ground so it would appear smaller, and virtually every millimeter of me jiggled when I moved. My triceps continued to "wave good-bye" long after I'd stopped, and I couldn't tell where my butt ended and my hamstring began.

I became very depressed. No matter what I tried to do to stay thin, I always failed. I remember thinking, after the *gazillionth* attempt at losing weight, "I might as well face it, I am a fatso and I am destined to always be a fatso." Nothing to do but eat, I guess. I was a "closet eater"—you know the type. No one ever sees you eat. You get phantom fat from phantom food. We think we're so clever. We think you believe air makes us fat! " I just don't get it, must be her thyroid." Yes, yes—that's it, my ole' dead thyroid. Darn thing just doesn't work. I was so disappointed in myself; I really didn't care what I did to myself. I smoked like a chimney, I drank with a vengeance, and I ate without any consideration for what I was sticking in my mouth. I abused my body so vehemently that it is a miracle I saw my thirtieth birthday.

And then came the car accident that was the last assault on my body that

I would endure. Our car was broadsided, and my right knee was history. Well, almost. The grand finale was performed by the surgeon. I was handed a cane, and movement, as I knew it, was over. I learned what and where my "femur" was because I could literally push into my thigh and <u>feel</u> it. That's how atrophied my right leg had become by dragging it around with a cane. I could actually feel the bone in my upper leg. That did it! Not only was I fat, but I was so soft I could feel my bones!

ONE LAST CHANCE

I was desperate. Desperate people do desperate things. So, I bought a subscription to "Muscle and Fitness Magazine." Radical, huh? The first time I looked through this "body-building" magazine, I was astonished by what I saw—hard, shapely, beautiful female bodies. I had never seen women like that. I didn't know it was possible. Muscle. Defined, sleek, gravity-defying muscle. Gluteals separated from hamstrings, biceps reaching out from under deltoids, triceps firmly inserted with all three heads etched against the skin, cleavage proudly displayed as pectoral muscle not breasts, abdominals carved out in sections...WOW!

I wanted muscles like *that*. But, to get them, I needed to join a (horrors) gym. It took almost a year before I had the guts to drag my demolished body into a public place that housed the bodies I saw in that magazine. Finally, clad in four layers of camouflage, I joined my first gym. Deja vu. Remember the gym class of my youth—how conspicuous and humiliated I felt? Well, here I am again, in

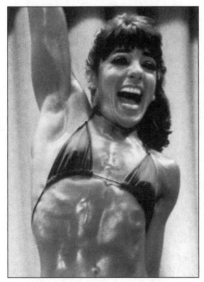

a place where I clearly did not belong, watching little hard bodies confidently strut around. But, this time —instead of feeling defeated—I silently vowed to myself that I would overcome my genetics, my lack of discipline and willpower, my addiction to food, my bad habits, my low self esteem—and I would become a *bodybuilder*.

AWARD WINNING ATHLETE!

Bodybuilding saved me. Not only did it save my metabolism by adding the muscle that my body so desperately

"My First Victory"

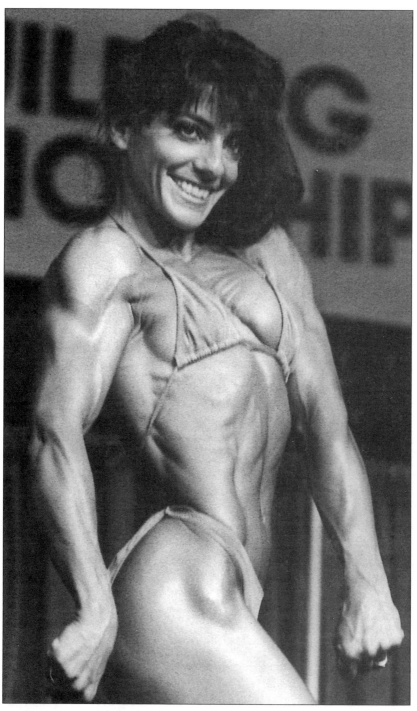

"Placing At The Nationals"

needed to stabilize, but, as my body developed, so did my confidence, my pride, and my sense of "self." I was finally an *athlete*. I was good at something. Encouraged by everyone at the gym who witnessed my metamorphosis, I decided to actually compete—to stand on stage in a bikini in front of an audience and have my body publicly judged! I placed second in my first competition. After that, I won everything for two years, and qualified to become a national competitor. But, at my first national event (held in Las Vegas that year), I had a little reality-check. My fellow competitors made me look like nothing more that a "fitness enthusiast." On a national level, the women looked like—well, men. The sport had gone in a direction that I had not, and I was left in the dust. But, I was determined to make a noise in bodybuilding without steroids, so for the next year of my life I ate steak every day, trained like an animal, *and gained 20 pounds*! Well, I was fat again. But under that fat was muscle. I had to diet down to that muscle and then get "shredded," so, four months before the USA Nationals that were being held in Texas, I began my contest diet. I knew I couldn't be the biggest competitor on stage, but I was determined to be the most *defined*. Bodybuilding is healthy, but competitive bodybuilding is not. It requires behavior and methods too radical to support a healthy lifestyle. You "bulk up," and then you "cut up." Here comes the *"Roller-coaster Ride From Hell,"* again. Didn't I get off this ride a few years back? Well, I bought another ticket and almost killed myself this time. I weighed in at 94 shredded pounds, and though I was emotionally elated, I was physically destroyed. I achieved this little "victory" by almost total caloric depletion, dehydration, constant cardio and caffeine. No drugs, but I still paid a big price. I did place at this event, then went back to my hotel room and hemorrhaged, and continued to bleed every day for almost a year. My hormones were completely whacked. I lost more teeth (no, I don't wear dentures, but I was headed in that direction), I shot out my thyroid, became hypoglycemic, broke out in a body rash that was out of control for months...but I was nationally ranked. I got in the magazines. I was a recognized athlete. The price tag for this dubious honor? A real steal—only my health. Obviously, it is not good to bounce around extremes.

Balance.

Did I finally learn that lesson? Hey, you don't have to hit me over the head with a brick...much. There are terrifying consequences to the kind of obsessive behavior that I indulged in. Tragically, one doesn't think of that at the time. I could be a candidate for flying jets with the magnificent hindsight that I now possess. I consistently robbed my body of so many vital nutrients during the twelve years before bodybuilding, and then again when I competed, that I nearly destroyed it. Fortunately, I went back to school to prepare for my American College of Sports Medicine exam (like the "bar" exam for my field), and I studied anatomy, kinesiology, physiology, and nutrition—and I am now the product of some clear choices I have made regarding exercise and food. It's no real trick to have a butt that defies gravity at the age of 24, but at twice that age, well, I have learned a thing or two about that.

But, I also know that transforming a butt the size of New Jersey into little melon balls is not all there is to life.

A woman, whether in South Beach or Seattle, is a creature of many lay-ers—each of which deserves to be acknowledged, nurtured, and appreciat-ed. After all, it is the *contents*, not the *container* that has any real value. So, let's celebrate our contents...as we begin the glorious process of restoring the vehicle that transports this precious cargo through life.

CHAPTER II

U n d e r C o n s t r u c t i o n

Upon crossing the piazza with a large piece of marble, Michelangelo was stopped and asked, "Hey, Mike, whatta you gonna do with that marble?"...to which Michelangelo replied, "Attsa no just marble...there's an angel in there."

I was a sculpture major my first go-round in college. I delighted in transforming shapeless masses of clay into beautiful human forms. I would look at this gray lump in front of me...and see my work of art.

Funny how later on in life I applied that same vision to...well, me. I just threw a tarp over my shapeless mass and pronounced it "a work in progress." Nobody got to judge it while it was "under construction." What artist displays an unfinished work? That's how you need to see yourself...as a work of art in progress. Remember...there's an angel in there.

This chapter will provide you with your sculpture tools.

Strength Training is one of them.

Many of the dramatic changes in the way your body looks are keyed into your muscle, so we cannot neglect this component and expect any drama. And the primary focus of many of my programs is on the *bain of every woman's existence*; THE BUTT, the hips, the thighs, the whole unruly mess below the Mason Dixon Line that seems to creep a little farther south with each passing year. Yes, we need to lose body fat and we naturally expect cardiovascular exercise to be the answer to that, but as you will learn in this book, it's not the *only* answer. Muscle is a huge determining factor in how lean you are. In my work, I have always encouraged and taught strength training to women. Determined to include this invaluable element in every client's program, I developed exercises and created protocols that were used in precise sequences that "fail" the muscle without heavy weights. This is the only

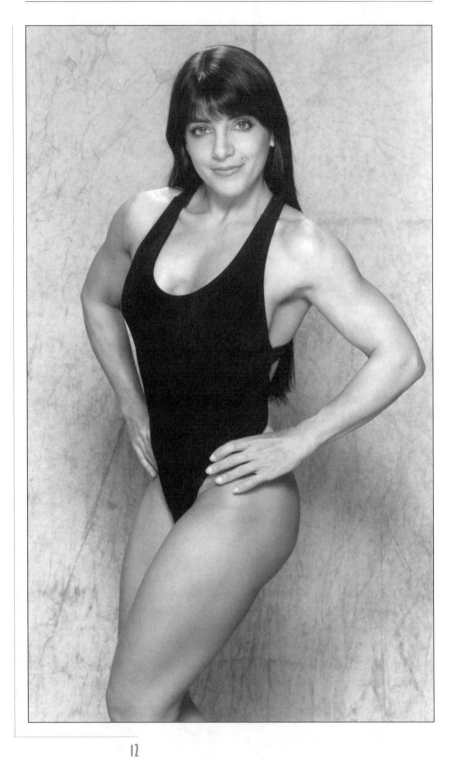

event where you must fail to win. It's our failure to "fail" our muscles when we train with weights that makes the whole thing seem like a waste of time.

BODY AWARENESS AND FUNCTIONAL STRENGTH
The Truth You've Been "Myth-ing" About Muscles...

Each woman has her own aesthetic that she aspires to...and the majority of us do not covet the look of today's "female bodybuilder." Instead, we want to look like the models in "The Sports Illustrated Swimsuit Issue." We want to be fit, but we want to be *slim*. We fear "bodybuilding" because we believe training with weights will translate to masculine muscularity. Unfortunately, as I said earlier, this is a myth that has been perpetuated by the competitive bodybuilding industry. The reality is, when a woman incorporates strength training into her program, it accomplishes a whole series of positive results. Our bodies shape and tone (aerobics alone cannot achieve this), we have more energy and vitality, our metabolisms elevate (thereby reducing body fat), our menstrual symptoms are much less dramatic, and we hold back the aging process.

Will it work for you? Look at me, I didn't come out of the box this way, remember?

But you have to crawl...before you walk...before you run...before you fly...and at one point, I never even believed I'd get up off the floor.

So, have patience with yourself. Enjoy the journey...it's fun (trust me)...rewarding (you'll see)...and best of all...you'll get there (I promise). Your angel will emerge.

Now, I do understand that you've probably been here before...*here* meaning about to begin yet another exercise program.

And I acknowledge that you probably began before with enthusiasm, and hope, all fired up to "really do it this time."

You may have joined a health club, and during your tour when you were brought to the "weight room"(in most traditional health clubs that's the dark, dirty room in the back where bats are flying, and sweaty animals are lifting and grunting)...you probably said "where's the aerobics room?"...you know, the place where they keep us girls...in a nice frigid environment so we don't spoil, or God forbid, sweat.

And in that aerobics class you might have put your right foot in when you should have put it out (managing to totally mess up the Hokey Pokey that Bambi is ecstatically teaching so she can get her own work out in) and you felt like a klutzy, overweight interloper who looked like something out of

"Fantasia" in the back of the class as you struggled to keep up...

("Hey you...shouldn't you be in a *walking* program...somewhere in Siberia?")

So much for gusto.

And another one bites the dust.

Okay...so instead, you decide to buy a video and try working out at home. Which one to buy? There are zillions! You could "sweat to the oldies" or "march to marching bands;" you have your choice of the infinite "rockin"..."steppin"..."boxin"..."leg liftin"..."ab crunchin"..."watch me's" on the market, and that's probably what you'll wind up doing...watching them.

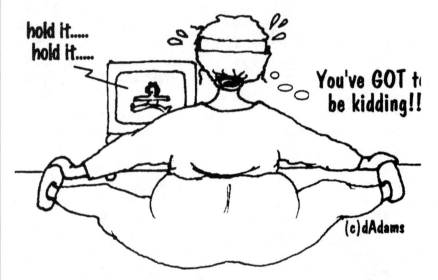

I must have heard; "I couldn't follow it so I sat down and watched it" a thousand times. Its some new passive exercise principle, I guess, and the workout video is about to become yet another dust collector on your shelf right next to...

The Books. All those books you've bought to learn new, newer, *newest* programs. More routines with no results.

15 Minutes to a New You...

3 Minutes a Day and You're Done (what are you, an egg?)...

12 Minutes 3 Times a Week...

Somebody out there is not being honest here! Granted, these efforts are better than no exercise, but realistically, how do you think you will look?

Or the routines are so complex...and require such an intense commitment...you burn out. On the shelf it goes.

Building quite a little library, aren't we.

And, of course...you might be one of those desperadoes who really "bit the bullet" and made 40 payments of $59.99 on a treadmill or stepper or bike just to have it wind up as an aesthetically offensive monument to your lack of commitment...a clothes rack that reinforces your guilt, and self-disgust. In the classifieds it goes...FREE-FREE-FREE...just get it the heck out of here!

Billions of dollars have been spent by women on exercise items. What are we doing with this stuff? Look in your closets, your attics, and your basements. Do you think the homeless could use any part of the collection—a "Thigh-Monster" perhaps or maybe that "Ab-Pulverizer" lying next to the "Bust-O-Sizer?"

And when there is no reward, no gratification, no light at the end of the tunnel, when you've tried everything and nothing works, you (once again) give up and resign yourself to your miserable existence.

Destined to be a fat person.

Might as well eat.

It's the only thing I get enjoyment out of anyway.

Why give up my pizza when this exercise stuff doesn't work for me?

Okay, why should you rally one more time?

Pour The Foundation...

Listen, you need to take this in stages. I did, finally. After throwing myself into situations I was not ready for (and feeling like an alien), injuring and embarrassing myself, and ultimately 86-ing myself...I realized I had to start from where I was. You can't start from over there when you're over here...you've got to get there from here and there ain't no one gonna miraculously beam you from one place to another.

I didn't start out in the weight room lifting heavy weights right next to the guys.

I started in my home.

Then, when I finally felt more confident, I joined a gym. And the boys.

And this is *my* idea of fun.

But, back to *your* particular stage. You will not get frustrated, or bored, if you approach this whole exercise thing in levels that are appropriate for you. And if you're at level *basement* (where I was when I started), then consider me the bearer of good news.

The elevator only goes up from there.

There is a distinct advantage to beginning an exercise program in your home with very simple tools as opposed to gym machinery. When you join a gym, what's the first thing they do? Those of you who have already gone that route know they put you with a floor instructor (usually some kid work-ing for minimum wage with little to no knowledge or education). This kid then sets you up on the designated "circuit" equipment—telling you what weight to use, how many reps to do, etc.—see ya. The reason they do this is, it's a numbers business, and they have to sell another membership and keep herding the cattle. The most efficient way to control a herd is to keep them going in the same direction—so you all sit on these machines, counting your reps, moving down the line, until your circuit is completed, and then you leave. No one needs to supervise you. You have been programmed, and you do your bit, no muss, no fuss, and no results. You haven't learned anything specific, you haven't been shown any free weight exercises, and you proba-bly haven't even been told what to avoid if you have any health issues (which in most cases they haven't screened for in the first place). Now, don't get me wrong, this is not how all health clubs or gyms operate. There are many excellent, responsible facilities around the country, but you need to know what to look for. You must be evaluated. You must have an educated indi-vidual take you through your first workout. You must have your special needs and challenges addressed in your program. *And you must get results.*

You're supposed to get something out of this! Two thirds of the people who join facilities drop out because they see absolutely no change in their physiques. Of course that's discouraging. Exercise is not something we're longing to do anyway, and if it gives us no return, we'd much rather do some-thing—*anything*—else.

What I am saying is that going through the motions on these machines with-out knowing what you are doing, what muscles you are working, may be bet-ter than lying on a couch eating a bag of chips, but it won't give you any drama. You are on that equipment because it's safe for you to use on your own.

When you are a beginner, there is no *Body Awareness* on machines. And without body awareness you can injure yourself...not just in sports or exer-cise activities, but in everyday life. So body awareness is something we must develop. Machines take this focus from you because it locks you into *it's* range of motion, *it's* lever system, which makes it possible for you to do the movement even if you were a *zombie*, because you don't have to think about what you are doing. Ask any woman on a machine in a health club what she is working. If it involves upper body at all, say a back machine, or a chest machine, or a shoulder machine, nine times out of ten she will say *arms*. Why? Because it's her arms that are moving, and she's not thinking about anything else. And no one's taken the time to educate her. And, my friend, if we are not thinking about the muscle we are working...*we are not fully work-ing it.* And when that happens...not much else does.

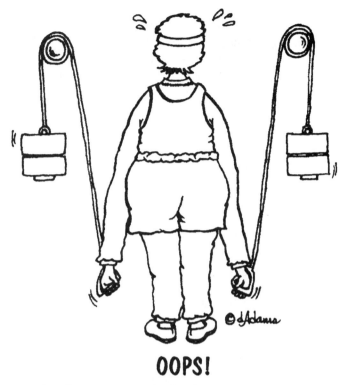

OOPS!

By mastering the exercises in this book, you will promote "core stability." When you maintain the stability of your core, the center—the foundation of you—is more grounded, more secure...less vulnerable.

This is so important, and it's usually the phase we skip right over. And without a strong foundation, how can you build anything that will stand?

So you see...it's a good thing you want to begin in your home. It's not a bad thing, it's not a wimp thing, it's a useful, wise, and helpful thing.

The techniques that you will learn from this book are ones that you will be able to take to a gym or health club anywhere in the world. And although you will need to be taught how certain pieces of equipment work, you will already know what those machines are working, and how it's supposed to *feel*.

The exercise routines in this book are exactly what you are asking for...they can be done at HOME. They are easy and, if you follow my instructions, they work. These exercises follow the basic principles of strength training: Form, technique, range of motion, resistance, and muscle failure...

FAILURE?? Hold it...are you telling me you want me to fail at this?
Yep. The whole idea is to fail the muscle..."till it won't go no more." Otherwise it will have no reason to change. If you don't push it past what it

is used to, a muscle will stay pretty much the same. You know those people who have been working out for years and never improve? You got it—they do not ever reach muscle failure. They stop when it starts to burn a little, or when they have reached their assigned number of "reps." Therefore, they have removed the necessary stimuli for their muscles to respond.

Now, since you will not have the heavy gym equipment to challenge your muscles, you have to do it another way. Some of the exercise routines in this book have been designed in a precise sequence to repeatedly affect a particular muscle until it fails. But, I'll explain more about this in a little bit.

First, I have incorporated some innovative (and inexpensive) pieces of equipment in my programs that you can purchase for your home. The "toys" that I introduce to you will greatly enhance your workouts while making the event different and fun. They greatly relieve the boredom that so quickly sets in when we exercise in our homes, and I am very excited about presenting this equipment to you. We need alternatives...solutions...fun. This stuff makes working out fun! Imagine that? I have done extensive research in this market. I have worked with just about every gadget ever invented in the fitness world. What I present here are small, compact, and effective items that will make the difference between "I'll exercise later" and "I want to play with that now".

At this point, you probably understand one thing about me...I need to derive some sort of pleasure out of what I'm doing or it just becomes another thing "I used to do." I have been training for almost 20 years. It's the longest relationship I've ever managed to sustain, and this is because it has never stopped giving me pleasure. One of the ways I make sure this "rapture" continues is to constantly invent ways to stimulate both my muscles and my imagination. I try out all the different paraphernalia that is introduced, and while some of them are just variations on a theme with nothing really new to offer, other pieces are novel, cutting-edge approaches to exercise that can significantly impact the benefits of training while holding your interest. And, they take up almost no space!

Just imagine actually looking forward to your workouts.

No psyche jobs. No guilt trips. No little "negotiations" with yourself.

The kids are in school...the husband's at work...

Forget the dishes, LET'S GET BUSY!

You can target your lower body and your upper body individually, or do a total body routine. How you choose to construct your personal game plan should be based on your goals, health considerations, lifestyle, and current degree of commitment. Don't approach this as an "all or nothing" situation. Adapt your workouts to your daily life, not the other way around. When it becomes a case of "life intruding on exercise"...life ultimately wins and you're back to square one.

I want to tell you about a client of mine that attacks fitness programs the way she does everything else in her life—200%! And every single time she begins a new program, she hits a wall six weeks into it. At this point she becomes weak, her energy drops, her motivation disappears, her attitude sours, her fat loss plateaus, she loses muscle instead of building it, and she is discouraged and frustrated. Then, she gives up. What happens? Does she just lack "the right stuff?" No, she is a very driven, goal oriented person. She just piles too much on top of an already stressful lifestyle, and her adrenal glands have had enough and become fatigued (see *What About Stress???*). Once that happens, there is a domino effect throughout the systems of the body, and the body remains in a tearing down mode (catabolism) instead of building up (anabolism). I had her cycle her workouts to fit more comfortably into her lifestyle, and I recommended that she begin more slowly this time, instead of like she was shot from a cannon.

So, first, I want you to realistically evaluate the time (and energy) you have to dedicate to this. If you can only commit three days a week at this time, that is fine. Start where you are...and take this in levels.

What Are Your Goals?

This is where you need to begin your program, by asking yourself what you really want from it.

What are your expectations?

Your hopes?

Your dreams?

Are you being realistic?

On the other hand...are you being so "realistic" that you are not indulging in a little reverie?

Is your goal to be a perfect size six—or to be perfect butt naked?

Take it from me, those are two different goals. And they require different degrees of commitment.

It's okay, however, to start with one, and graduate to the other. Remember, this is how I approached the whole deal.

When I finally forced myself to look at my body in the mirror, my evaluation was that a beautiful naked butt would be my reward—in my next life. In this one, I thought I would have to settle for looking cute in petite-sized clothing. But, tenacity, along with knowledge (and the motivating effect of consistent changes), rewarded me in this life. So, do not sell your dreams short.

Instead, set up a series of short-term goals leading to the big prize. This way, each little goal that you achieve will encourage your next level, and your "destination" will not seem impossibly far away.

Flexibility...Strength To Your Core

Before you do anything physical, your muscles should be prepared. That means awake, stimulated, and warmed up. Therefore, you need to do something cardiovascular for five to ten minutes to elevate core temperature and get all systems "on go" to prevent injuries. Warm up before you stretch. Do not stretch cold, because you can injure yourself. (Hot metal bends before breaking, but cold metal, well, you know what I'm getting at; you are simply more pliable when you're warm).

Once you've warmed up, either on some piece of aerobic equipment or by jogging in place, if your available surface is appropriate for jumping around (by that I mean *no concrete floors*), you can then stretch your muscles.

Some "experts" say you really do not need to stretch if you work all muscles throughout their range of motion when you train them. But, as you may have ascertained by now, the "experts" in my field do not agree on a lot of stuff.

Take it from someone who's trained both ways...STRETCH.

Okay...so it's boring.

But, you need to be flexible. Flexibility reduces the risk of chronic pain, and it complements your workouts by increasing your range of motion. Range of motion concerns both the natural movement of a muscle or joint, as well as your body's unique limits. For some people, it may be natural for them to touch their toes while hardly bending their knees. For others...well, let's just say some of us need to work at this. It is a useful endeavor, however, to routinely work at improving your range of motion.

Also, (and this gets back to foundation) stretching addresses your connective tissue; your ligaments and tendons—the unsung and oftentimes *unstrung*-heroes of the body that sustain the most frequent and the most bothersome injuries. Stretching helps to strengthen and protect where your muscles insert, and these insertion points (the points at which the muscles attach to bones via tendons) become less vulnerable and more powerful, supporting and propelling your movements more efficiently. Deplorably, the development of these supporting structures is often overlooked in workout programs.

Another point that needs to be made here is a situation that you and I are both facing: We are losing flexibility as we age. This is not good. Soon, we will be stiff little old people who need help tying our shoes. Nice picture, huh?

(A little perk from all of this stretching—not that you care, of course—is that this insertion points become more defined, more etched on your body's sculpture. This will intensify your definition and tone...not that how all of this looks will matter to you, I understand.)

Before you stretch, here are some guidelines for you to follow so you do not injure yourself. Contrary to popular belief, unfocused stretching is not a benign activity. Have respect for "flexibility training"...it can enhance your life, or interrupt it...so please pay attention:

- Think of stretching as relaxing your muscles, not forcing them to submit to your will. Have patience. Flexibility (like anything else) does not happen overnight.
- Breathe into the stretch. Key into your body and listen to its signals to stop. Then, take another deep breath, and as you exhale, gently ask it for just a tiny bit more.
- Stretch only to the point of mild discomfort, not pain. Going past an uncomfortable sensation into a painful one may cause small tears in the muscles, which will decrease their strength and flexibility, and initiate injury.
- Never, never bounce. Never. There will be no exceptions. Ever. (Am I clear on this point?)
- Do not stretch your lower back with your knees locked.
- Hold each stretch for 60 seconds (to really begin effectively stretching connective tissue).

There are actually some out-and-out dangerous stretches. The following are some of the more insidious of the offenders:

- The "Yoga Plow"—where you lie on your back—throw your legs over your body until your toes touch the floor above your head—and radically compress your cervical vertebrae constricting the airway.
- The "Hurdler's Stretch"—where your have one leg outstretched—and the other bent back at the knee in an awkward and unnatural position—stretching the tendons and the ligaments of the knee joint in a hazardous way.
- Deep knee bends—where you squat down so low that your butt almost touches the floor—opening the knee joint up and overstretching the tendons and ligaments.

I would have demonstrated the above nasty stretches in photographs, but, quite frankly, they hurt.

Cellulite: Can You Really Knead, Rub...Punch It Out?

What is Cellulite ?
It's FAT—right?!
So they tell me.
And, has it ever worked to manipulate, vibrate, or roll (remember those

old "fat jiggling belts," or the "fat roller machines" in women's salons years ago?) any of your other fat away? No.

Okay, what about these "cellulite cures" that involve everything from creams—to wraps—to massage—to pushing it around to loosen it up so it can be "absorbed"—everything under the sun except exercise? Do any of these "treatments" have any impact on our enemy at all? And, what about exercise? Is it enough?

The term "cellulite" is used to refer to that (ugh...need I describe it?) "dimpled" appearance on the hips, thighs and butts of a majority of adult women, (95%, statistics say) even if they only need to lose a "few" pounds. Some women may be genetically predisposed to this "condition" while others might not. I, of course, am—and had a fair amount of the stuff adorning my "other fat" until I became healthy and lean. As long as I stay at my "fighting weight," (and control my health issues), I am dimple-free.

There are some unique characteristics to cellulite, however. We have heard that fat "trapped" in the matrix of connective tissue gives the skin this unsightly texture. As we age, there may be a breakdown of the connective tissue, and this coupled with the fact that aging skin becomes thinner and less elastic makes cellulite a more common irritant to us "baby boomers." Now, when we gain body fat, the fat cells that are trapped in this "matrix" increase in size, causing this horrific effect to become more dramatic. But, trapped or not, is it still just plain old adipose tissue—stored body fat under the skin?

Well, yes...and no. If it were just "plain old body fat" it would behave like plain old body fat. But, as you might have noticed, it just *does not*. In *The Cellulite Solution*, written by Elizabeth Dancey, M.D., the argument is presented that cellulite is a "real medical condition rather than just a superficial beauty problem." Dr. Dancey (a British M.D.) spent years in Belgium studying cellulite, and wrote about the causes and treatment of cellulite that are accepted in Europe but not widely known in the United States. Why doesn't cellulite budge even when we get so thin you can virtually see through the rest of our bodies? Dr. Dancey says that cellulite is "primarily a lifestyle problem. In recent years we have become more sedentary, and we are consuming ever-greater quantities of processed foods or ready-made meals containing additives, artificial sweeteners, flavorings, colorings and other artificial products. Our way of life seems to be more stressful, and we are exposed to a greater number of free radicals in the form of pollution, sunlight, and smoking."

Also, women are getting cellulite at a younger age—as young as fourteen, Dr. Dancey writes. This is because of the "junk food" most young people eat, the fact that adolescent girls are taking birth control pills, and the decrease in exercise that is now, sadly, typical of our youth.

All of the many factors that cause damage to our bodies can contribute to the development of cellulite. Dr. Dancey says that we must bring our bodies back in "balance" to be able to battle our nemesis. Throughout this book you will read about the importance of keeping your body in balance, and the many factors that destroy that balance. Cellulite, being as unsightly as it is, might be just the catalyst you need to pay attention to these issues. Well, my friend, whatever it takes.

There have been some technological advances that have enabled scientists to examine cellulite (ultra-sound, X-rays, thermal imaging, Doppler techniques) and discover its unique characteristics. So, what is the difference between cellulite and fat? Dr. Dancey tells us that, "cellulite is, indeed, mostly fat, but it's not ordinary fatty tissue; it is fatty tissue that has been damaged by certain malfunctions of the body's systems."

You know, since I myself have been plagued by this "condition," I have tried to find as much information as I can about it. As in most things, I refuse to accept something that bugs me out before fully investigating the possibilities of doing something about it. Frankly, I am fascinated by Dr. Dancey's work, and I wanted to share it with you here. Basically, most of what I found in her book is completely allied with the recommendations presented in this book for overall health and conditioning.

But, back to orange peels.

Let's look under the microscope together at something we would all like to eradicate forever. In *The Cellulite Solution*, Dr. Dancey writes:

"Located on the surface of each fat cell are microscopic structures known as receptors, and it is these receptors that control the storage and removal of fat. Research has shown that there are several types of receptors; some enable the storage of fat and others enable its removal. The ones that control the storage of fat in the fat cells are known as alpha-2 receptors, and these are stimulated by insulin released when there is excess fat in the bloodstream, for instance after a meal. Sugar in excess can also be transformed into fat and stored via the alpha-2 receptors in the same way. (See, NOW WHAT DO I EAT?)

Receptors that control the release of fat from the fat cells back into the bloodstream are known as beta-receptors. These are stimulated by the hormones thyroxin and adrenaline, and other naturally occurring substances.

The distribution of fat-storing and fat-releasing receptors around the body influences where we store fat. Why is it that women seem to carry most of their weight on the bottom, hips, thighs and inner knees, yet when they try to lose weight, it seems to come off the top first—the chest, arms, face and neck?"

Time out. Haven't you always suspected that the fat on your lower body resisted the exodus along with the rest of your fat—even though you have been told that it all departs evenly? I know. They said that it just seems to leave slower from our hips and thighs due to a greater concentration in those areas. Is this true? Dr. Dancey continues:

"There is no doubt that when women gain weight they tend to gain it in the lower body, and when they lose weight it seems to fall off the upper body but remains stubbornly attached to the bottom, legs and thighs. In fact, the more they continue to diet, the more the weight seems to disappear from the top, and then when they stop dieting and regain the weight, the bigger the bottom and thighs become. And the more they repeat this lose-gain-lose-gain cycle, the more pear-shaped they become. Unfair, or just a fact of life?

The reason for this is that the fat cells in the bottom, thighs and the inner area of the knees—the most common cellulite trouble spots—seem to respond in a different way to fat consumed in the diet than fat cells elsewhere in the body.

Research has shown that in most women the fat cells around the bottom, thighs and knees have a greater proportion of fat-storing alpha-2 receptors and a lesser proportion of fat-releasing beta receptors than fat cells elsewhere in the body. Further research has enabled us to quantify this difference: In the bottom, thighs and knees there are approximately six fat-storing receptors for every fat-releasing receptor. This situation is exactly reversed on the upper body.

The fat cells in these cellulite-prone areas are therefore more avid, more hungry for fat and, hence more ready to store fat than fat cells elsewhere in the body. Yet, their capacity to release fat is reduced by a factor of six. In real terms, if we were to gain seven pounds of fat, six of these would be gained on the bottom, hips and thighs and only one pound on the upper body. Conversely, if we lost seven pounds, only one pound would come off the lower body and the other six pounds from the upper body. The more this lose-gain cycle is continued, the more this pattern is repeated. This is why the fluctuation of weight caused by repeated dieting—the yo-yo effect—will change the pattern of fat distribution and, hence, body shape.

Interestingly enough, a new fat storing receptor has just been discovered in men. Some men have a greater proportion of fat-storing receptors around the tummy and intestines—the typical fat storage site for men—than elsewhere in the body. So this does seem to confirm that the pattern of fat storage is determined by genetics and sex."

There are other issues that are believed to be at work here. One of the storage depots for fat-soluble toxins in the body is body fat. Your body may partially react to these toxins by "walling them off," which reduces the communication between that part of the body and the rest of it. This "wall" around the toxins is an additional reason cellulite might have its different look from other fat. But, we will get to that in a bit.

In order to mobilize body fat, an adequate blood supply through fatty tissue is necessary. Dr. Dancey says: "It is important that the arteries, veins and lymph vessels are working properly to keep the fatty tissue nourished and to remove waste products and tissue fluid. A breakdown in one or more of these systems allows cellulite to take hold. Cellulite tissue has poor circulation. The relative lack of oxygen and nutrients leads to a build-up of toxic waste products called metabolites. These toxic metabolites not only cause tissue damage to the existing tissue but also affect the way that new tissue building takes place. Within the tissues themselves are fiber-making cells known as fibroblasts. These fibroblasts make tiny fibers that form a supporting meshwork around the fat cells to bind the whole structure together. However, if the fibroblasts are deprived of oxygen and nourishment, instead of making fine fibers they make heavy fibers that surround and envelop the fat cells. It is the build-up of these thick fibers that is one of the reasons for that familiar 'tethering' effect seen in cellulite." So—a lack of oxygen in the tissues causes a build-up of toxic waste products which causes damage to the tissue, poor oxygenation of the tissues allows thick fibers to form around the fat cells, and poor blood supply prevents the removal of fat from fatty tissue.

Another key to all of this, according to Dr. Dancey, is lymphatic drainage. Dr. Dancey writes: "In a recent study at Brussels University, lymphangiograms (a medical investigation which determines the structure and flow of the lymph system) were performed on all women who presented themselves at the university's cellulite clinic. The results showed that the lymphatic system was deficient in all clients with cellulite." If the flow of lymph is disrupted, the lymph fibers become thicker and form a "honeycomb" around the fat cells (the "walled-off" effect). Fluid then becomes trapped between the fat cells and the fibers. Tissue pressure is increased, and this prevents the blood from flowing freely through the tissues. The blood now seeks the "path of least resistance," and it will tend to go around this mess rather than go through it. The lymphatic system is not removing toxins, the bloodflow has been re-routed so the cells are deprived of essential oxygen and nutrients, and fat cannot leave the fat cells, but it can continue to accumulate, making the area look even worse.

Yikes!

So, if this is how cellulite is formed, what actually causes it?

Dr. Dancey writes that cellulite (along with being a life-style problem, as well as an inherited trait) is caused by a combination of many different factors: Diet, (too much fat, too much sugar, yo-yo dieting, a diet poor in trace elements, too much alcohol) water retention (drinking excessive amounts of water is not a cure for cellulite; a balance of sodium, protein, potassium and water is necessary), artificial food products; flavorings, colorings, preservatives and pesticides (all of which can cause weight gain, fluid retention, tissue damage and circulatory disturbance), food allergies and intolerance (see, *TAKING CONTROL*), hormonal influences (according to research carried out in France, "any change in the normal functioning of the ovaries can encourage the formation of cellulite"—see, *The Baby-boomer Fat Cell*), and damage or restriction of the lymphatic or circulatory system (chronic pelvic infections, constipation, poor posture, abdominal bloating, very tight clothes and always sitting on your butt!—does this mean that the old "secretary spread" is not a myth? Do you know how long I have been sitting on my butt writing this book???).

So, how do we get rid of the stuff? One part of that answer is coming up in the section, *Cardiovascular Conditioning*. (Also, look for some insight into controlling toxic body wastes in *TAKING CONTROL*.) Dr. Dancey writes: "It is important to understand that treatment for cellulite has to take the form of a systematic, integrated approach. Every possible factor has to be addressed, regardless of the original cause. It is not enough to simply make changes to your diet and exercise regime, although this certainly should be the starting point. To treat cellulite effectively, we have to get the body to alter its cell structure through its own repairing mechanism, and that takes time."

Starting with diet, Dr. Dancey's recommendations are: Cut down on refined and processed foods, and all artificial food products, cut out artificial sweeteners, control sodium intake, drink the appropriate amount of water for you (see, *Live It Or Diet Lifestyle Systems*) but not an inordinate amount, remove excess fats (all bad fats), reduce sugar intake, limit alcohol intake (a glass of good red wine if you are not allergic to it is okay), limit coffee intake, eat plenty of fresh vegetables (raw veggies are valuable), eat fruit, but separate it from meals (see, *NOW WHAT DO I EAT?*), follow the food combining and separation principles (see, *NOW WHAT DO I EAT?*), eat an adequate amount of protein. Dr. Dancey also recommends protecting yourself against free radical damage with appropriate supplementation (see, *Live It Or Diet Lifestyle Systems*), and eliminating stress.

Regular exercise (aerobic/cardiovascular conditioning and resistance training) is a must, and your guidelines for this portion of your battle are coming up. However, along with all of this, Dr. Dancey also recommends certain types of aromatherapy ("a powerful form of treatment for cellulite providing the mixture is chosen correctly, and if used in conjunction with other measures") and creams containing key ingredients ("beware of those that are marked as 'miracle' cures").

I honestly don't know what to make of all of this. In some part of my psyche it makes sense, but my education has drilled into me that you cannot "spot reduce," that fat will "leave as it came," and "there is no such thing as 'cellulite'." I can tell you one thing—my lower body definitely clings to body fat more than my upper body, and once I put all of my puzzle pieces together, (see, *15 Rounds—My Championship Bout*) my lower body did become leaner. John A. McDougall, M.D., author of *The McDougall Program For Maximum Weight Loss* says that women are "slow losers." In his book, Dr. McDougall describes how women accumulate fat more quickly than men do, and burn it more slowly. He cites the following study: "Eight women were tested while walking on treadmills. They were in a special room called a 'whole-body calorimeter,' which measures energy expenditure during exercise. The scientists wanted to know whether the women could carry some additional weight without actually raising the level of calories they burned. Remarkably, each of these women was able to carry al least 20 percent of her own body weight before she increased her energy expenditure. Thus, a woman weighing 100 pounds could carry an extra 20 pounds without increasing her energy consumption above the level she burned when walking without a load. Her body reacted as if it weren't carrying any extra weight at all."

Dr. McDougall tells us that women's fat is stored in different places than men's to ensure that calories are available for pregnancy and lactation. (Once again, my friends, our aesthetic desires are challenged by nature.) Women are designed to carry fat on the butt and legs very easily (no kidding). This fat is also deposited below the surface of the skin—in fat cells that are larger than men's. Men are programmed to store fat as abdominal fat, which is mobilized and burned more easily than fat around the hips and thighs. Dr. McDougall says: "What all of this means is that even when women are watching their diets, they are still likely to put on extra weight. This causes many women confusion and frustration, especially if 'All I have to do is look at food to gain weight' is a common lament. Indeed, women are going to store some weight naturally no matter what they eat, but those who eat fatty foods are going to be overweight—by anyone's standards." Dr. McDougall recommends a low fat eating regime in his program, maintaining that fat in the diet translates to fat on our hips (see, *NOW WHAT DO I EAT*).

There has actually been a new procedure—direct from Europe and recently introduced in the United States—which is said to "break up" cellulite. There is a machine that manipulates the surface of the skin, pulling and prodding and breaking open fat cells. The fat is then "liberated" and off it goes into the body. But I caution you: Remember toxins are stored in this now released fat, and will wreak havoc in your system. A procedure like this should never be done without an accompanying detoxification program (see, *Get Rid Of The Stuff*), not to mention an individualized nutrition/lifestyle system.

I combat the enemy on several different fronts: Diet, aerobics, and resistance training. I am a firm believer (because of personal experience) in working the muscles that cross the hip joint very specifically and methodically (much like a ballet dancer) to dramatically alter the appearance of that area (see, *Do Women Need To Train Differently From Men?*). I have found some very effective techniques, and I have designed exercise protocols using them (see, *A Little Behind In A Big Hurry Lower Body Routine*) that have given me great satisfaction not only in my own results, but those of my clients as well.

So, is that spot reducing? Well, when you work the muscle in an area, you will affect the integrity (tone) of that muscle, which changes your shape. And, ultimately this does affect your fat (remember—increasing the size of your lean muscle mass elevates your body's ability to "burn" fat). Also, if Dr. Dancey is right—and stimulating the area encourages mobilization of the fat trapped there—then that could be why the relentless working of those muscles seemed to do the trick. But, along with all of the other components of this war, you must "liberate" your fat with an exercise that can use that fat for fuel—and that's aerobics.

CARDIOVASCULAR CONDITIONING... YOUR AEROBIC PROGRAM

Why do we do aerobics? (By aerobics, I do not mean just the classes, but any cardiovascular exercise). For a healthy heart? Longer life? Lower cholesterol?

Who are we kidding? Our first thought is to *lose fat*.

So we need to figure out the most efficient way to do that for ourselves.

Duration, Intensity, Frequency

Before we get on with your strength training program, (which will basically be an "anaerobic" activity, meaning it is not "in the presence of oxygen" so your body cannot use fat for fuel—I want to discuss "aerobic" activity, (exercises done "in the presence of oxygen"—where your body can use fat for fuel). You are working aerobically if you can sustain the activity endlessly (sitting around is actually "aerobic" but you are not working at a high enough intensity level to initiate significant fat burning). Which brings us to the intensity factor of aerobics, one of the "big three"...*duration, intensity, and frequency.*

At what intensity should you be working?

In 1993, The Federal Health Administration announced its relaxed guidelines for exercise required to maintain health. Where they had once recommended vigorous (intensity) exercise for at least 20 minutes (duration) three times per week (frequency)—they decided to recommend simply accumulating 30 minutes of "moderate" physical activity (which included gardening and housecleaning). They modified their guidelines because they couldn't get Americans to follow the original ones. (Kind of like lowering the river instead of raising the bridge, isn't it?)

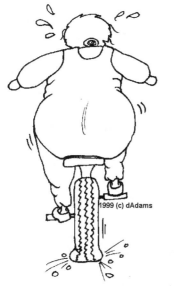

Many people misinterpreted this message and decreased the "big three" (most notably intensity), and subsequent research indicates this is a mistake. In fact, in 1996, the government officially announced "The Death of Exercise Lite" by releasing "The Surgeon General's (new) Report on Physical Activity and Health," and an official warning (reminiscent of the one issued in the 60's on cigarette smoking) that

NEXT TIME I'LL GET WIDETRACKS!

states, "The Surgeon General has determined that lack of physical activity is detrimental to your health." No more Mr. Nice Guy. Also, a recent study at the University of California at Berkeley demonstrated that if it is appropriate to the individual, aerobic exercises with increased intensity, duration, and frequency are associated with increased health benefits. The key word here is individual.

So how do you know what is the appropriate intensity level for you?

(Before we continue, I want to reiterate that the status of your health must be evaluated before you engage in an exercise program. In *Appendix A* you will find *The American College of Sports Medicine Guidelines and Checklist.* Please do not skip this step. As a Health Fitness Instructor who is certified by The American College of Sports Medicine, I never began working with a client—nor did any of my trainers—until we did a complete evaluation. As I have said before, anyone who does not do this is incompetent. So, don't do it to yourself, understand?)

Okay. Back to intensity. The intensity of your aerobic activity is determined by your heart rate. Not your friend's, not Jackie Joyner-Kersey's, not your 80-year old Aunt Edna's, but yours. You need to calculate what your heart rate should be, and then keep it within that range for the duration of your "aerobic bout"(the time between warm-up and cool-down). I promise I won't get too technical here...so stay with me. How do we figure this out? It's called *The Karvonen Formula*...and it's simple to calculate.

First, you will need to know your age. Your real one. Okay. Then you will need to know your resting heart rate. That is your pulse at rest, first thing in the morning when you wake before you even visit the bathroom. Using your index and middle finger (never your thumb, it has a pulse) press (but not too hard) along side your Adam's apple. Count the beats for a full 60 seconds. That's your resting heart rate. (You can take your pulse on your wrist, too.) The number, depending on your condition, might fall anywhere between 50 and 80. Below 50 generally indicates that you are really fit, or if you are unfit, there might be a problem. Above 80 could mean that you're just very unfit...or a signal to check with your doctor. In any event, do not be alarmed. Your resting heart rate, as well as your heart rate response to exercise, usually describes your level of cardiovascular fitness. (As I have said, I recommend you check with your doctor in any event before you begin an exercise program.)

If you know your age and your resting heart rate, you can do the Karvonen formula.

It is 220...minus your age...minus your resting heart rate=X.

Then you take X and multiply it by a percentage between 50% and 80%, and that percentage is determined by your level of fitness. So, if you have not been exercising regularly and you consider yourself unfit, you would choose a conservative percentage somewhere between 50 and 65%. (If you have high blood pressure, or any cardiovascular condition, consult your physician for your exercise heart rate recommendations. Typically, a very conservative exercise intensity of about 50%-55% is recommended to start.)

So...X times 50%=Y.

Then you take your resting heart rate, and add it back in to the equation...

Y + RHR = Z.

Z is your heart rate for your aerobic bout.

Let's take an example...me.

220 - 51 (my age) = 169 (my predicted maximum heart rate)

169 - 48 (my resting heart rate) = 121

121 x 80% (I'm very aerobically conditioned) = 97

97 + 48 (my resting heart rate) = 145 Beats Per Minute.

I typically like to keep my heart rate between 145 and 150 BPM when I do my cardio. Because I am so fit at this point, I feel I personally get the most benefit out of this intensity, and I enjoy the challenge of it. I could never, however, have sustained this heart rate when I began exercising. I used to suck wind two minutes into anything cardiovascular. But, as I explained before, one's level of exercise is very individual. You have to do what you can do—and what you should do is a topic of much debate.

Perhaps you have heard the conflicting views on how long your endurance workout should last, and how intense it should be. Recent reports from The American College of Sports Medicine suggest longer, lower intensity exercises burn more fat. This means that somewhere in the vicinity of 50 to 65% of predicted maximum heart rate might be the most efficient zone for liberating stored body fat to use as fuel. They also state, however, that with higher intensity you burn more calories. And, ultimately, doesn't that translate to increased fat loss? It's confusing, right?

Well, it goes back to your condition. The point at which stored fat becomes primary fuel for exercise is absolutely dependent on the training status of the individual. Elite athletes who have developed a more efficient enzyme system can start to contribute free fatty acids within five minutes of beginning an aerobic exercise. Untrained individuals, however, can require 20 minutes before their bodies start accessing stored fat for fuel. This is one of the reasons that it is universally accepted that the best exercise protocol for burning fat is lower intensity—longer duration. Another reason is the involvement of amino acids in endurance exercise. When we exercise for long periods at a high intensity (again, what that might be is individual), studies show that the energy from amino acid conversion to carbohydrate contributes an increased percentage of the total energy requirement.

In English? It means that long periods of high-intensity exercise could cause us to begin to tear down muscle for fuel. Also, another consideration in high intensity aerobic exercise is that, because it begins to border on "anaerobic," it becomes a more "acidic" event to the body. (I will explain more about this condition in *Taking Control*.)

Dean Ornish, M.D., in his book, *Eat More, Weigh Less*, states that moderate exercise may be better than intensive exercise for losing weight. He cites the following study: "Dr. John Duncan divided 102 sedentary women into three groups. Each group was asked to walk three miles, five days per week. One group walked three miles in thirty-six minutes, one group walked that distance in forty-six minutes, and one group strolled the same three miles in one hour. To the surprise of many, he found that the strollers lost more weight than the women in the other two groups. Why? The number of calories they burned was the same, but the type of calories varied. For short, intense exercise, your body tends to burn carbohydrates because it takes less time to convert carbohydrates into glucose, your body's fuel. Longer, slower exercise gives your body a chance to use body fat as fuel."

So, we go back and forth on this one in the fitness business. Although it is technically correct to say that "the contribution of fat to the oxidative fuel requirement is greater in a longer endurance mode," it is also true that "the direct expenditure of energy is linearly related to exercise intensity." Excuse me?

Well, the good news is, we are able to get pretty specific about exercise recommendations with *Live It Or Diet Lifestyle Systems*. There are several components that we consider, including blood type, metabolic type, and oxidative rate.

Peter J. D'Adamo, M.D., author of *Eat Right For Your Type*, contends that the type of exercise that is best for you depends on your blood type (see, *Blood Type*). I am blood type O, and the following is what Dr. D'Adamo recommends for me: "Type O's who want to lose weight must participate in highly physical exercise. That is because this type of exercise makes the muscle tissue more acidic and produces a higher rate of fat-burning activity. Acidic muscle tissue is the result of ketosis, which was the key to the success of our type O ancestors. I dare to say that there wasn't one overweight Cro-Magnon on the planet!" Dr. D'Adamo says that type Os should perform cardiovascular exercise at approximately 70% of our maximum heart rates.

Jay Cooper, M.S., author of *The Body Code*, offers exercise suggestions according to genetic body type (see, *Metabolic Type*). Using the evaluation method in Mr. Cooper's book, I am a "Nurturer," or gonadal type (I am actually the same type using all of the body-typing programs). Mr. Cooper says that my type needs lots of cardiovascular exercise in "the flow." He writes: "The flow is the level of intensity in the target zone that generates the release of beta-endorphin and enkephalins. To become physically and psychologically addicted to exercise, you must find the flow. Nurturers generally find the flow at an intensity level of 70 to 80% of aerobic capacity." Mr. Cooper says that the best time for me to do this is in the morning.

Now you see, I love this—because as I already told you, I thrive on intense aerobic activity. It is how I stay lean and energized. And, I am at my absolute best at this first thing in the morning. Both Dr. D'Adamo and Jay Cooper were right on about me!

Also, according to Live It Or Diet's research project studying the effects of exercise on oxidative rate, slow oxidizers become more balanced with cardiovascular exercise.

Anyway... what do I recommend for you?

Choose a couple of your aerobic workouts each week where you adhere strictly to a low-intensity/long-duration protocol (an example would be one hour of walking at a heart rate of about 50 to 65% of max). Then, a couple of times per week, do "interval training," which will take your aerobic workout and periodically push it above the "anaerobic threshold"(a point where you start to feel somewhat breathless). This is a method that effectively encourages adaptive changes in your cardiovascular mechanism and results in the ability to sustain higher workloads in your aerobic system. Higher workloads have higher energy requirements, so you become a more efficient little fat burner. (An example of this type of training might be a walk-jog where you intermittently break from your walk into a modified "sprint" to get your heart rate up, and then slow back down to your walking pace— remember to warm up and cool down).

(See *Appendix D* for information on heart rate monitors so you can track your heart rate.) When we build your *Live It Or Diet Lifestyle System*, we will be able to make the appropriate exercise recommendations for you.

Now, when to do your cardio? Well, if you are going to do it during the same time period as your strength training, there is a theory that you will burn more fat if you follow your *anaerobic* workout with your *aerobic* workout. Remember—your body *cannot* use fat for fuel during your anaerobic workout (strength training). Your body will use stored glycogen as energy. Once you've depleted those glycogen stores, it is believed your body will turn to its fat stores sooner during your aerobic workout when your body *can* use fat for fuel. In any case, it makes sense to prioritize your resistance training if definition, tone, and fat loss are your goals. With a pound of muscle comes an energy requirement of approximately 75 calories...but more on this in *The Beauty of Being Strong*. (Turn to *NOW WHAT DO I EAT?* for more information on glycogen.)

Possible Aerobic Activities

Question: What is the best type of aerobic exercise to choose when beginning a program? Answer: One you will enjoy and stick with.

In his book, *It's Better To Believe,* Dr. Kenneth Cooper (the "father" of aerobics) says that endurance exercises should not result in physical exhaustion. The following are a list of endurance exercises from Dr. Cooper's book that, when performed with the appropriate intensity, duration, and frequency, will improve your aerobic and cardiovascular capacity: Walking, treadmill walking, running/jogging, outdoor cycling, stationary cycling, swimming, and miscellaneous events such as aerobic dancing, stair climbing, stationary running, rope skipping, step aerobics, slide aerobics, rowing machines, and cross-country ski simulators. (I will add "Spinning" to this list.) I recommend cross-training aerobic exercises, which means you do not do the same activity every single day. This may result in "over-use" injuries. (I will go into cross-training later in this chapter.)

Dr. Cooper tells us that: "When you're participating in endurance exercise, you'll experience the greatest fitness benefits if you monitor how you feel about the effort you're putting out. When you first begin, a program should involve at least 'fairly light' effort, and then in later weeks you should move on to a 'somewhat hard' to 'hard' degree of intensity. This may seem a rather vague way to evaluate how much effort you're exerting. But actually, a scientifically tested scale known as the *Borg Rating of Perceived Exertion* has shown this subjective approach to work quite well. After they move beyond the first couple of weeks of a program, most exercisers who feel that they are working out somewhere in the range of 'somewhat hard, but still feels fine,' to 'hard and heavy,' will get all the endurance benefits they need. But if you feel you're working 'very hard,' you've gone too far—unless you're striving for a competitive level of training."

Is It Ladylike To Sweat?

If you are exercising aerobically at the intensity you need to be at <u>individually</u> to burn body fat, then you should be sweating. If you are not, you are not working hard enough. But *do not* bundle up in sweat clothes and rubber paraphernalia to accomplish this. When you wear all that stuff, you impair your body's cooling mechanism, and you will actually be burning *fewer* calories, not more.

△△**Note**: Drink 16 ounces

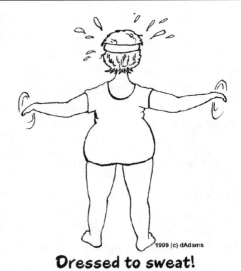

Dressed to sweat!

1999 (c) dAdams

of water before you do a cardiovascular exercise, and again after it. Most of what you lose during your workout is water, and you need to replace it.

STRENGTH TRAINING...YOUR WORK IN PROGRESS
The Beauty of Being Strong

The shape of your body comes from your muscle. The way you hold yourself, move yourself...project yourself involves the use and condition of your *muscle*.

Muscle burns calories, supports your skeletal system, and gives you confidence. It is the only tissue you can *shape*. You cannot shape fat, and although we usually associate aerobic exercise with eliminating fat, increasing your lean muscle tissue increases your body's need and ability to burn fat for fuel.

I love being strong. I love that I can lift things...sit up straight...run without jiggling. My body language changed 100% when I developed muscle. My attitude changed as well. And, ultimately...the way the world perceived me.

But, the best reward of all is that I look younger now than I did in my twenties!

I truly believe working to maintain my muscle keeps me young, and there is actually research to support this belief. An integral component of this phenomenon is the stimulation of the release of certain hormones. One of these hormones is *Growth Hormone*, and the release of this powerful hormone is responsible for "younger" skin and a more favorable body composition. Guess what? An intense anaerobic workout can cause your body to release that wonderful youth-enhancing growth hormone and, growth hormone is the most significant fat-burning hormone in the body, as well. So, if high-intensity resistance training stimulates its release, then this is yet another reason resistance training has an effect on fat burning (besides elevating metabolism), even though it does not directly access fat for fuel. (We will take a closer look at Growth Hormone in the *Food* and *Femininity* sections.)

In your programs, you will be performing movements with resistance, which will result in muscular integrity. The resistance will be supplied by weights (dumbbells). Hence the names; "weight training," or "resistance training," or "strength training." Women seem to like the sound of the phrase *shape* and *tone* better than the words build, or gain, or develop, which they find intimidating. Shape and tone sounds—softer, more feminine—just for us girls. Men *build* muscles, while women *shape* and *tone* them. Make no mistake, however, we are talking about the same thing—muscle—improving the integrity of the muscle. And muscle integrity is nothing more (or less) than the tone, definition, shape, and strength of a muscle.

I do not view strength training as black and white. There is a whole world between "mass" and "definition" that is a rainbow of colors. Fundamental, basic, "hard core" (if you will), exercises are not the only means available to effect change in the body. There are a myriad of refining and defining techniques and movements that address the intricacies of the physique. How they translate to a butt that defies gravity—that you will not need a leash for—that will end at your hamstrings and not at your ankles, well—that is what we're here to talk about.

If an exercise program is approached correctly, it will improve your performance in day-to-day life. This book's approach emphasizes balance, strength and flexibility, and will also help you develop neurological coordination—which will lead to more effective and extensive use of muscle fibers, and—bingo—more dramatic results.

And, keep in mind, my hungry friends, increased muscle translates to increased metabolism...so you can eat more without wearing it.

Bodybuilding saved me from starvation.

•Here are some facts for you to consider if you are still not sold on strength training:

For every pound of muscle we have on our bodies, we will require approximately 50 to 100 calories per day to maintain that one pound of muscle.

After the age of 35, most of us will lose up to 1/2 pound of muscle every year if we do not engage in some exercise that stresses our musculo-skeletal system (resistance training). Muscle is responsible for 25% of the body's caloric expenditure—even at rest. Non-training adults will experience a one-half percent reduction in metabolic rate every year of life. This gradual decrease in metabolism is closely related to the gradual increase in body fat that accompanies the aging process. So...again...one mo' time...otra ves, amigas, even if you weigh the same as you did in high school...you probably look different...don't you?

And, where do you think fat goes when it finally does leave your hips?

Does it evaporate?

Does it go down the toilet?

Do fairies come in the night and cart it away?

No. It goes to the muscles where it is burned up as fuel. *To the muscles.*

To review: The more muscle you have, the more opportunity, the more little furnaces, the greater the demand...for liberating your body fat to be used as fuel. Shall we continue?

The Music And The Mirror...And The Magic

The following is what you will need to get started:

• Number one...A POSITIVE ATTITUDE. Okay, that's the last I'll say about that.

• Second...a clear space in your home with a mirror. Now, don't get in a snit about this. Look around...you have room. You don't need much, and you have to take this seriously for it to work. If you don't create a designated area and you constantly have to move stuff around to do this, you'll blow it off, you know you will.

• Third...MUSIC. That's right...your favorite uplifting, motivating music that makes you want to move. Not that I want you dancing about with reckless abandon, but if you're like me, music gets you going...sets the mood...lifts you up off your butt...cha-cha-cha.

• Fourth...you'll need some light dumbbells...a set of three's, five's, and eight's should do it to start. Then, when you're ready to advance, you can run out and buy some ten's. Yea! (Well, it's the little things). Or, you can choose to buy the really compact and efficient weight set that I recommend. (Check *Appendix A* for where to find your "toys.")

• Fifth...a step of some sort about eight to ten inches in height that will fit your whole foot and won't move around. You can position a step stool against the wall, or if you happened to have ordered one of those "aerobic steps" from a past attempt with a Fitness Bunny video, dust it off...it's perfect.

• Sixth...(but this is actually 1A) check with your doctor to make sure you do not have any contraindications. It's vital that you do not engage in a program that might compromise any issues you may be dealing with physically.

The Negatives And Positives

I am talking about muscle contraction here. There are two phases of muscle contraction; *negative* (eccentric) and *positive* (concentric).

The negative phase of a movement is the actual stretching of the muscle. Most machines begin an exercise in a stretched position because putting a muscle on stretch before contracting it results in a more forceful, or complete contraction of that muscle. When using "free-weights," however, it is safer to begin in the position of completion of a movement (the point where you will end up) so you can set everything safely. Typically, the negative phase is performed in a count of four, so that it is slow and controlled. This might vary according to protocols and specific desired effect, but a four-count should be the rule for a beginner.

The positive phase of a movement is the contraction of the muscle. Do not bounce from the negative phase into the positive phase (or out of the stretched position). Typically, again, unless specific protocol indicates, the positive phase is performed in a count of two. Hold for a count of one between both the negative and positive phases to prevent the impulse to bounce.

It is important to accomplish *full range of motion* of the muscle. This is when the negative phase and positive phase fully stretch and contract a muscle to positions that incorporate complete action in the joint that the muscle is acting upon, without compromising that joint (do not hyperextend a joint, even if your genetics allow).

Breathing is also an important consideration. There is a tendency to hold one's breath when concentrating. Since oxygen is a requirement not only for life, but for exercise performance as well, inhale during the negative phase of the contraction and exhale in the positive phase. Breathing in this manner will assist the action.

Taking It Slowly

In the upcoming routines I emphasize "muscle failure," but I want to caution you regarding this concept, as you are probably a beginner, or someone who has not exercised these muscles for a while. The first two weeks that you perform your routines, execute fifteen repetitions to a slight burn as your body acclimates to this event. Otherwise, you will be tearing down too much muscle fiber, and that will result in a soreness that will make you miserable. I want you to stay with this, so ease into it. Learn the form, get comfortable with the movements and, two weeks into it, begin to challenge yourself to go past the burn to failure. Please do not do this from the start, or the resulting "crippling" effect will give you a handy little excuse to stop.

Your Personal Best

I hope by now you're getting that—in order to be the best you can be—there are many aspects and considerations that must be addressed. In *It's Better To Believe*, Dr. Cooper included a chapter he called, "The Secrets Of Becoming A

Superwoman." Among some of his recommendations in this chapter are the following: "Focus even more than men on total body conditioning, including strength work, to prevent the loss of muscle mass and functioning—limit running to no more than fifteen miles per week if you're a recreational exerciser—keep your body fat between 12 and 22 percent of your total body weight—to avoid back problems later in life, concentrate on strengthening the muscles of your abdomen and lower back." Dr. Cooper also mentions a special consideration for women is that; "most female knees are different from those of men, and exercise programs must be designed with this fact in mind. In women, the quadriceps tend to meet the knee at a wider angle than in men. As a result, the kneecap moves laterally and may be more subject to injury." So, should our approach to exercise be different from a man's?

Do Women Need To Train Differently From Men?

This is what I believe. I believe that women have special issues (besides the difference in our knees) that cannot be ignored if we expect to get the desired results from resistance training. Most men train for increased size, most women want to *decrease* their size, (and we especially want this result between the waist and the knees).

I have said that you cannot "spot reduce," and technically, this is correct when you are talking about mobilizing adipose tissue. In order for your body to perform the extremely difficult task of removing fat from fat cells, an intricate cycle has to take place that involves oxygen, enzymes, and certain other factors that are highly sensitive and complex. Conditions must be "just so" for the appropriate chemical reactions to take place that allow fat to be used as fuel by our muscles.

Of course, we females already know that we are programmed for more fat cells in our lower extremities than men are. But, I am talking about the muscles under those fat cells. Consider this; dramatically improving the integrity of those muscles will affect the overall appearance of that area.

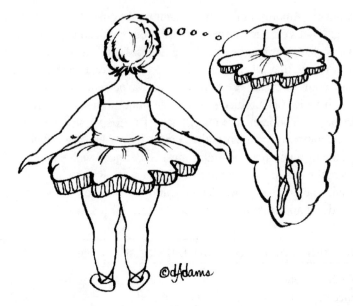

©dAdams

Think of ballet dancers and skaters for a moment. Picture their lower bodies—how narrow their hips are. Of course, the *structure* of the hip area is a matter of genetics—but, the *movements* that they employ in their events—the constant, relentless application of particular actions involving the contraction of the muscles that cross the hip-joint—that impacts the shape of the hip area.

Allow me to share my experience with you. When I first began bodybuilding, I trained hard and heavy in every muscle group. And, this resulted in increased muscle size, in every muscle group. This was terrific, except that it was not my intention to have wider hips and a larger butt. So, I went back to my dance roots when it came to my lower body routines. I incorporated movements and principles that worked targeted muscles in sequences with hardly any rest, much like a dancer would do at a ballet bar. I designed protocols that worked the muscle with a single joint action movement, immediately followed by a compound movement (other joints and muscles coming into play). Then, I worked these areas three times a week, and my other muscle groups twice a week. The results were incredibly dramatic! Performing ballet type movements with resistance to failure and a frequency that is usually associated with a dancer's regimen rewarded me with a little more muscular version of a dancer's lower body—exactly what I wanted.

When I began training other women, I used my protocols on them, with the same results. Three times a week, in one way or another, I included some lower body training in their programs. This may be translated in some exercise physiology languages as "over training" those muscles—but so be it, I say. If performed safely by individuals who are not already compromised in the hip joint, these protocols should not result in injury. After all, I am talking about very light resistance here, not heavy weights.

The following is a routine that stresses the lower body area. It is a series of movements that have been configured to train the muscles for definition, density, and shape—without increased size.

"A LITTLE BEHIND IN A BIG HURRY" LOWER BODY ROUTINE

This first routine is designed to affect all the muscles of the hip joint...(if we're talkin' butt...trust me, those are the ones you are concerned about).

Let's Talk Form...

It is important that you do the exercises exactly as directed...providing that what you are feeling is in the MUSCLE, not in the JOINT. Joint pain is never good. NEVER. So, do not ignore it.

Follow the form specifically as described. THE FORM IS VITAL. That's why you need a mirror. Never, NEVER sacrifice the form. The challenge here is not in how much weight you can lift—leave that to the muscle-heads in the gyms—it's how perfectly you can achieve the movement.

Hello Gorgeous...

Stand before your mirror sideways. Look at your posture. Don't worry, it'll improve.

Slightly bend your knees, roll your hips forward, and contract your abdominals to support your spine. Looks better already, right? Hang in there, kid, you're doin' great. You got this far, didn't you? And, if you feel stupid, you're in the privacy of your home, so who cares?

Now, I need you to release from your hip-joint...it's that little movement you may be familiar with—you know—picture a stripper "bumping"(tilting the pelvis backward and forward). Practice this movement a few times...release the hip joint...(you're sticking your butt out)...then, squeeze your butt...(you're tucking it back in)...bringing your hips forward so your back is straight again.

Do this a few times...RELEASE...SQUEEZE...(you should feel your butt muscles stretch and tighten).

Remember to keep your knees slightly bent at all times.

Pretty, huh? Anyway...you're alone. And, this movement is an integral part of the exercises in many of the following routines, so you've got to get it down.

THESE ARE IMPORTANT CONSIDERATIONS:

• Keep your chest up and your shoulders back throughout the routines.

• Keep your knees slightly bent...never lock them out.

• When picking up your dumbbells (or anything for that matter) bend at your knees, and don't reach for anything that is not directly in front of you.

• Whatever direction your toes are going in, your knees follow, so always keep your knees over your toes.

• Work the muscles through the burn (muscle burn not joint burn)...almost to failure (the point where they simply will not contract anymore—if you completely "fail," you'll fall down). Going to failure in resistance training is something most of us never do, because this is where it gets uncomfortable. But, remember...it's also where the drama comes from. This sequence was designed to bring you to muscle failure in your glutes by the end of the entire series of exercises.

• I will be making references to "releasing the hip joint," and "pelvic tilts," but I want to caution you that I am not talking about arching your back and compromising the integrity of your *center*. Hold your center strong by supporting it with your abdominals, and feel yourself being pulled up by a chord to the ceiling. Instead of arching your back, when you release from the hip joint, hinge forward a bit so you do not painfully compress your lower lumbar vertebra.

• *If your back or knees hurt, STOP.*

• *Always consult your doctor before beginning an exercise program.*

THE EXERCISES

1. LUNGES OFF A STEP
2. HAMSTRING DEADLIFTS
3. DUMBBELL SQUATS
4. SUMO SQUATS (PLIÉS)

These exercises will be performed in sequence...nonstop (i.e., no rest between them). Remember the reason for this is to insure muscle failure, which is how we stimulate the muscle fiber without resorting to heavy weights.

Let's take a look at each exercise individually before we put them together.

1. LUNGES OFF A STEP

The Lunge is a very difficult exercise to master. Most people do it incorrectly, so chances are, if you've seen it done, you've not observed the proper form. Let's begin by breaking down the basic lunge movement.

First, place your step where it cannot move. We are using a step in this exercise because when your front foot is elevated, less stress is put on your knee when you push off, and your buttocks goes through a fuller range of motion, which makes it work harder...(when you put a muscle on stretch you get a more forceful contraction). Your step should be about eight to ten inches in height. Stand the appropriate distance from the step that enables you to reach it with your entire foot landing on it. (Do not hang your heel off the edge—an unstable foot creates an unstable knee, which creates an unstable hip, and ultimately a very unstable and possibly injured you.)

Negative phase: Count of four

1. Lunge forward slowly and land with your whole foot on the step.

2. Drop down slowly keeping your front knee slightly behind your front ankle...both knee joints should be at 90 degrees in this position.

3. (Almost but do not touch the floor with your back knee.)

Positive phase: Count of two

1. Push off the step with your whole foot (concentrate on your heel) and come back to starting position.
Alternate legs

ΔΔ HOT TIPS

• Before you do this exercise with dumbbells, practice it with your hands on your waist, or resting on your front knee as you lunge. This will help you balance,

THE LUNGE MOVEMENT
OFF A STEP

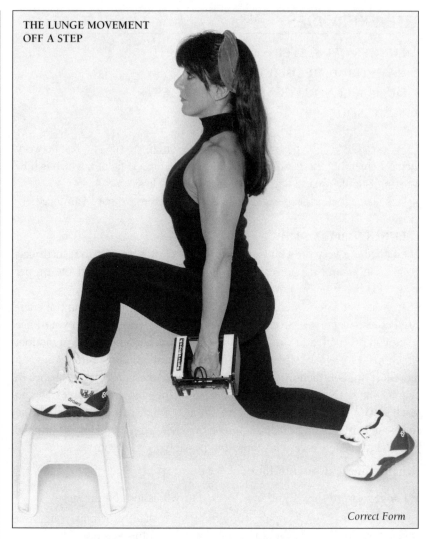

Correct Form

and the hardest part of this movement is staying balanced. But, conquering this aspect of it will help you develop balance and stability in general. When you are ready, hold a set of dumbbells that provide the correct resistance for you to perform twelve to fifteen repetitions.

•Keep your upper body straight...do not bend at the waist. All activity is below the waist.

•Use your abdominals to support your back.

•Move carefully and deliberately through the exercise...do not use momentum.

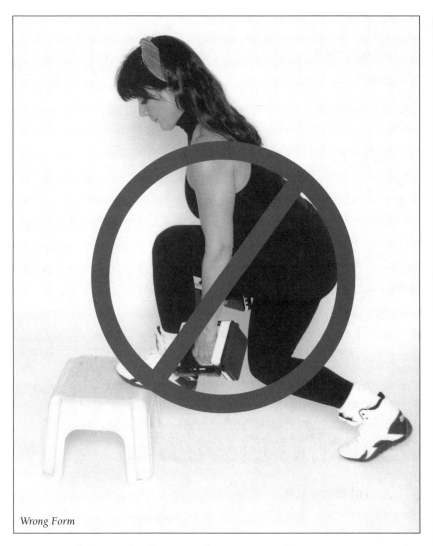

Wrong Form

- Keep your knees in the direction of your toes, and point your toes straight-ahead.

- Do not bounce your back knee off the floor.

- Do not jut your front knee out over your toes.

- Remember, your stability begins at the floor with a stable foot. Land on the step with your whole foot, and when you come back to the starting position, plant your foot firmly (but don't slam it) on the floor. Resist the impulse to do this little "cha-cha" step that every beginner does to get oriented before they lunge with the other foot.

• When easing down into the lunge after you've landed on the step, picture yourself going straight down, like an elevator. This part of the movement is completely vertical.

• Alternating legs in this exercise puts all the muscles involved through a full range of motion. When you stay on one leg for twelve to fifteen repetitions and then switch to the other, you will effectively fail the quadriceps (front of leg) on *that* leg, but the buttocks and hamstring on that leg are not fully contracting. Try it. Lunge forward and step back into position. Then lunge forward on the same leg again. You see...you've never completely <u>extended</u> that hip (this happens when that foot goes behind the standing leg as you squeeze your butt...as in a ballet move). A full contraction of the buttocks and hamstrings occurs when the moving leg winds up a little behind the standing leg, which it does as you lunge with your other leg.

• Breathe

LUNGE VARIATIONS

The following are other "Lunge" movements I will teach you: Walking Lunges, Back-Step Lunge, Lunge 'Mambo,' and Pulse Lunges.

Lunges are awesome for your butt! Please don't let the lengthy explanations intimidate you. The Lunge is worth every bit of the effort...believe me. It is one of the most effective exercises for conditioning your lower body, and promoting better coordination. But, I do have a healthy respect for what can go wrong, so I want to explain enough to let you visualize the exercises in this book, but not so much that you think they are impossible.

Anyway...one picture says a thousand words...as they say...(so see *page 44*)

2. HAMSTRING DEADLIFTS

The common name for this exercise is "Stiff Legged" Deadlifts...and they are usually performed the way they sound...which is dangerous. You might have seen this once or twice...or a thousand times in gyms...someone standing on a bench, with locked-back knees, a rounded back, holding a bar over the edge of the bench and *bouncing*. Sounds painful? It is...and it's the <u>wrong type of pain</u>. When done correctly, "Hamstring Deadlifts," which I like to call them, are excellent for the hamstrings and buttocks.

When done incorrectly, they can cause injury to your back, and to your hamstrings.

We'll begin once again by standing sideways in front of the mirror, and practicing first without dumbbells.

Standing straight with your feet and legs together, slightly bend your knees, release from the hip joint, and—keeping your chest and head up, your back flat, and your abdominals tightened—drag your hands down your legs as you stick your butt out and stretch the backs of your legs (hamstrings).

Negative phase: Count of four

1. Bend forward only as far as your flexibility allows with a flat back.

2. Your hands ride down the front of your legs, staying close, your arms are straight, your head stays up, and your knees stay slightly bent. Most people can only go as far as a little below their knees with their hands before their backs begin to round out.

Positive phase: Count of two

1. From this "stretched" position...squeeze your butt to come back up. Make sure your back stays flat, your head and chest are up, and you are pressing your heels into the floor. Do not bounce up.

2. Come up only as far as contracting your buttocks takes you. You should wind up just short of perpendicular with the floor. If you come all the way back up, you will use a lot of low back in the end of this movement.

Release from the hip joint, and go again.

∆∆Hot Tips

• When you use your dumbbells (ones that allow you to perform twelve to fifteen repetitions)—slide them down your legs—do not wave them out over your toes. (Keeping the resistance close to the "force"...in this case your low back, glutes and hamstrings...decreases the risk of injury.)

• Resist the impulse to round out your back to get more "stretch." By rounding out your back while holding weight, you are stretching your spine's ligaments, you are not doing a more effective job on your hamstrings and glutes, and you can hurt yourself. If you feel the stretch in the backs of your legs, then you've got it.

• As you descend, picture sticking your butt through the wall behind you. (Sounds weird, I know...but that phrase seems to trigger the image.)

• Keep watching yourself in the mirror to check your form: Back flat, stomach in, chest out, head up, knees slightly bent, feet parallel—facing forward, legs together, heels on the floor, butt through the back wall...Whew!

This exercise will further "pre-exhaust" your glutes on your way to failing them so they respond the way you want them to. By "pre-exhaust," I mean that we are working the butt again in this exercise, isolating it without working the front of your legs. After this exercise, we will add back in the front of the legs to further slam the ole' glutes! *Fun, huh?*

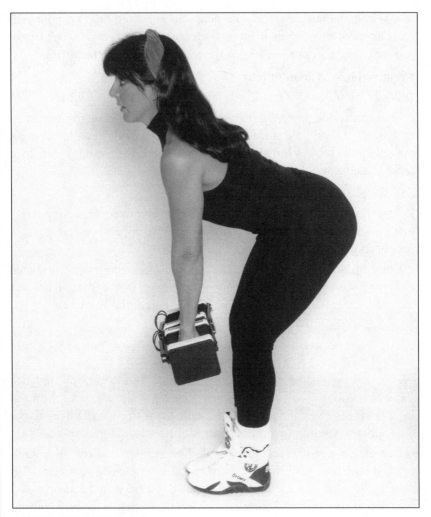

HAMSTRING DEADLIFTS   *Correct Form*

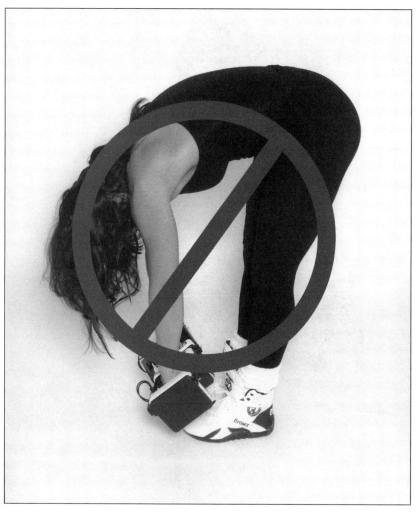

Wrong Form

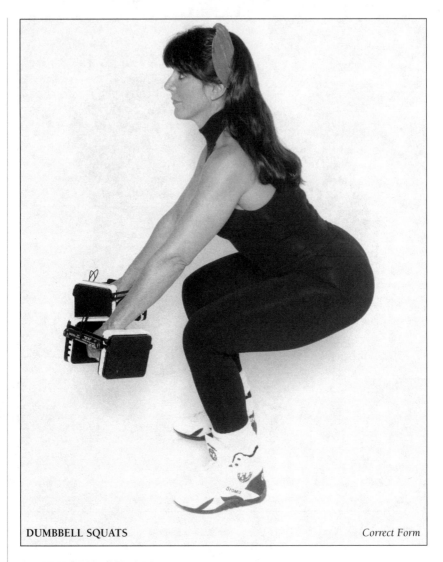

DUMBBELL SQUATS *Correct Form*

3.DUMBBELL SQUATS

When we think "squats," the usual picture that comes to mind is a bar across the shoulders, arched back, and knee joints stressfully opened.

But, that's not what we are going to do.

I teach "Dumbbell Squats" to beginners, and I've noticed—when integrating them into a sequenced event—that even light resistance burns the muscle.

Stand sideways in front of your mirror. Before using dumbbells, do the movement a few times just reaching out in front of you (like Frankenstein). Got it? This is to help you balance.

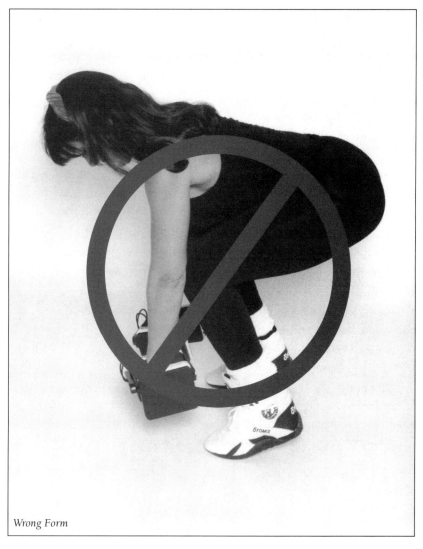

Wrong Form

Begin with your back straight, your head up, your arms outstretched, your knees soft, your feet shoulder width apart, only <u>slightly</u> turned out.

Negative phase: Count of four

1. Release from your hip joint.

2. Reaching forward to counter-balance your weight, squat down keeping your back straight, <u>your heels on the floor</u>...until the backs of your legs are parallel with the floor. Your knees and your hips should be at 90 degrees at the bottom of the movement.

Positive phase: Count of two

1. Coming back up, press into the floor with your heels.

2. Concentrate on the contraction of your buttocks to move you up.

3. Squeeze your butt at the top, and do not lock out your knees, and do not stand there resting for any length of time.

After the squeeze, release the hip joint again and go.

∆∆Hot Tips

•When doing this exercise with dumbbells, choose a weight that will enable you to perform twelve to fifteen repetitions. As you descend into your squat, allow the dumbbells to counter-balance you. You will really be able to "sit" into the exercise this way without falling on your butt.

•Keep your chest up, your back straight, your abdominals supportive.

As you descend, do not bend at the waist or round out your back.

•Control every aspect of this movement. Do not drop, or bounce out of the squat.

•Your knees and toes should face the same direction...always.

•Do not sit any lower than parallel with the floor.

•Remember to let your breathing help you (inhale as you lower your body, exhale as you ascend).

By now, your glutes should be worked to the point of almost complete failure. Squats have long been recognized as the premier exercise for the butt. By doing them in this manner, they are both safe and effective.

*Here are another couple of thousand words...**(On page 50)*

SUMO SQUATS

Begin this movement by standing with your feet wide apart, with a natural turnout in your hips and knees, and point your knees in the same direction as your toes. (For those of you who are familiar with ballet, this will resemble a "second position plie" stance.) Do not force your turnout. When you are ready to add resistance to this movement, hold one or two dumbbells in front of you between your legs—close to your body. Choose a weight that will provide you with the appropriate resistance to achieve twelve to fifteen repetitions to failure.

Negative phase: Count of four

1. Again, release from your hip joint while the rest of your body remains stationary (pelvic tilt backward, which sticks your butt out).

2. Descend slowly, keeping your head up, your back straight, your knees over your toes.

3. If you are in the proper position, with the correct distance between your feet, you should wind up with your knee joints at ninety degrees and the backs of your legs parallel to the floor at the bottom of the movement.

Positive phase: Count of two

1. After holding for a count of one, begin to tuck your pelvis forward, squeezing your butt to ascend. Do not round out your back, keep it straight, with your head up.

2. At the top of the movement, you should have fully contracted your glutes, your pelvis will be slightly tilted forward, your back should be straight, and your knees slightly bent.

3. Squeeze your butt, and descend.

<u>Do not stay up there.</u>

∆∆Hot Tips

• To accomplish the desired wide stance safely for your joints, begin by standing with your heels together, your feet turned out in a comfortable position for your hip joints. Lunge one leg out laterally so there is approximately three feet (depending on your height) between your heels.

• Stand sideways to the mirror so you can check your alignment.

• Concentrate on pressing your heels into the floor as you ascend.

Sumo squats not only work the glutes, but the inner thighs as well.

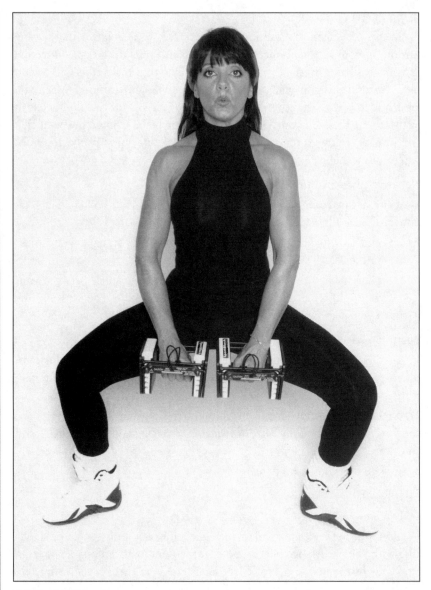

SUMO SQUATS   *Correct Form*

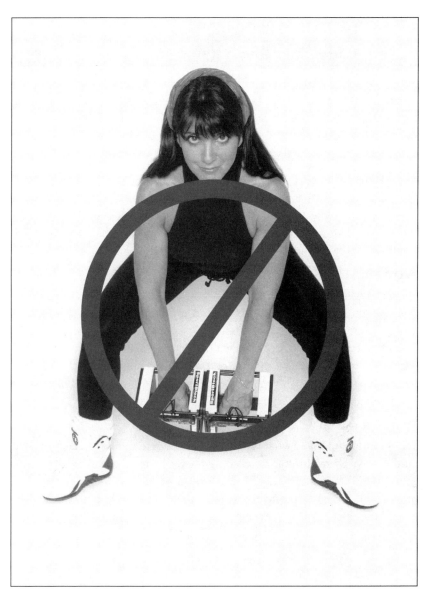

Wrong Form

WHEN EXERCISE BECOMES FUN
Playing With Your "Toys"

Yes—Toys! that's what I prefer to call the home exercise equipment that I recommend to get you started. First of all, the names alone suggest fun rather that work. A Ball. How intimidating could that be? Power Blocks. You see—not so bad, right? The pictures in this book have been taken using these two extremely versatile, inexpensive, and effective toys.

EXERCISE BALL

How many exercises can you do with a ball? About 60! It's a concept that is so simple, it'll blow your mind. This looks like a beach ball, but the movements you perform with it take old familiar exercises (like crunches) and sends them a quantum leap in effectiveness. It's also inexpensive.

"POWERBLOCKS"

What a great investment for a home gym! These weights go from five to forty-five pounds, and are designed to take up no more than one square foot of space. There is a woman's version that starts lighter and goes up to 23 pounds in smaller increments. Perfect for women beginning a strength-training program! PowerBlocks are state of the art, affordable, and attractive. They are so cool looking, you'll want to keep them out! (The exercises pictured in this book are being performed using PowerBlocks.)

HEART RATE MONITOR

It is important to know what your exercise heart rate should be...and to make sure it stays there during the exercise. Many people have difficulty taking their pulse during exercise, so I recommend a heart rate monitor. This tool allows you to know your heart rate at all times, increasing both the efficiency and the safety of your workout.

See *Appendix D* for where to purchase your "toys."

EXERCISES FOR THE REST OF YOU

Exercises For Your Upper Body

As we now know, resistance training, (i.e., strength training, weight training, etc.) is for everyone—and a necessary component of your health and fitness quest. I have given you a lower body routine, and here I want to give you an exercise for each upper body muscle group. These will get you started on your exercise regimen, with additional exercises to follow on video.

(See, *Appendix F* for audio and videotapes)

For these exercises, you will need an exercise ball and a chair (unless you have a weight bench at home).

EXERCISE FOR CHEST:

Chest Press

• Position your weights by your ball.

• To start—lie back on your ball with your feet firmly planted on the floor. Get stabilized on the ball.

• Reach down and <u>carefully</u> pick up your weights.

　1. Starting position—Bring your weights close to your armpits, your palms are facing your feet, and your elbows are sticking out to your sides. Your head is on the ball, but bending back just a bit so that your whole torso is on the ball as well. This is the *stretch* position of the exercise. The chest muscles are now on stretch. Take a moment to feel that. Count one. Breathe.

　2. Press the weights up in an "A" until they almost touch over your chest. Do not bang them together. Your arms should be straight, but do not lock out your elbows. Do not bounce out of the stretch position. Feel the *contraction* at the top of this movement in your chest. <u>Keep your shoulders on the ball.</u>

• You should start to feel a slight "burn" in your chest between 12 and 15 repetitions. This is good. Choose a weight that makes your feel that.

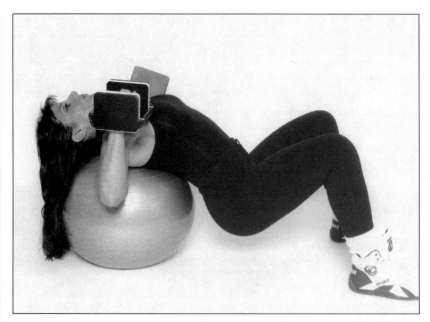

CHEST PRESS   *Starting Position*

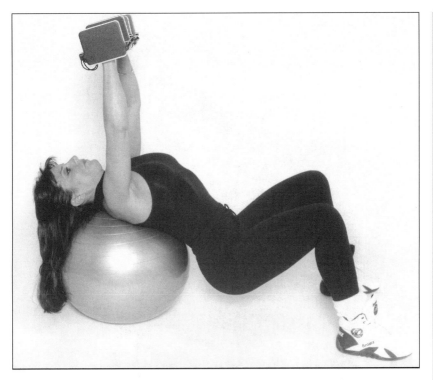

Ending Position

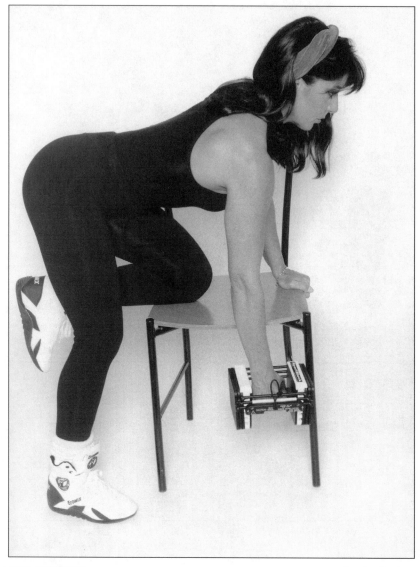

ONE ARM ROW   *Starting Position*

EXERCISE FOR BACK :

One Arm Row

•Position your weight on the floor by your chair (or bench). If you are starting on your right side, put the weight on the right side of the chair.

•Put your left knee on the chair, and your left hand on the edge of the chair
in front of you.

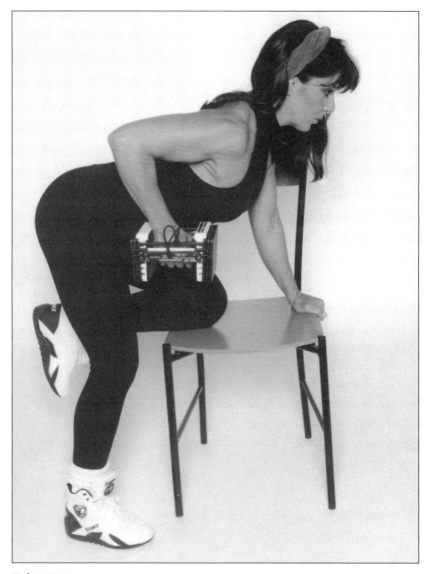

Ending Position

•Flatten your back—sticking your butt out. Look in the mirror. Is your chest parallel to the chair seat? Is your back as flat as a table?

1. Pick up the weight. With your palm facing in, and your arm straight, stretch your back <u>without rounding it out</u>. This is the *stretch* position.

2. Squeeze your back muscles to bring the weight up to just below your breast. Your palm should be almost touching your side, your arm should

be close to your body, and your elbow should be pointed toward the ceiling. <u>Do not bounce out of the stretch position</u>. Count one between the *stretch* (dumbbell is close to the floor) and the *contraction* (dumbbell is close to your side).

•Perform the movement until you feel a slight burn in your back—between 12 and 15 repetitions.

•After completing movement on right side, immediately switch to left.

EXERCISE FOR SHOULDERS:

Shoulder Press

•Perform this exercise sitting on a chair. Keep your back supported and flat throughout the movement.

1. Start with the dumbbells positioned just above your shoulders. Your palms should be facing in front of you, and your elbows are pointing toward the floor. The dumbbells should be just a couple of inches from the top of your shoulders.

2. Press the weights up in an "A" until they almost touch over your head. Do not bang them together. Your arms should be straight, but do not lock out your elbows. <u>Do not bounce out of the stretch position.</u> Feel the *contraction* at the top of this movement in your shoulders.

•You should start to feel a slight "burn" in your <u>shoulders</u> between 12 and15 repetitions.

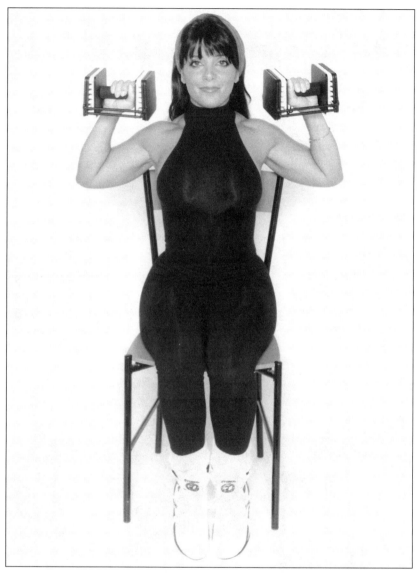

SHOULDER PRESS   *Starting Position*

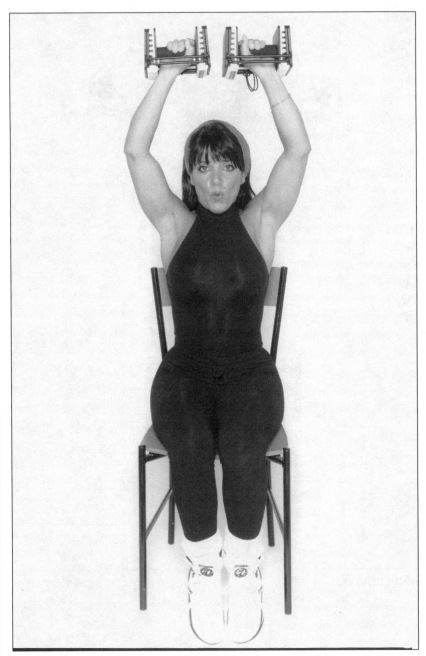

SHOULDER PRESS   *Ending Position*

EXERCISE FOR BICEPS:

Seated Bicep Curl

• Perform this exercise sitting on a chair. Keep your back supported and flat throughout the movement.

1. Begin by holding your dumbbells with your arms straight at your sides, your palms facing in.

2. Squeeze your biceps to bring the weight up, and as you do, immediately turn your palms towards the ceiling instead of in."Palms up" is the most efficient angle for your biceps. Bring the weight up past a 90-degree angle in your elbow joint to about 40 degrees. Do not take the weight all the way up to your shoulders.

• You can perform this exercise alternating arms, or both at the same time. Hold for a count of one at the top to squeeze your biceps. Bring the weight down slowly to starting position.

•Perform 12 to 15 repetitions to a slight burn in your biceps.
(See *page 66*)

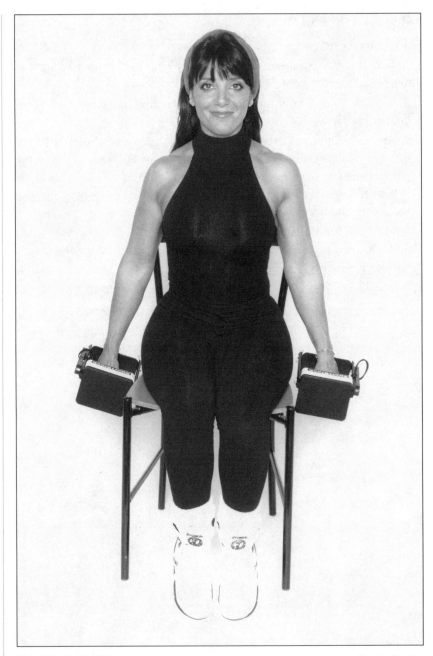

SEATED BICEP CURL   *Starting Position*

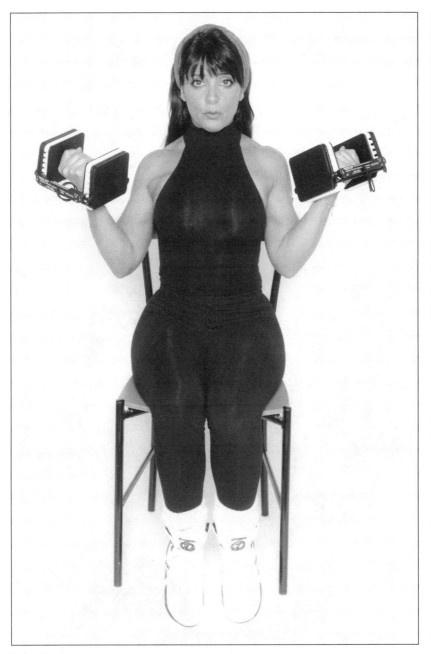

Ending Position

EXERCISES FOR TRICEPS:

Lying Tricep Press

•You can do this exercise on your ball, or lying on the floor. If you are on the floor, keep your feet on the floor, your knees up, and your back flat against the floor.

1. Holding your dumbbells, begin with your arms close to your head, your elbows pointing toward the ceiling, and the dumbbells by your ears. Your triceps are now on *stretch*.

2. Contract your triceps, moving the dumbbells until your arms are straight (perpendicular to the floor), and the dumbbells are over your head. This time I want you to lock out your elbows (unless they are severely hyper-extended) and squeeze your triceps. Make sure to keep your arms in throughout the movement.

• Perform 12 to 15 repetitions until you feel a burn in your triceps.

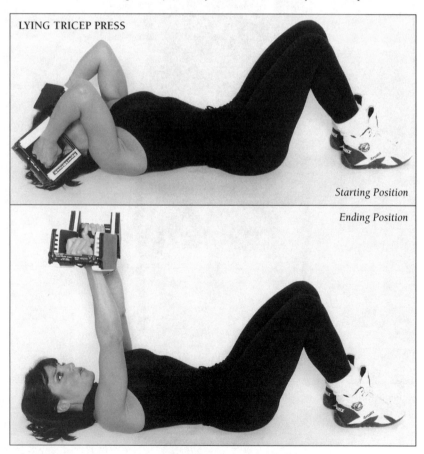

LYING TRICEP PRESS

Starting Position

Ending Position

EXERCISE FOR STOMACH

CRUNCHES

•You can use your ball, or use a chair to put your feet up on.

Crunches On The Ball:

1. Keep your feet on the floor, and, if you are a beginner, most of your body stays on the ball. (As you get stronger, your head and shoulders can hang off the ball for more stretch and a more intense exercise.) Support your neck by putting one hand on top of the other under your neck, not your head. Keep your elbows pointing out laterally, not up towards the ceiling. Keep your chin up, and look to the ceiling. Do not pull your head.

2. Squeeze your stomach muscles and crunch up. Hold for a count of one. Exhale as you crunch, inhale as you stretch.

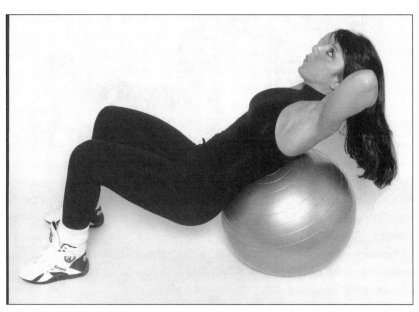

CRUNCHES ON BALL

Crunches On Floor:

1. Lie on the floor with your feet on a chair so that your knees are at 90 degrees. Support your neck by putting one hand on top of the other under your neck, not your head. Keep your elbows pointing out laterally, not up towards the ceiling. Keep your chin up, and look to the ceiling. Do not pull your head. Crunch up, and hold for a count of one.

•Again, abdominals do not usually fatigue easily. Keep going until they burn.

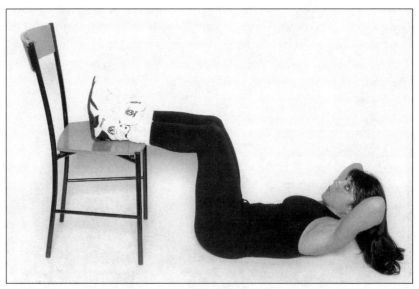

CRUNCHES ON FLOOR

•A note on concentration: When strength-training, it is essential for you to be thinking about what you are doing. Remember, do not just flail your arms around. Put your mind in the muscle that you are working. When you are performing a chest movement, you should feel it in your chest—a back movement, you should feel it in your back, and so on. Stay in control of the motion. Breathe, and do not bounce. Let the muscle that you are working fatigue, and then rest it. *Never work the same muscle groups two days in a row.*

CIRCUIT TRAINING
"Super-Circuit Training"

This event integrates "aerobic" with "anaerobic" exercise to accomplish not only strengthening and toning, but fat-burning as well. This is a very efficient way to address both issues if time is a problem. The idea is to <u>keep moving</u>

from one exercise to the next—without rest. It is not unlike the "super-sets" I have presented here for the lower body. The difference is, between sets of resistance movements, you insert a cardio interval. The purpose is to keep your heart rate up, so the cardio (aerobic) interval should be between one and three minutes in length. The following is an example of a total body workout, using marching in place as your aerobic portion.

Do not do this routine two days in a row.
Music, maestro!

1. March for 5 minutes	10. Dumbbell chest press
2. Stretch	11. March for 2 minutes
3. March for 2 minutes	12. Dumbbell shoulder press
4. Dumbbell squats	13. March for 2 minutes
5. March for 2 minutes	14. Seated bicep curl
6. Lunges	15. March for 2 minutes
7. March for 2 minutes	16. Tricep press
8. One arm rows	17. March for 2 minutes
9. March for 2 minutes	18. Abdominal crunches

March again for 2 minutes and repeat all of the above. End with another 5-minute aerobic interval. If you have a heart-rate monitor you can tell if you are staying in your "zone" for fat burning. This entire event should take you about an hour.

Don't forget your music!

"CROSS-CONDITIONING" OR "CROSS-TRAINING"

When you are training frequently, it is a good idea to vary your exercises to reduce the risk of injuries. Choose two or three exercises that you enjoy (such as power gliding, swimming, and cycling), and alternate them so you do not do the same thing two days in a row.

"POWER-GLIDING"

This is an exercise I invented for myself that is somewhere between "race-walking" and running. The difference is, it moves low and long, rather than short and "hippie" like race walking, or "jumpy" like running or jogging. I will go into this in more detail, but for now, just picture the cartoon character associated with the phrase "Keep on truckin." Remember his stride, with that big foot coming toward you? (Wow, you *are* as old as me!) Well, believe it or not, he is what I visualized when I created this movement. The reason I developed this stride, (which also has a fast pace and arm movements), is because the pounding of running (which is my favorite thing to do) was not only contraindicated after my knee surgery, but it also ages the face, (and who needs any help with *that*).

CHAPTER III

<u>Now, What Do I Eat?</u>

Have you noticed how society accepts a "thin" woman more nonjudgementally than it does a fat woman? Since I've been both, I can tell you from experience that this "observation" is, unfortunately, true.

How I envied the waifish girls like Twiggy, my hip-less high school friend, Pam, and especially my genetically skinny sister, Joanne.

Ah...but there's the key. Genetics.

We are individuals whose body types are determined by our genes.

Really?

Dr. Neal Barnard in *Live Longer, Live Better*, tells us if we come from pears, we will be pears, and if we come from apples, we will be apples.

Period. End of sentence.

And it would also be "end of chapter" if there weren't a whole lot of encouraging words to be shared on the subject. We can't control our genetics—we are dealt that hand at conception—but we can adapt our eating patterns to "leanfully" coexist with our genetics. And you *can* modify your shape. I've done it!

The important thing to realize here is that we are all *different*. I am not my sister Jo. Same family, yes...but we are not *twins*...so we are not the same. Which explains why we grew up eating the same food, at the same time, in the same amounts, *and I wore it*...while everyone thought we *starved* her.

As I might have mentioned, I am 100% Italian. Now, Italian food may be completely harmless to that genetically gifted 25% of the population that (according to research) can eat all they want and never gain an ounce. You know these people. (Didn't you always want to give them their own planet?) But I, of course, exist in that miserable 25% that has to negotiate with everything we eat. According to this same research, 50% of the population has normal responses to food (whatever that is).

STOP THE FATNASY!

I'm really not talking here about food per say.

What I am talking about here, specifically, are <u>refined and processed carbohydrates.</u>

And what is an Italian meal primarily composed of? You got it. We have at least three starches (usually refined carbohydrates) in a meal. Well, you gotta have Italian bread (a refined carbohydrate usually served with butter) and, of course, pasta (refined)...and then beans (if you're having Pasta Fagioli). Then, Eggplant Parmesan (my favorite—my mom's is the best on the planet!)—but do you know how it's made? Coated with bread crumbs, fried, and layered with sauce and cheese, sauce and cheese...

And then...how about a canoli or a tiramisu (refined to the *tenth* power) for dessert?

Oofa. Thatsa five...(not to mention the sugar!). And...we eat this stuff at <u>night</u>.

It has a lot to do with our individual response to this stuff, and with hormones (I don't mean just estrogen, either—we already know how yanked around we are by *that* one). In this book you will learn about several other hormones, the significant roles they play in the way our bodies process food, and the profound way we are all unique in this respect.

And this is just one issue.

Does it ever seem like you are controlled by food? And doesn't that make you feel guilty, weak, and undisciplined? Well, I have news, my friend—we are not pathetically weak-willed gluttons. We *are* controlled by food. There is no drug more powerful. (Just watch a child on sugar, or someone who's had too much alcohol). So, if we take a look at this little factoid, we realize that everything we eat has a consequence. It could be positive, it could be negative, but it will *be*. So, there is never a time when..."aw, come on, one won't hurt ya." Not when you walk the metabolic tightrope I do. When I'm out of balance...I fall, and in this chapter you will see why.

Anyway, back to pasta. Now, this isn't about "pasta bashing," so don't call the Pasta Police. But, a New York Times article a few years ago was headlined,

"Bye Bye Pasta, It's Been Fun." Now, what was that all about?

Hadn't we been told to eat more carbohydrates? Hadn't they proven that *fat* was the dietary villain here?

There are more "fat-free" products on American supermarket shelves today than ever before, but what has happened to America? It's fatter than it's ever been! We are the most obese people on the planet; 35% of our female population and 32% of our male population are dangerously fat, and one quarter of our country's children is overweight. And we are eating fat-free! Well—are we? Or, are we now just combining these seemingly benign foods with some remaining dietary fat—and what fat we have eliminated we've replaced with—<u>refined carbohydrates</u>? Refined carbohydrates plus fat equals a larger fruit in the fruit bowl—no matter its shape!

We have been told in the past to eat lots and lots of carbohydrates (and, let's face it, our choices have been, at best, unfortunate), eliminate fat, and "don't worry about protein—we get enough of that one way or another."

Do we know what we are doing?

THE REAL DEAL
The Good Old Days

To better understand what refined and processed foods do to us, let us now take a look at how people ate "way back when." Our ancestors were hunters and gatherers. They ate meat when they managed to kill an animal (and if they were lucky enough in the hunt to not become the hunted), so primarily they lived on fresh fruits and vegetables, and lean wild game. Humans seemed to have been designed for this type of diet. In fact, there is evidence to support the theory that our ancestors were very fit precisely because their diet was appropriate for the continuation of our species. Robert Pritikin, in his book, *The Pritikin Weight Loss Breakthrough*, hypothesizes: "Perhaps there is a diet that humans are designed to eat, one that promotes health and protects us from most diseases. Logic pointed directly to such a possibility, since a major part of our evolution included the process by which human biology adapted to foods that were available in our environment. Certain foods dominated the diets of our ancestors. The challenge early humans faced was to adapt biologically so that they could extract maximum amounts of nutrition from these foods, and thereby survive. Scientists today know that the diet we evolved on is made up largely of plant foods, such as vegetables, beans, grains, and fruit, coupled with relatively smaller quantities of animal foods. This diet was extremely low in fat, because even the animal foods our ancestors ate were lean."

Progress?

Then, along came technology. We began "refining" grains, which removed the germ (and the essential fats) so they wouldn't spoil during storage. But, one of the problems that resulted from the development of this "process," is that the food we now consumed had its vital nutrients stripped away. Compounding this issue, by existing on a diet where the staple component had all the nutrient value of cardboard, we were developing many "third world" type diseases. When this reached epidemic proportions, "the powers that were" passed "The Enrichment Act," which forced companies to put nutrients back into their products. Hence..."enriched" rice, "enriched" pasta, etc. But these "enriched" carbohydrates (does anyone know what Uncle Ben Converted his rice to?) are still too far removed from the way nature intended them to be, so they are absorbed into the blood stream faster than most "whole" foods. Also, they are calorically more dense. And, the significant issue with high-density, refined carbohydrates, is the response of the hormone insulin. Genetically speaking, most of us are not equipped for this relatively new food on the scene, and it will probably be several hundred thousand years before our digestive systems adapt to it. So, in the meantime, research now indicates that 75% of us have an insulin response to excess carbohydrates that will prevent us from being as lean as we would like to be, and evolution won't be able to solve that little problem in our lifetime.

Now, *why* is too much insulin undesirable in fat control? *And how much* carbohydrate is *too much* at one time? And *what time* is the *wrong time* to eat it? *How much* protein is too much? Do I eat protein *with* carbohydrates? And what about *fat*?

And you thought you were confused before...right? Wait...it gets better.

Certain carbohydrates get into your bloodstream faster than others. This is undesirable because the faster your blood sugar elevates, the more dramatic the insulin response.

What does this all mean?

It means that you could not only store those carbohydrates as fat, but you might be unable to use already-stored fat for energy, and you might not be able to access the glucose stored in your liver to feed your brain. And then your body will send out a cry for more...

CARBOHYDRATES.

And around and around she goes...and round she does become.

"Wait a minute...you're telling me that even if I eat no fat...and count my calories...and exercise my face off...I could still have trouble losing body fat? This is not only unbelievable, but unfair."

You said it.

And, here's the kicker. You know those elegant little social events that take place every evening commonly referred to as "dinner?" Well, depending on your daily schedule (which affects the rhythm of certain hormones) if they occur after six p.m., and they are comprised of mostly refined carbohydrates (with some dietary fat)...guess what?

You got it. Stored as fat.

Also, you know that bagel, or energy bar that you might typically grab before an aerobic event for "energy?" It could shut down your body's mechanism for burning fat!

How can this be?

Well, the human body was designed in this fashion for very specific reasons. And, understanding *how* the body works, and *why* it works this way, will illuminate these complex issues for you and give you more control. It did for me. They say that "knowledge is power." Well, I still don't know who *they* are, but for once, they were right. Education is powerful stuff.

Now, if you're wondering why you needed this education—why you can't just turn to page "such and such" and get your "menu"—well, I want you to finally realize that *you will have more power over your body when you understand how it works.*

Allow me to digress here with a little car analogy.

If you're like me, you've left the mastering of the complex machinery in your life (like your car) to your significant other..."Honey, it's making this loud kachunk noise and it shudders when I stop like it's cold, but it's actually hot, I think, because the little light that says 'hot' came on and there's steam coming out of where the engine is..."

Helpless, aren't we?

We cannot sort out how to keep our cars running efficiently without *knowledge.* "What do you mean it's out of oil? It had oil when I bought it." Has your car ever broken down on the road, and have you lifted the hood (after someone came over to show you how to do it) and stared at this massive metal *thing* without having a clue about what you were looking for, or at?

"It just won't go anymore, that's all...it's stopped and I can't make it go."

Do you want the same helplessness with your body? Wouldn't you like to know how it goes so you can keep it going more efficiently, and beautifully? Wouldn't it be nice not to be at the mercy of the millions of opinions that are being passed off as "scientific facts," all of which confuse the daylights out of you?

Wouldn't that be terrific?

Also, consider this—if we were cars, we would acknowledge that we were all *different types of vehicles!* So we would require different fuel mixtures and amounts. Some of us are racecars, some of us are all-terrain vehicles, some of us are delicate classics, and some of us are diesel-powered Mac trucks! Got it?

I rest my case.

Now that I have your attention...

Read on...and wonder no more.

EVALUATING THE "BIG THREE" MACRONUTRIENTS:

Carbohydrates, Proteins, and Fats

First of all...we really have to begin at the beginning here.

Hardly a day goes by that I'm not asked..."Well, what is a protein? Meat, and what else? Okay, I got tuna fish, what else?"

People are really confused.

You all do understand that bread and pasta are carbohydrates.

But what are fruits and vegetables? Lots of people think they are their own little nutrient. There are proteins, carbohydrates, fats...and fruits and vegetables.

Hello. Fruits and vegetables are *carbohydrates*.

Okay, that's a good place to start. So let's look at carbohydrates.

Carbohydrate

This class of foods is commonly known as sugars and starches, but what all carbohydrates basically are is sugar. Sugar molecules that are chained together—and some of those chains are longer or more "complex" than others.

Carbohydrates—along with fats—are usually referred to as "fuel foods." Protein can also serve as a "fuel food" (contrary to popular belief), but we will get to that in a bit.

It is a fact that carbohydrate is the preferred "fuel food" (even though both fat and sugar [glucose] provide energy at a rate that meets the demands of specific physical activities) because dietary fat is perceived to be more "fattening" than carbohydrate (we'll also get to that later).

How do carbohydrates actually become fuel for our activity?

Let's examine what happens to carbohydrates when we eat them. Some—the ones called "simple sugars"—can be absorbed into the bloodstream right from the mouth, stomach, and intestine—while the more "complex" carbohydrates need the digestive enzymes to break them down into "simple sugars" so they can enter the bloodstream. Only glucose, however, can be used by the cells, so the liver has to convert the other simple sugars to glucose.

Once we have glucose in the blood, it needs *insulin* to enter the cells, so the pancreas (which is the factory for insulin) releases it. Some of this glucose will be used for energy, and some of it will be stored as *glycogen*. Now, just as your car's gas tank has a limited capacity for fuel storage, so your body has a limit as to how much glycogen it can store (about 1500 calories of energy from carbohydrates can be stored in our muscles and liver). When your glycogen stores are full, whatever excess glucose remains will be stored as fat.

Muscle glycogen is actually stored where it is used—and can only be used as fuel for that particular muscle—which won't share. Not even with the brain—"The Big Kahunna."

Now, the brain depends on glucose for fuel, but it cannot store it. It also will not readily use fat for fuel. So, when we skip a couple of meals, our ability levels drop significantly because our nervous system is deprived of its fuel. That's when we become "hypoglycemic" (i.e., low blood sugar), as well as dim-witted. This is not a good time to play "Jeopardy."

The liver can convert *glycogen* back into glucose and release it back into the bloodstream. This is where glucagon comes in (another hormone that is released by the pancreas). Glucagon's primary function is to release stored glycogen from the liver. Remember, however, that we only have a limited capacity for glycogen storage here (about 60 to 90 grams), so it's important to maintain these storage sites. And we do that by eating carbohydrates. How often should we eat them? There is no simple answer to that question. To merely say—eat three times a day, or eat every five hours, or three hours—is misleading. It depends on the composition of the meal, your individual metabolism, your activity level, a whole slew of variables. Some food can sit in your stomach for as long as four hours. Then, the intestines have to deal with it. And, depending on the situation, you may not want to consume more food until you've digested the last meal. The concept of frequent feedings should address the fact that eating frequently needs to be proportionate to the complexity of the meals. When we "snack" on the small "meals" that are recommended in some books, what we usually turn to is some type of carbohydrate. Well, if you keep giving your body sugar (which all carbohydrate is ultimately converted to), why would it break your fat down? On the other hand, if you wait too long, your next meal could cause an insulin spike—which will inhibit fat utilization. There is *so much* to consider. Throughout this book I present research that supports many arguments in this and other issues—but ultimately it is what is appropriate for you that is the bottom line. In your *Live It Or Diet Lifestyle System*, we will address meal spacing, as well as the issue of hypoglycemia.

As far as "to eat or not to eat" just prior to aerobic exercise, I asked Bach McComb, Ph.D., N.D., D.O., to elaborate on this issue. (Dr. Bach is a friend of mine in Fort Lauderdale who is an Osteopath, Naturopath, and nutritionist. Dr. Bach does nutrition counseling and product formulation, and he continues to educate himself in this complicated and ever-changing field.) Dr. Bach said:

"It really depends upon what your goals are, both short term and long term. For example, if your goal is to burn fat stores, then eating will be counter-productive. If your goal is to have maximum energy for your workout, then it depends upon your body's energy stores (glycogen and fat) and its biochemical efficiency at utilizing those stores. Unfortunately, many people in our society have down regulated their biochemical energy utilization enzymes by constantly snacking on "junk food" and related sources of quick sugar. These are the people who get weak and spacey when they go very long without ingesting food/junk food. Under normal conditions, the average person will have way more than enough energy stores (glycogen and fat) to see them through just about any workout (including a marathon) provided they do not exceed their aerobic capacity (by aerobic capacity I simply mean that their cardiovascular-respiratory-circulatory systems' capacity to deliver sufficient nutrients and oxygen to the heart and the specific muscles performing the work to allow for efficient conversion of energy stores to energy that runs the body).

The idea that a person 'needs' to eat prior to exercise is really pretty absurd. They need to eat properly each and every day, day in and day out, in order for their bodies to be properly nourished and able to replenish energy reserves and rebuild muscle, connective, and other vital tissues. A meal just prior to exercise will have little, if any, positive impact upon their performance and recovery. In fact, it is more likely to hamper performance, digestion, and ultimately recovery, rather than help it.

Think about it in terms of survival and digestive physiology. Do you think that it would be in our best interest from a survival perspective if we needed to eat in order to be able to run fast and far? Or to fight off an enemy attacking unannounced? Of course not! Our bodies are designed to be able to respond to a threat or stressor at any time, pre or post meal. Exercise is a stress stimuli that sets off a chain reaction in our bodies that mobilizes energy stores. It is part of the basic stress response known as the 'fight or flight' response, which is mediated by the sympathetic nervous system (see, *Metabolic Type*). When this system is activated it prepares our bodies to respond to a perceived threat by heightening our attention and awareness, increasing the blood flow to the muscles, mobilizing energy reserves to increase blood sugar levels, etc. At the same time, our parasympathetic branch of the autonomic nervous system (see, *Metabolic Type*) becomes suppressed. This system helps to run the digestive, maintenance and repair departments of our bodies. So you see, if we exercise shortly after eating, and we do so with sufficient intensity, our digestive abilities will become impaired, thereby making that meal much more of a liability than a help.

Besides the stress response activation of energy stores, there is also your body's normal homeostatic response that will help to maintain energy/blood sugar levels. When you exercise on an empty stomach and begin depleting blood sugar, this is sensed by the hypothalamus at the base of the brain. The hypothalamus then sends a message that ultimately reaches the pancreas, causing it to release glucagon (see, *Insulin and Glucagon—The Critical Balancing Act*). Glucagon is a hormone that travels through the blood stream to all the tissues of the body, including the liver, where it stimulates the mobilization of glycogen stores, which can readily be broken down into glucose (blood sugar). It also stimulates gluconeogenesis, which helps to produce new glucose from other stored materials, as well as the breakdown of fat for energy production.

So, the bottom line response to the question of whether you should eat something before exercising is: No. Since most people who exercise are interested in burning fat stores, eating will be counter-productive. Even if you are already quite lean and simply want to maximize the intensity of your workout, I still think that the vast majority of time, you'll perform better if you don't eat anything prior to exercise. Your body should have more than enough energy reserves to get you through just about any workout within reason. If, on the other hand, you are an elite athlete who pushes him/herself through long, grueling workouts everyday, this does not apply. Elite athletes who are maximally stressing their bodies' performance and recovery boundaries are a whole different story.

Many people, as previously mentioned, have symptoms when they miss meals (see, *Hypoglycemia*). This may indicate a blood sugar problem and should be evaluated by a physician who is knowledgeable in nutrition and metabolism."

Other nutritionists recommend eating a little something before exercising aerobically. They maintain that some people might feel fatigued all day if they do a cardiovascular event in the morning without eating. If you are one of those people (and again, everyone is different) eat a very light serving of a complex carbohydrate; something that enters the bloodstream slowly—like a small serving of high fiber cereal, or half of a grapefruit. Never try to exercise right after a big meal. Remember, digestion will be compromised, as well as your workout.

Dr. Ornish, Dr. McDougall, and Robert Pritikin, among others, all advocate frequent feedings. Dr. Ornish and Mr. Pritikin both cite (what seemed to be) the same research project. Dr. Ornish writes: "A study in the New England Journal Of Medicine by Dr. David Jenkins and his colleagues at the University of Toronto reported that grazing is good for you in a remarkable variety of ways. The researchers randomly divided people into two groups. Both groups ate the same type and amount of food. However, one group ate the food divided into three meals a day, whereas the other group ate it divided into seventeen meals a day (what the researchers called ëthe nibbling diet'). After only two weeks, they found that the nibbling diet: Reduced blood cholesterol levels by over 15 percent, reduced cortisol levels by over 17 percent (which indicates less stress on your body), and reduced blood insulin levels by almost 28 percent (by nibbling throughout the day, your blood sugar stays more constant, so you don't need to make as much insulin)."

While reporting on Dr. David Jenkins' study in his book, Robert Pritikin writes: "Dr. Jenkins had volunteers, all of whom were diabetic, eat three meals a day consisting of 30 percent fat—then he took the same people, placed them on the same diet, but portioned out the food in thirteen small meals, taken every hour. The people who ate thirteen small meals throughout the day produced 30 percent less insulin per day than those who ate the three large meals each day, even though they were both on the same exact diet."

Dr. McDougall advocates eating six or more small meals a day, and snacking frequently on recommended foods. He says: "Studies have shown that obese people tend to eat fewer, but larger meals than lean people."

The whole subject of digestion requires an entire library of books. The active digestive process is a very stressful event. The highest priority the body has on a long-term basis is the intake of nutrients. If you eat too soon after your last meal, that new food may impede the digestive efficiency of both meals. Most people eat under stressful conditions anyway (on the run, thinking about something else, etc.) and what should be a relaxed event in the first place is further compromised.

While researching this book, I came across many conflicting views on carbohydrate and protein requirements, meal patterning, macronutrient ratios— in fact, about the only common thread I have found is that it's good to *eat*.

The views on carbohydrate requirements range from:

"The actual amount of carbohydrate required by humans for health is zero" (Doctors' Michael and Mary Dan Eades in their book, *Protein Power*).

To:"When the body has to deal with a high-protein, low-carbohydrate diet, it says, 'Hey, I didn't fall off the turnip truck. The brain needs carbohydrate to function, so I'll start ripping down muscle mass, and I'll turn much of the protein in that muscle mass into carbohydrate.'" (Dr. Barry Sears in his book, *Enter The Zone*).

I will try to put all of these disputes in a row for you, and once it quacks, we can finally pronounce it a duck and get on with it.

Protein, The "Under-rated" Nutrient

"Proteins are the building blocks of life"...have you heard this expression?

Believe it.

Your muscles, ligaments, tendons, organs...your body is made from proteins.

And enzymes (the stuff that controls all the chemical reactions in the body) are also made of proteins.

Without protein, we could not manufacture hemoglobin or red blood cells (which need to be replaced every 90 to 120 days) and our internal transportation system would be shut down. Also, if we do not consume balanced protein, and we do not make an adequate number of red blood cells, even if we have sufficient iron in our diets, we could still become anemic. (I will explain "balanced protein" shortly.)

We would not grow, repair damaged tissue, or regulate our daily body functions without protein in our diet.

Sounds like a pretty important nutrient, doesn't it? Something we might need to pay attention to, wouldn't you say?

Proteins are long chains of amino acids. There are 20 different amino acids that make up protein. Your body can make twelve of them. The other eight (Essential Amino Acids) have to come from your diet every day. In fact, two of the twelve amino acids your body can make may be "essential" as well, since the body cannot make enough of them under certain conditions. So those too, at times, must come from the food we eat.

Proteins wear out, and—if any of the amino acids are missing—we cannot make new ones. This, as you can imagine, would be a disaster.

Let me give you an example.

You've no doubt heard of the immune system?

This exists all throughout your body and has specialized cells that float around whose job it is to recognize foreign invaders. When they see one, they mount a defense that is designed to neutralize the invasion. Without a working immune system, you are susceptible to infection and—like a terminal AIDS patient—you succumb.

So, a strong, healthy immune system is a very important part of *living*.

But, your immune system cannot work unless it has the necessary raw materials to accomplish "cell division." One immune cell that recognizes a foreign invader cannot do the job itself, so it has to recruit an army of additional cells to do that job. When the foreign invader initiates a signal, an immune cell takes that signal and starts dividing, making more and more cells. To divide rapidly enough to produce the number of immune cells needed to fight infection, it must be able to make DNA, which is the basic foundation of all life. To make its DNA, it needs certain raw materials. It has to get those raw materials from either the diet, or from the only part of your body where the raw material is stored, and that's the muscle.

The muscle in your body is a "savings bank" of raw materials that are necessary for certain life sustaining functions. For example, when your body is in "crisis" from a severe illness or injury, your muscle could be broken down in order to provide those raw materials that are necessary to boost the immune system. Muscle will surrender these raw materials without a fight, but when it does, it shrinks in size.

So, visualize your muscle mass constantly, day in and day out (albeit imperceptibly), shrinking and struggling to build back up if you do not have protein balance in your body.

This is just one example of the importance of protein. It is a very busy nutrient.

In addition to all the building and repairing that protein is contracted to do, it can also be used as a "fuel food."

But, before protein can be used as fuel, it must be converted to carbohydrate. There is only the addition of a nitrogen molecule that distinguishes protein from carbohydrate, so the body can make carbohydrate from protein, but not visa-versa. The body does this by removing the nitrogen, typically as urea in the urine. This could, however, tax the liver and kidneys if done on a regular basis.

Because of the fact that scientists were unable to detect increased nitrogen in the urine of exercisers (until a few years ago), they concluded that amino acids were not being used as energy. With scientific advancements, however, new techniques have shown that protein is converted to carbohydrate during exercise. In fact, research indicates that with increased intensity and duration of an exercise, the contribution of amino acids is increased. Recent studies show that If you are exercising intensely for more than an hour, energy from the conversion of protein to carbohydrate may contribute as much as 12% of the total energy requirement!

This protein use could, however, deprive the body of the amino acids necessary for repairing tissues, as well as developing enzymes, hormones, and muscles. It could also mean that you are breaking down your *existing* muscle for fuel. Therefore, once again, this issue of *balance* comes in. We must have a diet that includes an appropriate balance of proteins and carbohydrates (and some fats) so the body can function as it was meant to. What that particular balance is depends on your individual requirements. When you know your oxidative rate, you will learn your appropriate ratio of protein, carbohydrate, and fat (see, *LIVE IT OR DIET LIFESTYLE SYSTEMS—A Holistic Approach*). But, in general, from all of the research and the books that I have read over the past several years, the average recommended dietary ratio appears to be: 15-30% Protein, 40-65% Carbohydrate, and 15-30% Fat. Wide ranges, right? (For those who are fortunate enough to not be concerned with the issue of unwanted body fat, fat intake could be at 30%, as long as the majority of that fat is not saturated.)

When I studied nutrition, we were taught that the "RDA" for protein was .8 grams of protein per kilogram of body weight (a kilogram is 2.2 pounds). So, using myself as an example, at approximately 48 kilograms (105 pounds) the "traditional" RDA of protein for me would be approximately 38 grams of protein a day. And that's what I used to teach my clients. Over the past several years, significant data has appeared that supports the argument that living in this "modern age"—with all of its characteristics: Stress, pollution, pesticides, preservatives, etc.—demands higher protein requirements than the RDA's specify. Also, the old recommendation does not take the individual into consideration. The fact that I am a bodybuilder and tear down my muscle tissue on a daily basis, in addition to my other life stressors, along with specific information regarding my oxidative rate and thyroid function—these factors are not considered with the old method.

One of the current means of calculating protein requirements factors in individual considerations, and are determined by the amount of lean body mass you have (as opposed to total body weight). According to *Protein Power*, the following are appropriate protein guidelines: If you are sedentary, you need .5 grams of protein per pound of lean body mass. If you are moderately active, you need .6 grams; active, .7 grams, very active, .8 grams, and if you are an athlete, you need .9 grams of protein per pound of lean body mass. (See *Appendix D* for Accumeasure Personal Caliper.)

Dr. Barry Sears, author of *The Zone*, concurs, except he takes the requirement for "athletes" up to one gram of protein per pound of lean body mass. Again, using myself as an example: At 15% body fat, I am 85% lean body mass, which means approximately 89 pounds of me is lean body mass. I would put my activity level somewhere between "very active" and "athlete" because I do some form of strenuous exercise six, or sometimes seven days a week. So, that puts my individual protein requirement at approximately 80 grams per day—more than double that of the old RDA for me!

The biggest problem, I have learned, is not that we are actually eating too little protein, but we are not <u>efficiently</u> digesting the protein we are eating. The solution to this is not to just eat more protein. In fact, Dr. Bach McComb says that hypoglycemia (see, *Hypoglycemia*) could in some cases be more than a blood sugar issue—it could actually be a result of inefficient protein digestion. Dr. Bach says: "Your body needs certain protein constituents (specific amino acids) in order to replenish stored glucose reserves (glycogen). If a person doesn't consume, properly digest, absorb, and assimilate sufficient protein, they will not be able to properly restore blood glucose levels when needed. Protein is the most complex and difficult macronutrient to digest, and there are a number of things that people typically do to interfere with its optimum digestion, such as: Overcooking, poor food combining, eating under stress, taking antacids inappropriately, being inadequately hydrated, drinking too much and/or the wrong liquids with meals, etc."

Be careful as you read all of the recommendations for higher protein. I have been tested, so I know what my personal needs are, and I know if I am in "protein balance" and "calcium balance." I mention calcium balance because ingesting more protein than your body needs might increase your risk of osteoporosis (see, *15 Rounds—My Championship Bout*). In the book, *What Your Doctor May Not Tell You About Menopause*, written by John R. Lee, M.D., he says: "If one eats more protein than required for nutritional purposes, it is not stored in the body (as fat is, for example) but must be excreted. Excess protein waste products are excreted in the urine. The excretion of protein waste products through the kidneys increases the urinary excretion of calcium. The ratio of calcium ingested and calcium lost in the urine is called the "calcium balance." A high intake of protein creates a negative calcium balance (i.e., more is lost than was ingested). A negative calcium balance will cause it to be pulled from the bones." This is obviously undesirable!

(See, *Osteoporosis*).

It is also important to note that you must <u>not</u> try to meet your daily protein requirements in <u>one</u> meal, but spread your protein intake throughout the day. A good guideline for most people is to not exceed 30 grams of protein in one meal. Also, please keep in mind that there are many other sources of protein apart from animal (see, *Help-I'm A Vegetarian!*).

Another issue is your thyroid function (see, *Thyroid Hormone*). Broda O.

Barnes, M.D., in his book, *Hypothyroidism—The Unsuspected Illness*, warns us about the following: "It seems clear that diet quite high in protein utilizes available thyroid hormone. Two studies in the medical literature indicate that excess protein lowers the basal metabolism. This may explain why so few people have been successful in losing weight on standard types of diets. With extra thyroid needed for utilization of protein, the metabolism could fall to the point that 800 calories a day would maintain existing weight, rather than lead to weight loss. It would appear that a rational and natural approach to overcoming obesity should employ a slightly modified diet containing approximately one gram of protein for each kilo (2.2 pounds) of body weight and a minimum of fifty grams of carbohydrate to avoid ketosis. Enough fat should then be added to keep appetite satisfied and still not quite enough to satisfy the body needs, thus allowing a weight loss of one to two pounds a week. It may take a short time to adjust to the absence of excess carbohydrates previously consumed, but one can live on such a diet comfortably for long periods if some extra vitamin B is added. <u>Those who do not care enough about their health to follow such a diet program will probably suffer less damage by remaining overweight than by following crash diets.</u>"

Dr. Atkins, in his book, *Dr. Atkin's New Diet Revolution*, tells us ketosis is something we should consider "one of life's charmed gifts." Dr. Atkins writes: "The term ketosis, when it applies to the benign diet-induced type we're talking about, is really a shortening of the term ketosis/lipolysis. Lipolysis means 'the process of dissolving fat.' There is no lipolysis without ketosis, no ketosis without lipolysis. Being in ketosis simply means that you are burning your fat stores and using them as the source of fuel they were meant to be."

Hold the phone.

This is not dangerous?

Neal Barnard, M.D., wrote in his book, *Food Is A Wonder Medicine*: "Some weight-loss plans, such as Dr. Atkins' Diet Revolution, promote diets that eliminate carbohydrates and push high-protein products like meat and eggs. There are several things wrong with that. First, they are not a formula for permanent weight loss. High-protein diets will cause a loss of water from the body, and fairly quickly, too. High-protein foods release by-products that act as diuretics, forcing the kidneys to work much harder than they should, gradually wearing out the 'nephrons,' which are the kidneys' filter units. High protein diets also cause calcium to be lost in the urine, and may be the principal reason for osteoporosis in the United States."

As you can see, when we go back and forth between "traditional" views and "cutting edge" arguments, it becomes, at best, confusing. Research is constantly being conducted in this arena, however, so the controversy, no doubt, will continue to rage.

There have also been recent studies that suggest eating protein can stimulate the use of fat for fuel. The connection? Once again, *Human Growth Hormone*. (Growth Hormone is mentioned in several places in this book because it applies to many different aspects of the body's mechanisms.)

You might also find this interesting...

There have been numerous experiments investigating the compulsive eating of sugar. The outcome of these studies is the following: Animals have demonstrated an "addiction" to sugar under unnatural circumstances. They will not consume an excess of sugar when their diet is "balanced;" however, on a <u>low protein</u> diet their reliance on sugar becomes excessive.

Let's see now, protein was the nutrient we were once told we didn't have to think about, wasn't it?

In order for your body to perform all the necessary jobs with it's protein tool, it must have all the amino acids present in the tool box, so, once again, it is important to eat high quality <u>lean</u> protein in your meals throughout the day. How much protein you need to consume on a daily basis, once again, boils down to who you are, and what you require as an individual. Your *Live It Or Diet Lifestyle System* will evaluate what your macronutrient requirements should be. (Right now, however, it sure seems like some folks would have the old "Food Pyramid" turned upside down—(see, *Fat Free-Fat Chance.*)

We've covered two macronutrients, and we've touched on a few concepts that I'll be going into more detail on in the next chapters. But first, it's time to get to know the remaining nutrient...the one you cower from in fear. Hide your hips, we are going to discuss...

Fat, The Misunderstood Nutrient

For almost two decades fat has been getting a very bad rap. Conventional wisdom would have us believe that it is solely responsible for the out-of-shape bodies we are so ashamed of.

And so, if we cut it out of our lives completely...we eliminate the enemy, right? Well, to begin with, we should not be so phobic about fat. Our bodies need certain fats. To just focus on fat as the only bad guy in your dietary dilemma (unless it is, of course, the bad fat) might prove disappointing (and even harmful).

Fats have many important jobs in the body; among them, making hormones. Fats make you feel satiated after a meal. They keep you warm. And fat, along with fiber, slows down the absorption rate of carbohydrates into your blood stream.

In fact, you cannot even burn fat unless you consume certain fats.

(I knew that one would get you.)

To sum all of this up: For optimal health, the human body needs dietary fats. Again, I am referring to a balance of these fats, and I am not referring to *unnatural, partially hydrogenated fats*, which should be avoided and/or eliminated.

"Essential fats" are fats that your body needs, but cannot make itself. You have to get them in your diet. *Linoleic Acid* is actually the only essential fat, and unless you go on a totally "fat free" diet, you will get it from the food that you eat. One of the important lessons here is, *fat does not necessarily make you fat.* If the fat content of your diet is too low, you could experience the following symptoms: Compromised immune system (resulting in frequent illnesses), dry skin, brittle nails, dull hair (or worse, hair loss), gastrointestinal disorders, bad PMS, depression, headaches—the list goes on and on. Does any of this sound familiar? If you are like me (and have tried at least one of the "fat-free" diets out there), you probably recognize several items on that list. I will go into more "gory details" on this subject in *Fat Free-Fat Chance.*

THE OTHER ESSENTIAL NUTRIENTS: VITAMINS, MINERALS, WATER AND OXYGEN
Vitamins and Minerals

There are seven nutrients required by your body for life—Protein, Carbohydrate, Fat, Vitamins, Minerals, Water, and Oxygen. The first three, or Macronutrients, are the energy nutrients—that is, they contain calories and break down to yield energy the body can use. Vitamins and minerals are *Micronutrients.* They do not contain calories, therefore, they do not supply your body with energy. Without the presence of vitamins, however, your energy will be compromised because you cannot efficiently convert the macronutrients to energy. (In fact, every single process in your body requires the presence of vitamins.) But, please do not believe claims that say you will boost your energy just by taking certain vitamins. Vitamins are <u>supplements</u> and are supposed to be taken with food (in order to be absorbed properly). Also, certain vitamins and minerals actually interfere with one another, so they should not be taken together. There are four "fat-soluble" vitamins (A, E, D, and K) and nine "water-soluble" ones (C, and B-1, B-2, B-3, B-5, B-6, B-12, Biotin and Folic Acid—the "B Complex" Vitamins). Fat-soluble vitamins can be toxic if overdosed because an excess will be stored by the body in fat cells.

Minerals are smaller than vitamins and are vital components of most constituents of the body, but they, like vitamins, supply no energy. The minerals that the body needs are: Calcium, magnesium, iron, zinc, copper, chromium, selenium, fluoride, manganese, sodium, potassium, phosphorous, and molybdenum. These are vital to the construction of the body (bone, teeth, tissue and blood), as well as the function of the body (hormones, enzymes, chemical reactions, etc.). Our bodies do not make them, so we must get minerals from our diet. Earl Mindell, R.Ph., Ph.D., and author of *Earl Mindell's Vitamin Bible*, wrote in his "Keats Good Health Guide," *The MSM Miracle*: "Minerals are known for their role as catalysts, speeding up chemical reactions in the body. As catalysts, minerals reduce the energy required for formation or breakdown of substances, so that processes such as digestion and healing occur more quickly and efficiently. Minerals perform in the body like worker ants in an ant colony, making sure everything that is needed for the colony to function properly gets handled efficiently.

Maintaining good health and preventing disease through adequate mineral intake should be a natural result of eating the proper foods. And, up until the industrial expansion of the 19th century, the cycle of minerals was mainly undisturbed, as vegetables, meat, fish and dairy foods remained reliable sources of most minerals. Today, however, increasing air and water pollution, intensive farming, deforestation, the refined and highly processed foods we eat, along with the use of prescription drugs (see, *Drug Depletion*), have the cumulative effect of depleting the natural availability of dietary minerals. It is my belief that mineral depletion so evident in today's crop-growing soils is reflected in the depleted state of health of people all over the world.

I don't want anyone fooled by those nutrition tables you see listing the amount of vitamins and minerals in foods. They don't reveal if produce was grown in a mineral-balanced soil or comes from an over-farmed or polluted soil. Nor can they give any indication of naturally occurring variations in soils from different geographic areas. What's more, I can tell you that some nutrition tables haven't been updated in over twenty years! As long as practices exist which continue to rob the soil of mineral content, even one year can make a difference to food values. For this reason, food that might have been nutritious at some point in the past may well prove to be totally devoid of any food value by the time you eat it."

Talk about a raging controversy! The need for vitamin and mineral supplementation is not only disagreed upon, but opposing parties are downright passionate about their differing opinions. "**To supplement or not to supple-**

ment" certainly seems to be the question, and the answers range from:

"Normal people eating a balanced variety of foods are likely to consume more nutrients than they need. Of course, 'health hucksters' won't tell you this because their income depends upon pushing products. The RDAs are deliberately set considerably higher than virtually all-normal people require in order to encompass the range of individual variations and provide for storage of safe amounts. In other words, bioindividuality has been taken into account." (*The Vitamin Pushers*, Stephen Barrett, M.D. And Victor Herbert, M.D., J.D.) to:

"How much supplementation do we need? This is a crucial—and irrationally controversial—question. The answer is very simply that we often need far, far more than the RDAs indicate. They are way off the mark for a number of reasons. First, let's consider again the 'average, healthy American' eating a well-balanced diet on whom those RDAs are based. We've already seen that the 'average American diet' is hardly adequate—if such a diet even exists. What about that 'average, healthy American?' He (or she) doesn't exist either...we have come to identify and respect the existence of something quite different in nutrition—biochemical individuality." (*Food Allergy & Nutrition Revolution*, James Braly, M.D.)

And back and forth this issue goes. Confusing, right?

Also, since studies show that we habitually eat the same ten foods over and over again in our diets, we probably aren't getting the variety of foods necessary for balanced nutrition, so we take vitamins to compensate for that. (We will get into the concept of "Food Rotation" later in this chapter.) Another reason for swallowing supplements might be, since we feel we have destroyed our environment, the nutrients just aren't there in the foods we eat.

Doctor Barrett and Doctor Herbert contend that the very fact that you have an orange on your plate means that the nutrients are on that plate as well..."If an essential nutrient is missing from the soil, a plant simply doesn't grow." (*The Vitamin Pushers*)

But Doctor Braly, in his book, takes this matter another step and says, "The actual RDAs of two different specimens of exactly the same food item can vary considerably. Two oranges, for example, can vary as much a 100 percent in their Vitamin C content, depending on: The time of year they were picked, total sun exposure during growing season, the age of the orange when it was bought and consumed, distance between orange trees in the orchard, amount of rainfall and wind during growing season, the quality of the trees, the site on which they're planted, how well the trees are maintained, and the handling factors."

In *It's Better To Believe*, Dr. Cooper states the following about what he calls the supplement issue: "In the past, a basic principle underlying many nutrition programs has been that a proper diet should make supplements unnecessary, but recent research findings suggest that certain supplements can provide some additional health insurance. In particular, if you are a woman past the age of menopause, you should consider taking calcium supplements. Also, it's important to take in sufficient amounts of the antioxidant vitamins—especially vitamins C and E and beta-carotene, the precursor of Vitamin A." (In fact, Dr. Cooper wrote a book called *Antioxidant Revolution*.)

What do *you* think?

I can tell you that I think there is a reason why so many M.D.'s and Ph.D.'s have departed from traditional medical practices and mind sets, and have explored the realm of "alternative" medicine, using nutrition (including supplementation), as well as other more "natural" approaches to "wellness." And I don't believe it is because they are getting on the "vitamin bandwagon" to make more money. Insurance companies still prefer to pay for an expensive medical procedure instead of a comparatively inexpensive alternative approach (one that addresses the *core problem* and not just the *symptom*).

Drug Depletion

There are many reasons why most of us take (or should take) vitamins and minerals. One is for nutrient insurance because we know we are eating poorly, and we want to compensate for that. Another really important reason to take certain vitamins is, if you have taken or are taking prescription or over-the counter drugs and other preparations. <u>Drugs deplete the nutrients in your body</u>. Different drugs cause different nutritional deficiencies. (See *Osteoporosis* for some real drama!) Most people are unaware of the nutrient deficiencies caused by drugs. Ask your pharmacist. Chances are, if he has an independent pharmacy (not part of a big chain), he has been educating himself in the area of drug depletion, as well as weight management and natural alternatives to harmful synthetic drugs.

Pharmacists are one of the most respected and accessible professionals in the community. We look to them for all kinds of answers, at all hours of the day or night. With the threat of the huge pharmacy chains gobbling up the market, our nation's beloved Corner Drug Stores are being put out of business. Rather than become a pill counter for one of these huge conglomerates, "Doc" has decided to turn his neighborhood drug store into a "wellness center." Hundreds of these pharmacy wellness centers use *Live It Or Diet Lifestyle Systems* as their schematic for determining an individual's needs.

I have had the privilege of speaking at LifeSpan conferences attended by independent pharmacists, doctors, nurses, and fitness professionals. (LifeSpan is a division of Health Trust Alliance.) I was thrilled to listen to (and co-lecture with!) Derrick DeSilva Jr., M.D., author of *Ask The Doctor* and host of a nationally syndicated radio show of the same name. Dr. DeSilva is touring the country, vigorously and passionately alerting health professionals to the hazards of conventional medications. He is currently writing a book about drug depletion with Dr. Jack Hinze, a clinical pharmacologist and a naturopathic physician (two seemingly opposing fields). Dr. Hinze has brilliantly converged his apparently endless knowledge of these fields, and develops natural formulations to heal the body. He too is committed to educating our country's pharmacists on a healthier approach. (Dr. Hinze also collaborated with Dr. Gary on *Live It Or Diet's* Nutritional Support Line.)

How the body is depleted of nutrients is information you *must* have, and I urge you to look for Dr. DeSilva and Dr. Hinze's new book, *Drugs That Kill.* (see *Appendix C* for Live It Or Diet Center locations.)

I am completely blown away by what I have learned about drug depletion. As a health and fitness professional, I now realize how critical it is to know exactly what drugs (and other non-prescription stuff) people are taking to make *any* determinations about them. This changes the complexion of *everything!* For example, let us look at some of the more common drugs people take. The following information is from LifeSpan's workbook:

Antibiotics deplete: *Probiotics/Enterobiotics*, (the "friendly" bacteria that is essential for immune function and defense against allergic responses and dysbiosis), all *B-vitamins* (which, when depleted, will cause fatigue, anemia, impaired immune function, and impaired metabolism of protein, carbohydrates, and fats), *Vitamin C* (depletion will cause a weakened immune system, susceptibility to some forms of cancer, prolonged wound-healing time, and damage to nerves, eyes and vascular system), and *Vitamin K* (which is needed for blood clotting). For additional depletions related to bone loss, see *Osteoporosis.*

Antidepressants deplete: *Coenzyme Q-10* (depletion will lead to more cell damage from free-radicals, compromised immune system, a faster aging process, increased fatigue, and possible increase in asthma, allergies, respiratory disease, decreased brain function, heart disease, weight gain, yeast infections, multiple sclerosis, gum disease, and diabetes) and *Vitamin B-2* (which is needed for the formation of cells, antibody production, breakdown and metabolism of starches, fats, and proteins, and healthy eyes).

Synthetic Female Hormones deplete: *Vitamin B-6* (depletion can lead to increase in; fatigue, carpal tunnel syndrome, water retention, irritability, increased PMS, symptoms, allergies, arthritis, asthma, and a compromised immune system) and *Magnesium* (which is needed for healthy bones, muscles, and nerves, along with defense against weakness, depression, high blood pressure, and heart disease—an estimated 75% of Americans are Magnesium deficient!). The list goes on and on: *B-2, B-6, B-12, Vitamin C, Folic Acid, and Zinc* are also depleted!

Aspirin depletes: *Vitamin C, Folic Acid, Iron, and Potassium.*

NSaids (such as Ibuprofen) deplete: *Folic Acid*

Laxatives deplete: *Vitamin A, Vitamin D, Vitamin E, Vitamin K, Calcium, Potassium, and Vitamin D.*

And these are just a few examples! I guess you get the picture.

Dane Woodruff, President and CEO of Health Trust Alliance, tells us that: "It is estimated approximately 70% of the prescriptions filled deplete the body of some nutrient that needs to be replaced in order to prevent a nutritional deficiency. Many of the problems that develop with long term drug use are related to drug-induced nutritional depletion rather than as a direct side effect of the drug itself.

In depleting the body of certain nutrients, drugs can induce weight gain by disrupting metabolic pathways and increasing appetite. Most overweight people have some type of homeostatic disruption, or nutrient imbalance/deficiency. Many over-the-counter and prescription drugs can initiate or contribute to these imbalances. In addition, nutrient depletion can cause the gastrointestinal tract to become inefficient, interfering with nutrient uptake and absorption. This can result in weight gain as well.

Problems that develop from long-term drug use are often related to nutritional depletion caused by the drug's effects on assimilation of nutrients. Unfortunately, food processing, poor food choices, dieting, alcoholism, smoking, and drug addiction will all contribute to susceptibility to nutritional depletion. A vicious cycle has appeared here. First, we are not getting the amount of nutrients we need in our diets. In addition, we are taking medications that further deplete our bodies of the few nutrients that we have been able to obtain."

Your *Live It Or Diet Lifestyle System* will take into account any drugs you may be taking. As you now know, this is a vital component!

I could go on and on—(actually I do in *Taking Control*).

Water

Water forms the major part of every body tissue, yet we often ignore it, and take it for granted. And, although water yields no energy, it does provide the medium in which practically all of the body's activities are performed. How much water do you need? (A lot...but for a simple guideline see *K.I.S.S.*) In your *Live It Or Diet Lifestyle System* we will help you determine how much water you need. There we will factor in body weight and activity level. In general, you need approximately half your body weight in ounces of water (pure, filtered, reputable spring water) per day. (A tip—drink eight ounces of pure water thirty minutes before each meal. This will accomplish two things: First, it will signal your system to start releasing digestive enzymes and second, it will calm down your appetite.)

Dr. Carolyn L. Mein (a Chiropractor with a degree in Bio-nutrition) discusses water in her book, *Different Bodies—Different Diets*. Like with everything else I am presenting to you in this book, there are conflicting opinions on what kind of water to drink. Dr. Mein writes: "The water that comes out of your tap generally comes from surface sources such as streams, rivers and lakes. The original water usually contains at least a moderate amount of pollutants. They include pesticides and fertilizers, as well as exhaust residues and bacterial pollution. When the water comes into the filtration facilities of cities and towns, it is treated to remove these pollutants. To accomplish this, various chemicals including chlorine, fluorine, phosphates, sodium aluminates, and other chemical elements are added to the water. While some of these chemicals have been implicated as cancer-causing agents, they continue to be widely used in municipal water systems."

Dr. Mein continues by warning us to not drink water that is completely void of minerals. "Minerals are the body's foundation. If a food, or even water, does not contain the necessary minerals to be assimilated, minerals are leached out of the body. This is the problem I have with distilled water, and reverse osmosis systems."

Dr. Mein ends her chapter on water with this: "Finally, it should be noted that anything to excess, including drinking water, can be harmful to the body. Drinking too much water can leach out mineral stores in your system and result in vitamin and mineral deficiencies.

Once again, the goal with everything is moderation, neither too much or too little. We want to achieve <u>balance</u>."

A little known fact is that hydration must take place on a cellular level (See, *The Importance Of Hydration* in PHASE I: *Starting The Process*). Just drinking tons of water may not insure that this is happening. We could drink water, and actually still be *dehydrated*! Also, just replacing your lost water without concern for lost electrolytes and electrolyte balance will equally not serve you. We lose sodium, potassium, and other minerals when we perspire—especially when we exercise. In addition, Dr. Gary wants us to know that for every 12 ounces of soda we drink, we lose (or urinate) 14 ounces of water!

In his book *Your Body's Many Cries For Water*, F. Batmanghelidj, M.D. tells us that water regulates the body's processes, and solids respond to the amount of water in the body. It is a primary regulator of the functions that occur within us, and must not be overlooked.

Oxygen

We all know we need oxygen to live. Which means your muscles need oxygen to function, and your blood has to supply the oxygen. You can't burn fat without oxygen. Your most efficient energy production systems are shut down without enough oxygen. But, you need an adequate blood supply to transport the oxygen, and this will be an inefficient event if your blood is deficient in certain nutrients.

It may seem dumb to discuss something as fundamental as breathing, but I would like to take a moment to call your attention to how you breathe when you are doing something physical. Is it through your mouth, or through your nose? If you are breathing through your mouth, your breathing is too shallow and you are supplying your cells with less oxygen. Breathe through your nose to get an adequate supply of oxygen to your cells, which enables all systems (including fat mobilization) to function more efficiently. It may take some practice at first if you are not used to it, but keep trying.

INSULIN AND GLUCAGON...THE CRITICAL BALANCING ACT

When our diets contain too many carbohydrates (particularly refined and processed ones), and not enough protein, we tip the delicate balance between two very important hormones in fat control—insulin and glucagon. Both of these hormones are released by the pancreas, but two different macro-nutrients stimulate their release—insulin is stimulated by carbohydrate (and high blood glucose levels), and glucagon is stimulated by protein (and lower glucose levels). Even though these two hormones are "opposing forces," they work in harmony with one another when it comes to metabolic functions of the body. When we talk about "the storage and release of energy" in our bodies, we must acknowledge what *Protein Power* calls "The Yin-Yang of Metabolism."

There has been a great deal written lately about our metabolic hormones and how they affect fat storage. The big culprit indicted in all of this is insulin, which affects every cell in the body. We know it regulates blood sugar, but it also controls the storage of fat, among dozens of other functions it performs in the body. It is called "the master hormone of metabolism" because without it we would die, but like everything else in life, if there is too much, or too little, in other words—an absence of "balance" in insulin production, we're in trouble. Eating a lot of carbohydrates—especially refined and processed carbohydrates—produces a lot of insulin. We always thought of just sugar producing this response, but keep in mind that all carbohydrates, once broken down by enzymes, enter the body as *sugar.*

Insulin is a storage/anabolic hormone. Studies show that insulin might be a vital instrument in the regulation of testosterone levels and sex-hormone-binding globulin in "normal-weight and obese humans" (Pasquali, et. al. 1995). Only one of its jobs is to take dietary excess and store it as fat. (Let me inject here that a rise in insulin doesn't mean that you automatically increase body fat stores—please do not leap to conclusions yet. Remember your responses are unique to *you.*) Insulin also initiates the response of an enzyme that inhibits the release of fat from fat cells. Therefore, when you have a carbohydrate snack (particularly a <u>refined</u> carbohydrate) before aerobic exercise looking for energy for your event, you could actually prevent the utilization of the very thing you are intending to burn for energy—your *fat.*

So, if we think of insulin as the "Yin" in the energy controlling behavior of the body, then the "Yang" is glucagon, which is a "mobilizing" hormone. When the presence of insulin decreases, the presence of glucagon increases, and when glucagon is at the helm, the body's metabolism is steered toward fat burning. While insulin stores, glucagon burns; while insulin stimulates the "fat-storing" enzyme, glucagon stimulates a fat-releasing enzyme, relieving the "gatekeeper" from his post and allowing fat to "escape" from the fat cell. Doesn't that sound great?

Here I want to briefly discuss *insulin resistance.* As a child, when your pancreas released the amounts of insulin necessary to deal with the sugar that you ate, your young cells were "sensitive" to that insulin. However, after years of eating "reward foods" (which then became "comfort foods," such as candy, cake and ice cream—see, *Sugar Sensitivity*), your cells' sensitivity might have become damaged, which would make them *less sensitive* or *resistant* to insulin. That means that it might now require more (lower quality) insulin in your system to make your cells accept the sugar from your blood. More insulin—possibly more body fat. But, there is a more serious side to this. In an article on diabetes published in the September 1st, 1999 edition of USA Today, we are told that there are millions of cases of insulin resistance, which they call "a precursor to diabetes" (see, *Can I Give Myself Diabetes?*). Ira Goldfine of the University of California at San Francisco (who is conducting research on genetic causes of diabetes), states in the article: "About

60 million Americans are estimated to have insulin resistance, and about 25% will go on to develop diabetes."

Now, of course, there are those genetically gifted individuals who have not developed *insulin resistance*, even after years of eating garbage. Ah, but how do they feel?

Although some of the books I have read recommend lowering carbohydrate intake to control insulin, others advocate the opposite. For example, Dr. McDougall writes: "In general, high-carbohydrate, high-fiber, low-fat foods make insulin work more efficiently and reduce the amount of insulin needed by the body. On the other hand, high-fat foods dramatically increase insulin production. Refined foods, like white bread, white pasta, and white rice move rapidly into the blood and cause a surge of insulin production, too." Robert Pritikin states: "In general, minimally processed plant foods keep your insulin levels low because they are slowly broken down by your intestines, which means their sugars are released slowly into your bloodstream, and you can keep burning fat."

It seems we might never get to the bottom of all this controversy and conflict. One constant I have observed (and so will you as you read this book) is that *refined and processed carbohydrates* are the ones that most of the experts nail as the "insulin instigator." Beyond this dietary no-no, your hormonal responses to more natural foods is unique and, as you will see in your *Live It Or Diet Lifestyle System*, you can have a game plan that works for you.

"CALORIES IN-CALORIES OUT"...AND OTHER FAIRY TALES

Everywhere we turn we are told, if "the calories you consume equal the calories you burn, you will maintain your current weight." At some point, scientists decided that energy was like a "seesaw." On the one side there is the energy that you take into your body, and the other side there is the energy that goes out via physical activity and metabolic function. So, a formula was developed that says: "If the energy input on this side of the seesaw is equal to the energy outgo on that side of the seesaw, your body weight stays the same." You're in balance. And, when you do the math on paper, or with calculators, or using the most sophisticated computer software available, it looks like a "done deal." The problem with it is...it just doesn't work out that way in real life.

Somewhere between the "calories going in and the calories going out" is a whole mysterious world that might as well be "Oz" for all the sense it makes from person to person. There is an enigmatic "unknown region" between the two sides of this equation that has to do with the way each of us *uniquely processes food*. Most people, however, still believe that if they want to weigh less, then the thing to do is to eat less, sometimes a lot less. In fact, the more they'd like to lose, the less they'd probably eat on a daily basis to get the body to burn up its stored fat to supply the energy it needs. This logic is guaranteed to fail them every time.

Some of you may have figured this out the same way most of us figure it out; you simply looked in the mirror and thought, "I don't look so good." Then you compared yourself to another who, for all intents and purposes could be a carbon copy of you in terms of age and physical activity—and you're *starving* yourself, but every time you look at this person, he or she has a cookie in their hand—and *they are skinny!* Well, what's up with that? You're being good, and this person's gone *wild*, or at least that is your perception. The fact is, they are not eating more than they require, and they are probably not eating more than you, it just seems that way.

This is a real biological fact. You can take two people who are exactly the same age, the same sex, who have the same physical constitution and engage in the same activities (basically "carbon copies"), and the number of calories that one person could require day in and day out can be totally different from the other person's need, even though they are almost copies, almost twins. So, what's different between them?

Their genes, for one. They are not identical twins.

And each person has their own "metabolic mystery."

There are some basics here, though. Being sedentary is a very good way to gain fat. You do need to expend calories above your daily basal metabolic requirements to efficiently lose body fat (see, *PUTTING IT ALL TOGETHER*). Robert Pritikin writes in his book, *The Pritikin Weight Loss Breakthrough*: "The muscles of an average woman can store about 1,000 calories in the form of glycogen; those of an average man, about 1,500 calories. The amount varies depending on the size of your muscles (men tend to have bigger muscles than women) and whether or not you have exercised. If you exercised vigorously, the reserves of glycogen in your muscles will be low, which means that you'll have more room to store more blood sugar. If you haven't exercised today, then your muscles will be full, which means there will be no more room." So, what happens to the food that you eat when your storage tanks are full? Well, if you are a couch potato, and you eat a refined and processed food that includes both concentrated carbohydrates *and* fat, the incoming fat will be forced into storage so the sugar can be burned off quickly. And what about your existing body fat? It stays right where it is.

Mr. Pritikin does offer that: "Exercise alone is not a very efficient way to lose weight. You burn about 100 calories per mile of walking or jogging. There are 3,500 calories in every pound of fat. That means you have to walk thirty-five miles just to burn 3,500 calories, and only half the calories you burn are from fat. The other half are from carbohydrate." You must couple a responsible eating regime with exercise for optimum results.

But, what do we usually do? Because most of us are not biochemists—and since there is so much conflicting advice out there—we take the course that seems the most logical to us. We cut our calories and hit the stairmaster. Most of the low calorie diets out there restrict calories by as much as 50% of what is needed for maintenance. But, we tell ourselves, that's okay... 'cause we won't do it forever; just until the scale comes up with the winning number.

So, every morning we wake to one thought: "What do I weigh?" Then we hop on the scale. And if the needle has moved in the wrong direction, we don't read a number, we read failure. Not good for the mood of the day. And we will probably eat even less that day...or else binge out of despair. In either case, the scale has done a fair amount of damage without contributing one bit of useful information. Scale weight gives no insight into the composition of the body (what is fat and what is muscle), and that is the key here. Think about it. John Lollar, my friend who developed the personal caliper, Accumeasure, puts it this way: "If you went into a market and saw a sign that read *12 lbs for $1.99!* you would want to know 'twelve pounds of what?' before you made a purchase. But you'll get on a scale and ecstatically exclaim <u>I lost twelve pounds!</u> Twelve pounds of <u>what</u>?"

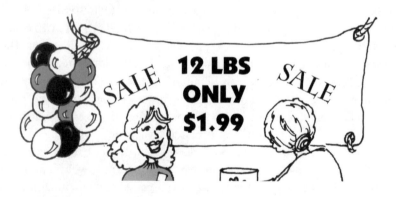

Most of us who desire to change our shapes to a more aesthetic, pleasing one, will have little success if we focus on just scale weight. Muscle weighs more than fat, and it's fat that you want to lose, not muscle. (Remember, a pound of muscle requires approximately 75 calories of energy per day for maintenance, and for every pound you lose, your caloric requirements decrease by that amount.) So, throw out your scales—get them out of your environment to remove the temptation. How will you monitor your progress? I find it interesting that we can test for such complex events as pregnancy and AIDS in the privacy of our homes, but we have to join a health club to have our fat pinched and measured by a stranger. No wonder we opt to go through life without this knowledge. But, even if you do not have your body fat *professionally* measured, you can still find out what it is—in your home—all by yourself. I just mentioned how—the Accumeasure—an accurate, user-friendly little tool you can use to test your body fat *personally*. (See, *Appendix D* for this convenient and inexpensive device. I recommend it if you really want to know where you're at, where you're going, and where you've been. The protocol has been tested against the most sophisticated methods of evaluating percent body fat, and it compared reasonably well.) In any event, it is not the *number* that you should concern yourself with when you test yourself, but the *descent* of that number.

Your body fat to lean tissue ratio is one of the most important bits of information to have when you begin a program. For now, however, you can use a tape measure, and a mirror. Personally, I use a mirror...and it tells me everything. We all know our bodies pretty well, and we have those little barometers, those particular *spots* on our bodies that indicate we've gained fat. I know where mine are. Also, I have a vein that runs down my stomach; when I can see it, I know I'm as lean as I like to be, and when it's not visible...uh oh. But what I simply won't do anymore is a diet that focuses on calorie deprivation. I know it's a no-win situation, and it will leave me in a bigger mess than having just gained a pound or two.

FAT FREE?-FAT CHANCE!

It is true that the typical western diet is still comprised of 40% fat, and that's too much. Especially since most of this fat is the "bad fat," or *saturated fat*. A saturated fat is solid at room temperature, like the fat you see on red meat, or butter, or—remember "Crisco?" I just ask people to imagine that stuff in their arteries, or under their skin. We really need to eliminate these fats from our diets, as well as "partially hydrogenated" ones. *Partially hydrogenated* basically means that a potentially good fat has been perverted in a process that allows it to be used in a product. This is also something to be religiously avoided. But, remember, *do not* aim for a *fat-free* diet. What you will be replacing those banished fat calories with to fill the void in your diet (as well as your stomach) will wreak havoc with your nutrient and metabolic balance.

When you eat whole grains and certain types of fish (like salmon) you will get the "good fats" that your body needs. But the boxes of "fat-free" products that are stacked to the ceilings in grocery stores are loaded with lots of little gremlins that will still make you fat. Read the labels. Bring your glasses to the supermarket so you can read the fine print if you have to. If the ingredient list reads as long as *Ulysses,* put the box back on the shelf. That product has been refined down to a drug, and your body's metabolism will just be out of control (and so will you) if you eat it. We think; "well, I have too much fat in my fat cells, so if I reduce the fat in my *diet* I'll reduce the fat on my *hips.*" Although this seems logical, this deduction is flawed because it does not take into account the aforementioned *metabolic hormones,* and how they respond to the "big three" macronutrients. *Balance, Grasshopper.*

High Fat Vs. Low Fat

Dr. Broda O. Barnes, in his book, *Hypothyroidism—The Unsuspected Illness,* writes the following: "For centuries, farmers have reduced protein intake, eliminated most of the fat, and shoveled in cereals to fatten animals for market. Unfortunately, physicians seldom go to the farm for medical information or we might long ago have had the answer to obesity." Dr. Barnes continues by wondering if it is possible to include more fat in the diet to help control obesity effectively and safely. He says: "For the past twenty-five years, the alleged danger of fats has been highly publicized. The time has come to correct the erroneous allegation." Dr. Barnes cites several studies, and concludes: "It appears from many studies that weight loss is more rapid and patients are better satisfied with a high-fat diet. There seems little doubt that a high-fat diet reduces the appetite through the slower release from the stomach of a fatty meal and by avoiding the excessive rise in blood sugar so common with high carbohydrate intake."

Okay.

But, in a recent issue of *Muscle And Fitness Magazine* (which, by the way frequently features insightful articles), Jose Antonio, Ph.D. writes: "A recent study by Horton, et. al. (1995) supports the contention that the composition of calories clearly influences fat deposition. Numerous studies show that diets with a greater percentage of their total calories derived from fat result in greater fat accumulation than an isocaloric diet of less fat. Glycogen and protein stores—unlike fat stores—are closely regulated, and increasing the intake of these fuels seems to stimulate their oxidation proportionately (as opposed to being converted to fat). Conversely, if too much fat is consumed, it's more likely to be stored as fat."

In the Horton study, the observations were the following: When subjects were overfed 50% above their normal energy requirements, carbohydrate overfeeding resulted in 75%-85% of excess energy being stored as fat, while fat overfeeding resulted in 90%-95% excess energy being stored as fat. It is studies such as these (and the conclusions that are drawn) that provide us with the foundations of many of the dietary recommendations that are being delivered to the public. In fact, it is the absence of such clinical studies to support his program that made Dr. Barry Sears and his book, *The Zone*, such a target for critics. Dr. Sears' sequel, *Mastering The Zone*, addresses some of the criticisms, offers some data, and basically stands by the original book and its arguments.

In *Dr. Atkin's New Diet Revolution*, by Robert C. Atkins, M.D., we read the exact opposite conclusion in another study. Dr. Atkins introduces us to two British researchers, Professor Alan Kekwick and Gaston L.S. Pawan, whose experiments provided: "The breakthrough concept, the mechanism and rationale, and the irrefutable experimental evidence that a low-carbohy-drate—yes, even a high-fat—diet has a significant metabolic advantage over balanced or low-fat conventional diets. Kekwick and Pawan did a study on obese subjects and found that those on a 90% protein diet, and especially on a 90% fat diet lost weight, but when they were given a diet of the same num-ber of calories, 90% of which came from carbohydrate, the subjects did not lose." The Atkins Diet contains: "Most vegetables, nuts and seeds, some grains and starches to the extent that your metabolism allows, occasional fruits, a variety of delicious protein foods, and some high-fat foods like but-ter and cream that you'll find stricken from nearly every other diet." Dr. Atkins has been accused of advocating a potentially dangerous "high fat diet." He maintains, however, that his diet is lower in fat than the typical American diet, and it results in "health improvement" because it eliminates "junk car-bohydrates."

Ookaay...

I have mentioned Dr. Dean Ornish, Dr. John McDougall, and Robert Pritikin elsewhere in this book. They are three of the better known advocates of very low fat diets. Dr. Ornish, in his book *Eat More, Weigh Less*, states: "Your body easily converts dietary fat calories into body fat. It is the exces-sive amount of fat and cholesterol in your diet—that is, more than 10 per-cent of calories as fat—that lead to excess weight, heart disease, and other ill-nesses." Dr. Ornish cites many studies, including one conducted at Stanford where the researchers found: "Overweight men and thin men ate the same number of calories. However, the overweight men ate more fat, and the thin ones ate less fat and more complex carbohydrates." Another study cited by

Dr. Ornish is one published in the American Journal of Clinical Nutrition by nutrition researchers at Cornell University that concluded: "Body weight can be lost by merely reducing the fat content of the diet without the need to voluntarily restrict food intake." (See, *The Set Point Theory* for more on this study.) Dr. Ornish's Life Choice Diet recommends that we eat foods that are very low in fat (no more than 10 percent of daily calories are to come from fat—and no saturated fat), high in complex carbohydrates and fiber—and avoid foods from animals. On July 21st, 1990, Dr. Ornish presented the results of his break-through disease-reversal study. 82% of his patients showed a reversal in coronary artery blockages. (Dr. Ornish's work is factored into *Live It Or Diet Lifestyle Systems*.)

Dr. McDougall, in his book, *The McDougall Program For Maximum Weight Loss*, writes: "Fat is easier to store than it is to burn as fuel. Your body will burn all the available carbohydrates before it burns significant amounts of fat. Regardless of the kinds of fats you eat, all are easily stored. Thus, even though fat is considered a high-energy food (as it supplies more than twice the calories of carbohydrates and protein), it is really a high-storage food, because in real life your body tends to store much of the fat you consume in your diet. Since more than 90 percent of the fat you eat is being stored, it means you need to consume only 3,765 calories of fat to make one pound of body fat."

Dr. McDougall does maintain that we do need "essential fats," and these must be obtained from the diet. However, he says: "Your need for essential fat is less than 2 percent of the calories in your diet. Even if you stopped eating fat entirely—a virtual impossibility, since all natural foods contain some fat—there is still a large supply of essential fat stored in your adipose tissues. Interestingly, essential fats are synthesized only by plants, not by animals. Therefore, a diet composed of plant foods—even those very low in fat—provides an abundance of essential fat to meet human needs."

Dr. McDougall's *Program For Maximum Weight Loss* advocates a diet comprised of whole grains, potatoes, squashes, legumes, yellow and green vegetables, and limited fruit. It eliminates all animal foods, oils, high-fat plant foods, and flour products.

We generally think that foods that contain fat satiate better than foods that don't, thus we eat less—but Robert Pritikin, in his book, *The Pritikin Weight Loss Breakthrough*, cites a study done by Dr. Susanne Holt and her colleagues at the Human Nutrition Department at the University of Sydney that demonstrated: "The foods that had the least capacity to fill people up were foods that were rich in fat and sugar. The foods that created the greatest feeling of fullness were natural plant foods (especially fruit), and the starchy carbohydrate-rich foods (with the exception of french fries, which are loaded with fat and have no fiber). By far, the most filling food was the potato, followed close by oatmeal." Mr. Pritikin's *The Pritikin Program* <u>does</u> allow some animal protein (limited to 3 1/2 ounces of animal foods per day), along with a large variety of vegetables, beans, fruits, whole grains, and low fat.

Dr. Ornish, Dr. McDougall, and Mr. Pritikin all tell us that it is dietary fat that is converted to fat—*not* carbohydrate. They maintain that the conversion of sugar (carbohydrate) to fat requires too much energy from the body (for not enough return) for the body to bother with it. All three authors also cite studies concluding that high fat diets increase the risk of heart disease and other diseases.

Who's The Villain?

In *Food Is A Wonder Medicine*, Dr. Barnard writes: "While extreme thinness may be a twentieth-century fashion perversion (amen to that!), overweight is not just a cosmetic issue. It is clearly linked to cancer, diabetes, heart disease, and other health problems. It is not 'natural' to be overweight. The fatty diet consumed in Western countries is not 'natural.' Being overweight is primarily due to the high fat content of our foods." Dr. Barnard also cites evidence that links many kinds of cancer (including colon and breast) to high dietary fat intake. In his book, *Foods That Can Cause You To Lose Weight*, Dr. Barnard states: "Carbohydrate-rich foods are power foods for weight control. They provide a 'negative-calorie effect' because they have ways of counteracting the storage of some of these calories as fat, and also encourage the burning of stored calories" (see, *Metabolism*). Dr. Barnard recommends that we eat a diet high in complex carbohydrates (as represented in our "Food Pyramid"), moderate in protein (with the majority of the protein coming from vegetable sources), and *look out for all fats!*

But...Dr. Rudy Rivera and Roger D. Deutsch, in their book, *Your Hidden Food Allergies Are Making You Fat*, write the following: "Who came up with this food pyramid? It is interesting that the official USDA food pyramid recommends a large sampling of grains and fruit each day. This pyramid may represent a way to assure adequate nutrient intake in the form of vitamins and minerals, but it is certainly no way to lose weight. As noted by Barry Sears in his book, *The Zone*, the food pyramid closely resembles the proportions of fat, protein, and carbohydrates fed to cattle in feedlots to fatten them for slaughter. I suggest you rethink the food pyramid. If it fattens cattle so well, why would it make us thinner? Americans aren't getting thinner; they are getting fatter."

Ooookaaaay...
Fat makes you fat.
Carbohydrates make you fat.
Protein cannot be converted to fat.
Excess anything can be converted to fat.
Fats curb hunger and cravings.
Eating fats make you crave more.
All right, class. Is that clear?
?????

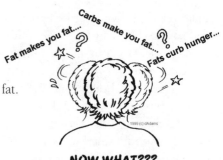

NOW WHAT???

Another *other* side to this issue is that *all calories are not created equal*. The "thermic effect" of fat, carbohydrate, and protein is different (and I go into detail on this in the section called *Metabolism*). Also, there is another underlying truth here—*all carbohydrates are not created equal, either*. Take a deep breath—and read on.

GLYCEMIC INDEX VS. "EFFECTIVE CARBOHYDRATE CONTENT"

Numbers, numbers. I'm so sick of keeping track of numbers, aren't you? First, we counted calories. Then, we counted fat grams. Then, carbohydrate grams, followed by protein grams. Then we were presented with a <u>new</u> chart to consult before any nutrient passed our lips—"The Glycemic Index Chart." The "glycemic index" of a food indicates how quickly that food gets into your bloodstream. The higher the glycemic index, the faster that food is absorbed into your bloodstream. Typical foods that have a high glycemic index are: *White rice, puffed rice, rice cakes, most commercial breakfast cereals, white bread, wheat bread, quick rolled-oats, instant potatoes, white potatoes, bananas, carrots, and corn.* Now that you know something about insulin, you know that a quickly elevated blood sugar will signal the pancreas to release high levels of insulin. This will lower your blood sugar, but it could also facilitate fat storage. So, even if what Dr. Ornish, Dr. McDougall, and Robert Pritikin say is true, and *carbohydrates will not be stored as body fat*, we do not want to eat a lot of high glycemic index foods if we are looking to lose body fat because of the insulin response. (See, *Insulin and Glucagon—The Critical Balancing Act.*)

Certain factors lower the glycemic index of foods. These factors are: Fiber content, fat content, and meal composition. Refined carbohydrates have very high glycemic indices, so they can make you fat even if they are "fat-free." Certain refined carbohydrates, such as fat-free cookies and rice cakes, actually have higher glycemic indices that regular ice cream. (Not that I'm recommending ice cream—please let me be clear on that—I am just using it as an example to show how fat can slow down the absorption rate of a food.) Dr. Barry Sears uses "glycemic index" as a tool in his book, *The Zone*. His charts break down foods into the following categories: "Rapid inducers of insulin, moderate inducers of insulin, and reduced insulin secretion." Keep in mind, however, that certain nutritious foods (such as brown rice, millet, potatoes, carrots and corn), with relatively "high" glycemic indices, will have their absorption rates (and thus the secretion of insulin) controlled by combining them with other foods in meals.

Doctors Michael and Mary Dan Eades use another indicator in their book, *Protein Power*, that they call "Effective Carbohydrate Content." They explain that: "Because the fiber content of foods is not metabolically active, you can subtract the grams of dietary fiber from the total carbohydrate content of foods you eat. We call what's left, the Effective Carbohydrate Content of food (ECC)." Although the authors of this book have a program that recommends lowering carbohydrate intake, when they count carbohydrates their ECC chart shows only the "metabolically active" grams of carbohydrate in a food. They contend, therefore, that by using this guide you will naturally choose foods that contain more fiber and less starch, and those will be healthier carbohydrate choices. They use the following example: One cup of broccoli, one cup of cabbage, three celery stalks, one cup of green beans, one cup of lettuce, 1/2 cup of mushrooms, one cup of zucchini, one cup of spinach, one cup of raspberries, and two slices of whole grain bread, spread out over a day, will give you only 40 grams of "usable" carbohydrates, and 21.3 grams of fiber, which they maintain is "almost 100 percent more than the average American diet—hardly stringent in terms of amount of food, vitamin content, mineral content, volume, fiber, or any other parameter." The authors of *Protein Power* feel that the whole concept of glycemic index gives people the inappropriate impression that there are "good" and "bad" carbohydrates depending on their number, and that this concept becomes "meaningless metabolically." When they developed their ECC charts, they removed the fiber component and left only "the pure, *metabolically* active carbohydrate for you to count so the whole concept of good and bad carbohydrates becomes meaningless *metabolically*."

Kathleen DesMaisons, Ph.D., author of *Potatoes Not Prozac*, calls her take on the whole subject "The Carbohydrate Continuum," and recommends staying away from "White Things" (quickly absorbed carbohydrates), and choosing from "Green Things" and "Brown Things" (which are absorbed more slowly). She tells us to eat foods high in fiber, and that "we will never get a sugar high from broccoli." (See, *Sugar-Sensitivity* for more on Dr. DesMaison's work.)

Dr. Bob Arnot in his book, *The Breast Cancer Prevention Diet*, makes a strong case against high-glycemic index foods. He warns that a diet composed of high-glycemic index foods raises glucose load, thus increasing insulin levels, hunger, body fat, and triglycerides in the blood. He further warns us that a recent study demonstrated that *women with elevated triglyceride levels had an increased risk of breast cancer*. Dr. Arnot recommends 30 to 50 grams of fiber per day, and at least 5 grams of fiber per serving, with no more than 5 grams of sugar.

I, of course, found all of this very interesting, so I went to another reference, *The Complete Book Of Food Counts*, by Corinne T. Netzer, and looked up a few foods. The following is what I found:

FOOD	CALORIES	CARBOHYDRATE	FIBER
Apples	80	20 grms	3.5 grms
Apple juice	80-90	20-23 grms	none
Wonder Bread (1 slice white)	70	13 grms	none
Whole Wheat Pita (small)	70	12 grms	2 grms
Saltines (1/2 oz)	70	9 grms	none
Rye Vita Crackers (1/2 oz)	50	12 grms	3 grms
Basmati Brown Rice (1 serv)	200	44 grms	3.1 grms
White Rice (1 serv)	200	44 grms	none
Rice Cakes (1/2 oz)	60	11 grms	none
Quinoa (1 serv)	200	38 grms	4.3 grms
Rolled Oats (1 serv cooked)	145	25 grms	4 grms
Steel Cut Oats (1 serv)	230	41 grms	6 grms
Pasta (1 cup cooked)	183	36.6 grms	none
Whole Wheat Pasta (same)	174	37 grms	6.3 grms
Sweet Potato	118	27.7 grms	3.4 grms
Sweet Potato (canned 1/2 cup)	90	20 grms	none
Carrot (fresh, raw, 2.8 oz)	31	7.3 grms	2.2 grms
Carrot (canned 1/2 cup)	35	7 grms	none

Now, using carrots and sweet potatoes (two nutrient-packed, extremely valuable foods) you can see the difference in the values between what God made and what remained after man processed and canned them. *Always buy a carbohydrate product with the least amount of processing and, therefore, the most fiber. Never settle for less than 2 grams of fiber in a product.* There is a great deal of evidence to support that appropriate fiber intake fights disease. (Some companies do a better job than others, and their foods retain more of their nutrients than with others, but <u>fresh</u> and <u>unprocessed</u> is always a better choice).

Back to carrots and sweet potatoes—they both fall under the "Unfavorable Category" in Dr. Sears' book, as they have high numbers on a glycemic index chart. But, according to *Protein Power's* "ECC," they are called carbohydrate "bargains," and are recommended. Dr. Atkin's *New Diet Revolution* recommends no more that 20 grams of carbohydrate per day on his "Induction Phase," and his book contains a carbohydrate gram counter from which you choose your daily carbohydrates. *Protein Power's* "Phase One" recommends no more than 30 grams of carbohydrate per day, chosen from their ECC chart. Dr. Sears wants to keep you in *The Zone* by consuming a diet that is 40% carbohydrate, which is portioned out in meals and calculated as "carbohydrate blocks," using the "glycemic index" as a reference. And then we come full circle with Mr. Pritikin, Dr. McDougall, and Dr. Ornish. Their very low fat, high complex carbohydrate "disease reversing" diets recommend approximately 20% protein (mostly vegetable), 10% fat, and 70% carbohydrate.

Two of the more recently published books on the subject of the body's response to carbohydrates are: *The Carbohydrate Addict's Diet* by Richard F. Heller, Ph.D. and Rachel F. Heller, Ph. D., and *Sugar Busters!* by a whole bunch of people (H. Leighton Steward, Morrison C. Bethea, M.D., Sam S. Andrews, M.D. and Luis A. Balart, M.D.). Both books became best sellers, (which proves that we are still searching). There is some good information in both books, especially <u>regarding the elimination of refined carbohydrates.</u> Both books discuss the studies linking an excess of insulin to high body fat and disease (see, *Insulin And Glucagon...The Critical Balancing Act*). *Sugar Busters!* gives you "acceptable foods" and "foods to avoid" (which have a high glycemic index). *The Carbohydrate Addict's Diet* shows you how you might be "addicted" to carbohydrates rather than just "indulging" in them. They offer "craving-reducing" foods, and allow a "reward meal" that includes the very things you might be "addicted" to (that's actually the part of the program that confuses me).

Are you dizzy yet? The one thing that all of these doctors do agree on is that most of us are fat because of *metabolic disorders*, and each approach attempts to control this condition by manipulating macronutrient ratios. It does, however, get confusing. But, listen—the starting gate is the same for each of us—*eliminate, or at least limit, refined and processed foods.* And, remember, you will know what is appropriate for you when we build your *Live It Or Diet Lifestyle System.* (By the way, if you still want to know the glycemic index of some foods, turn to *Appendix B.*)

ENZYMES...YOU ARE WHAT YOU DIGEST

Refining and processing foods not only destroys many vital nutrients (along with reducing valuable fiber content), but it also annihilates food enzymes. Food enzymes are naturally occurring enzymes that exist in every natural, raw food.

Enzymes are complex proteins that act as "catalysts" (substances that speed up the rate of chemical reactions without being used up in the process). Our bodies produce several thousand different types of enzymes that literally orchestrate every function in the body. No metabolic process can happen without them; they are the "link" in every chain reaction of our bodies. Digestive enzymes are produced primarily by the pancreas, and their job is to aid in the digestion of foods. When you consume certain foods that also naturally contain enzymes, these enzymes function as digestive aids as well. Overcooked and processed foods may not be fully digested when they leave the stomach, which means <u>you have just been malnourished</u>. Also, when this partially digested food continues on throughout the rest of the digestive system, it can become toxic. In her book, *Different Bodies, Different Diets,* Dr. Carolyn Mein tells us that: "When your food does not contain essential enzymes, your body must manufacture them. If the demand exceeds your body's ability to supply them, your digestion is inhibited. Consequently, the undigested food is stored as fat and you eventually notice a weight gain. Knowing this about enzymes, it might seem that the best diet would consist of eating only raw foods. However, totally raw diets put too much stress on most digestive systems. Balance is the key. Generally, everyone's diet should contain both whole and raw foods."

So, eating foods that contain "alive and well" enzymes will not only dramatically increase the efficiency of digestion (while reducing the work required by the body), it will also decrease the risk of disease. Many conditions have been associated with poor digestion, and you will learn more about this in *Taking Control.* But, for now, understand that you are not simply what you eat; instead, *you are what you ingest, break down, absorb, and utilize.*

ALCOHOL AND BODY FAT

Alcohol is a *drug*. And, being card-carrying members of "the Woodstock Generation," we all know what *that* is. For some of us, the fact that "the drink takes a drink" holds more significance than for others, but when we drink socially, most of us usually have more than one. And there are many undesirable consequences associated with this behavior.

First, let's talk calories. Alcohol contains seven calories per gram, compared to the four calories per gram of carbohydrates and proteins. So, when you do not figure it into your daily caloric requirements for maintenance, your conveniently boggled math could cause you to gain fat. If you do figure it in, those seven calories are empty nutritionally, and you will deprive yourself of your daily requirements of nutrients.

Also, alcohol disrupts every organ in the body, primarily the liver. Liver cells are the only cells in the body that can process alcohol, and in the presence of alcohol, liver cells must use it as fuel instead of fatty acids, which is their usual fuel of choice. Fatty acids, therefore, build up in the liver when we drink alcohol. When we abuse alcohol, fat accumulation in the liver becomes a serious problem.

Dr. Ornish writes: "Alcohol suppresses your body's ability to burn fat. When you drink alcohol, your body burns up fat much more slowly than usual. In one study, researchers found that three ounces of alcohol reduced the body's ability to burn fat by about <u>one third</u>." And, Dr. McDougall writes: "Alcohol accelerates the absorption of sugar from the intestine, increasing the level of insulin in the body. By activating an enzyme called lipoprotein lipase, insulin causes fat cells to accumulate fat. Insulin also blocks the breakdown of fat from these same cells, keeping them, and you, plump."

Dr. Bob Arnot writes in *The Breast Cancer Prevention Diet*, "Alcohol consumption is the most solidly established dietary factor related to cancer of the breast and one of the most powerful. The more you drink, the higher your risk."

On the other hand, you have, no doubt, heard of the research studies linking wine consumption to the low levels of heart disease found in France and other European countries. There are many factors that are involved in this observation of the benefits of wine drinking: Reduced stress, proven antiviral effects of grapes, high potassium content of grape juice, which could lower blood pressure and (as cited in *Protein Power*): "Several recent studies have shown wine to be an effective agent for increasing the body's sensitivity to insulin." The authors of *Protein Power* say that it might actually help reduce body fat to add a glass of <u>good</u> red wine to your meal. Now, I am going to qualify this all over the place here. *Good red wine* means *not cheap*, sweet wine with a high sugar content. And, *moderation* (a word I myself only recently learned) means we do not suddenly jump on this discovery with the zeal that we have been known to typically employ. This is truly another case of "more is definitely not better." Further, no one is talking about *distilled alcohol* here. Distilled liquor elevates insulin levels, and might damage your cells' sensitivity to insulin.

Dr. Barnard adds in his book, *Food Is A Wonder Medicine*: "Alcohol's reputation continues to decline in health circles. The findings that alcohol increases the risk of breast cancer and birth defects, and contributes to many other serious health problems, has cast a long shadow over the idea that a glass or two of wine might be good for your heart. For some people, at least, alcohol adds to the padding on the waistline. Six ounces of wine adds about 130 calories to your dinner. One beer contains about 150 calories (light brands about 100). A 1 1/2-ounce jigger of typical 100-proof liquor has 124 calories. In addition, <u>alcohol temporarily alters body chemistry to impair the body's ability to burn fat.</u>"

Add all that up, my friend.

HELP...I'M A VEGETARIAN!

If you consider yourself a vegetarian, you may fall into the following three categories: "Vegan," someone who only eats grains, vegetables, legumes, fruits, nuts and seeds; "Lacto-ovo Vegetarian," someone who doesn't eat any animal meat, but will consume milk products and eggs; and "Semi-Vegetarian," someone who is not technically a vegetarian, but considers him or herself one because they stay away from "red" meat.

As you can probably imagine, it is easier to insure that you are getting adequate amounts of all of the vital nutrients if you fall into the last two categories, but this is also possible even if you are a strict "vegan." Many grains and vegetables are good sources of these nutrients, and—if the food has not been compromised in any way—it should supply you with adequate amounts of what your body needs (provided, of course, that you are ostensibly healthy).

The main issue for vegetarians, however, is protein. Some of you might have heard of the book, *Diet for a Small Planet*, which was written by Frances Moore Lappe and published in 1971. Although Lappe's book made a significant contribution to the growing vegetarian community, it perpetuated the myth about "protein combining." Lappe wrote that, in order for a plant protein to be "complete," it had to be combined with another carefully chosen plant protein *in that same meal*. We now know that, while combining plant proteins does improve their efficiency, eating them in the same meal is not necessary.

Plant proteins have always been considered incomplete because their "amino acid profile" may be deficient in certain essential amino acids. The protein quality of these foods *is* affected by this deficiency, but—technically—all of the amino acids are *present*, so it is not as challenging as one would think to consume complete protein from plant sources. The American Dietetic Association recommends that we eat different types of proteins that "complement one another" throughout the course of the day. Most cultures already instinctively do this, i.e., "rice and beans," "pasta fagioli" (pasta and beans), and so on.

If you have heard that "plant proteins" do not have the impact on the human body that "animal proteins" do, this is probably because one is more "digestible" than the other. This is often referred to as "Biological Value," or "B.V. Rating" ("the amount of protein nitrogen that is retained from a given amount of protein nitrogen that has been digested and absorbed, i.e., a measure of protein quality"). Animal protein is rated at 95% digestibility, while plant protein is rated at 85%. In order to compensate for this ten-percent difference, you need to eat more protein in your diet if it only comes from plant sources.

Certain plant foods have higher protein than others—for example: Firm tofu (made from soybeans) contains twenty grams of protein for a half cup, most beans (including kidney beans, black beans, etc.) contain about seven to eight grams of protein per half cup, while lentils contain nine grams per half cup. One cup of soymilk provides ten grams of protein, and certain grains such as Quinoa and Spelt are relatively high in protein (approximately 5.5 grams of protein per half cup). A meal that includes Quinoa and lentils will provide at least 14 1/2 grams of protein, and one that contains firm tofu and rice will provide approximately 25 grams of protein. Also, remember that the Cream of Wheat you have for breakfast will rendezvous with the beans you have for lunch, and make both protein meals more "complete." Virginia Messina, M.P.H., R.D., and Mark Messina, Ph.D., in their book *The Vegetarian Way*, sum it up by saying: "Meeting protein needs doesn't require any particular meal-planning approach other than this: Eat enough calories to maintain ideal weight, and include a variety of plant foods in your diet."

As far as calcium is concerned, you will find that many plant foods have a bountiful supply of this mineral. We worry that if we cut milk products out of our diet, we will become calcium deficient. But, it is important to realize that many humans are *lactose intolerant* (which means we have trouble digesting milk products—mostly because of the way they are processed). In general, calcium is most plentiful in soy products, dark green leafy vegetables, and beans. There is, however, much concern (and debate, of course) over the calcium requirements for women. The issue here is osteoporosis, but many other factors (such as hormone levels) are involved besides calcium. In *The Vegetarian Way*, the authors present studies to support their argument that, "...throughout the world people who consume the most calcium actually have the poorest bone health."

And, just when you thought you had the answer to something!

CAN I EAT OUT?

I know, the "food police" have said a lot about dining out lately, and I am horrified at some of their suggestions. First, the answer to the above question is yes....absolutely. It's nice being taken care of for a change. We deserve it. But what are some of the "authorities" saying about eating out?

Recently on the "Nutrition Tip Of The Day" segment of a South Florida news program, the following "tips" were offered to keep you from "wearing" your restaurant meal:

*"Upon arrival...eat plenty of the bread that's brought to the table. Bread has no fat, and it will cut down on your appetite so you will eat less of your meal."

*"When eating at a Chinese restaurant, eat plenty of white rice. White rice has no fat, and it is safer than the mysterious dishes on the menu."

????

OHMYGOSH.

Oookaaay...

I have some different tips.

*First...that "authority" needs to brush up on some of the alternative information in the weight-management department, like something that's been published after 1985.

*Second...when the wait-person arrives at your table...*refuse the bread* and ask for your salad to be brought to the table right away, along with ingredients below. If you have read any of the preceding data in this chapter...you know why.

*When eating at a Chinese restaurant...*eat little to none of the white rice*. If they offer brown rice, order it as an alternative...but it too will be refined, so eat very little of it. Order your dishes *steamed* (there are many dishes on the menu that can be prepared that way), and make your own sauce from mustard and the (lite) soy sauce (most Chinese and Japanese restaurants offer "lite" soy sauce now).

Although it may seem challenging to stay on a food plan when you eat out (especially if your favorite establishment offers only fried foods, subs, and pasta), it is not impossible. All it takes is knowing how to order, and cooperation from the restaurant. Most restaurants are happy to make adjustments to accommodate health issues. You do not have to always order off the menu.

For example: Breakfast. If the menu offers egg dishes, vegetable dishes, chicken dishes, or turkey sandwiches—there is a good possibility that the kitchen has eggs, vegetables, chicken, and sliced turkey. So, order a 4 egg-white omelet stuffed with available vegetables and diced grilled chicken (or turkey). Hold the cheese (not like Jack Nicholson) and pass on the bread. 99% of the restaurants in this country have only refined and processed breads (even if they call it whole wheat). If you "need" a carbohydrate, order oatmeal with your eggs instead (without the milk and sugar, of course).

When you are having dinner in a traditional restaurant, order a *grilled* protein dish like fish or chicken, and ask for it *dry* if it comes with a sauce. Have the sauce put on the side if it sounds interesting and not too dangerous, and ask for lemon, mustard, olive oil, and parmesan cheese to create your own sauce if you need to. Have a salad with your "sauce." Pass on the starch—especially at night—and order double steamed vegetables (again, you can use your "sauce"). You may have a glass of good red wine with your meal if you choose (and if this isn't a no-no for your issues). In *Protein Power* the doctors even say that there have been studies that indicate that red wine increases your body's sensitivity to insulin.

If you are starving when you are seated, order bottled water with lemon slices. Drink a glass *before* your meal, not *during* it. Drinking while eating dilutes gastric juices and impairs digestion. Also, digestion starts in the mouth, and the habit of gulping a drink while you are chewing washes away the digestive process. Having some lemon before your meal is good because it stimulates digestive enzymes. Sushi is great—but not white rice. Some sushi restaurants offer brown rice; otherwise, order mostly sashimi (do have the sea vegetables—alkalizing and very healthy!).

I feel it is important for you to be comfortable dining out. It is one of the great pleasures of life. And if you are like me, and find it is a frequent occurrence in *your* life...you'll need to know the territory so you are not sabotaged. Avoid dishes in cream sauces. Avoid pasta dishes at night. Never have anything fried. *Ask questions* if you are unsure what the ingredients are. Tell servers you are allergic, or tell them you are sick, or *tell them nothing* because you don't have to...you're the customer, remember?

Keep your meals simple in strange restaurants. Don't let yourself be tempted by exotic titles and chef "specials." No matter where I go in the country, I never have a problem. I always order the same way, and I really enjoy the experience. No, I do not feel like I'm sacrificing my "evening out." I can taste my food, not its disguise (which is some chef's fantasy, not mine). I never look longingly at a companion's gooey, creamy, greasy plate and wish I could eat anything I wish. *I am eating anything I wish.* I wouldn't trade how my meal is going to make me feel compared to how theirs is going to make *them* feel for all the Miel De La Foret Vierge Tropicale on the planet (not to mention how mine is going to allow me to *look*.)

THE LINK BETWEEN BODY FAT AND EMOTIONAL PAIN

I would be remiss if I did not acknowledge this subject while discussing possible saboteurs of health. This component may very well be a large puzzle piece for you. If it is, it certainly needs to be addressed.

Most of us have heard of "stuffing," which is a response to an emotional trauma that manifests in mindless, continuous eating, even when we are not hungry. Here as well, though, we can consider that the emotional stress caused a biochemical imbalance that triggered this "sabotage" reaction. Listen, my friends, since I too am a victim of this behavior along with some of you, can we make a pact right now? As we reach for something that we know will harm us, throw us off track, *set us back*, let's stop for a moment and think of each other—joined in this struggle to love ourselves enough to not want to *inflict punishment on ourselves.* What did we do anyway? Chances are, someone's done something to us. And, wouldn't attaining our goals be the best revenge?

Dr. Doreen Virtue, a psychotherapist specializing in eating disorders, has written several books on this complex topic. In her book, *Losing Your Pounds Of Pain*, Dr. Virtue writes the following:

"Every extra pound you carry on your body equals a pound of emotional pain you carry in your heart. Pain is neither normal or acceptable, and the human response to pain is to seek relief. Many people use food as relief from such pain. A happy, content person eats moderate amounts of food and keeps physically fit. Anyone who has suffered through an abusive relationship, a life trauma, or excessive stress automatically seeks a way to feel better. Food can provide shelter and a way to block out awareness of painful memories and uncomfortable emotions. But food is a tool that revictimizes the victim. Being fat carries social consequences that are painful in themselves. The overweight person is in a cycle of pain."

Does this sound like you? Dr. Virtue contends the following:

"If you: Struggle with your weight, sometimes feel hopelessly drawn to eat something even though your mind is screaming, "Don't eat it!" and diet and weight-loss programs don't work for you...then there is some part of your life that is unresolved."

Dr. Virtue cites many research projects that "point to overeating as the chief coping mechanism for depressed sexual abuse survivors." Actually, there is so much to say on this subject, as with most of the subjects I have presented in this book, that there is a virtual library of information available. In Dr. Virtue's book, she helps you identify if abuse or stress (tension) is an underlying cause for overeating. She says:

"Tension is also a major factor leading to compulsive overeating due to psychological and physical forces. New studies point to brain chemistry changes in response to tension. These changes increase our craving for certain foods, especially those loaded with carbohydrates such as rice cakes or muffins."

Dr. Virtue identifies four primary emotions that could lead to overeating: "Fear, Anger, Tension, and Shame (FATS)." She recommends that: "When you're hungry, it's vital that you resist the impulse to automatically reach for food. Instead, ask yourself: 'Could I be feeling Fear, Anger, Tension, or Shame?' Just by asking yourself that question you'll feel more in control or your eating."

In *Appendix H* you will find a referral list of doctors, clinics, and programs that address food allergies and addictions.

SWEET *REVENGE*

No matter who we are, and how we process this information intellectually, there are times when we just have to have something *sweet*. We know that this desire, this sometimes overwhelming craving for a sweet thing, will come with consequences—but when we are in the throws of our body's calling, we don't seem to care. Then it happens—weight gain, fatigue, brain fog, headaches, gastrointestinal distress, impaired digestion, depression, anxiety, CRASH, and then craving again! Was it worth it?

The truth is, the desire for something sweet (besides being the result of imbalances) is innate. Humans have a strong natural instinct to consume sweet foods because of the need for our mother's sweet milk. One of the problems is that we carry this instinct into our adult life, and associate sweetness with comfort and reward. We turn to simple, refined sugars to satisfy our biological need, and set up a whole series of metabolic catastrophes that worsen with age. In some paradigms, the "sweet taste" is considered part of a balanced meal because it is one of the "Five Tastes" that nourish the body and support it's organs and systems (see, *The 5 Phases Of Food*).

I'm sure you've heard people say, "Sugar is sugar—your body uses it all the same." Well, this is not really accurate. Natural sugars are usually complex carbohydrates, and refined white sugars are simple carbohydrates. Natural sugars enter the blood stream more slowly and do not cause a dramatic insulin response. White sugar never even reaches the intestines! It is so refined and broken down that it is absorbed into the blood stream directly from the mouth and stomach lining—spiking your blood sugar and jerking you around like a marionette! When you eat complex carbohydrates, your body receives a more even sugar supply. And, whatever you do not need for immediate energy, your body stores in the liver as glycogen.

A brochure entitled, *Alternative Sweeteners*, published by Wild Oats Community Market, contains the following information:

"White sugar is a human invention, not a gift from nature. In 1795, Louisiana farmers devised a way to granulate sugar on a large scale, which sent once exorbitant sugar prices plummeting and brought white sugar to the masses. Unfortunately, our bodies weren't designed to process refined sugar—of which the average person today consumes the equivalent of 139 pounds a year (and if converted by the body would make 79 pounds of fat)!

Overindulging in sweeteners of any kind, whether natural or refined, is not advised. Any excessive amount of sugar will eventually weaken your pancreas and other sugar-processing organs. Here is the good news: Some natural sweeteners are better than others because they are gentler on your body and your blood sugar levels. Most natural sweeteners contain minerals and other nutrients that (while not providing a major nutritional power-house) make them easier to digest.

White sugar production is a notorious polluter and resource depleter. Sugarcane is a mineral-hungry plant, known for depleting soils (as well as people). Cane farming also requires massive amounts of chemical fertilizers and pesticides.

Refined sugar is a naked carbohydrate. Whole sugarcane is stripped of the minerals and nutritional elements (needed to properly digest it) to make refined sugar. Eating a naked carbohydrate forces your body to use its own vitamins and minerals for digestion. Over time, excessive consumption of refined sugars can lead to nutritional deficiencies and serious problems like osteoporosis and gum disease.

Your body can't produce enough digestive enzymes without the right balance of minerals. But, compensating for your sweet tooth with extra-healthy foods may be a losing battle because your body is no longer digesting or assimilating food as efficiently.

Did you know that food allergies are often caused by poor digestion? Refined white sugar can weaken your gastrointestinal tract and lead to leaky gut syndrome, a phenomenon where your gut allows undigested food molecules to escape into your blood stream (see, *Your Food Must Become You*). Your immune system tries to protect you by releasing strong chemicals like histamines, but this unfortunately also causes inflammation (see, *Food Allergies And Addictions*).

Over time, a flood of white sugar will strain your pancreas, liver, and adrenal glands (one of their jobs is to help regulate blood sugar levels—see, *The Endocrine System*). Your body may respond in two ways:

1. Hypoglycemia: Symptoms include exhaustion, depression, irritability, vertigo, mental confusion, anxiety, headaches, and blurred vision. If your blood sugar levels dip too low, too fast, less oxygen flows to your brain and uncomfortable symptoms are created (see, *Hypoglycemia*).

2. Diábetes: Or hyp<u>e</u>rglycemia, a disease that strikes when a damaged pancreas can no longer produce insulin to bring blood sugar levels down.

Excessive sugar consumption has been linked to everything from frequent colds to serious diseases like cancer, heart disease, candida, and Alzheimer's. Health experts have recently made another connection: Type II Diabetes—an insidious form of the disease that threatens to become a worldwide epidemic. In the last thirty years alone, the incidence of Type II Diabetes in the U.S. Has tripled! Unfortunately, victims may detect complications like heart disease before they detect the diabetes itself. People inherit a tendency toward Type II, but it's excessive weight, poor diet, inactivity, and age that cause it to surface. According to scientists, there are three ways to control or prevent Type II Diabetes: Healthy diet, weight loss, and exercise."

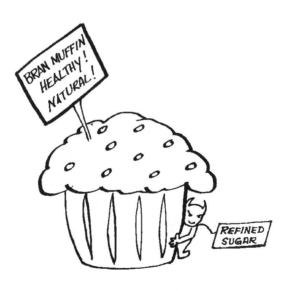

A Wolf In Sheep's Clothing

Refined sugar is disguised as many things in the marketplace. Do not be fooled. Just because a label *doesn't* say, "Contains refined white sugar—poison—beware," it doesn't mean that it doesn't contain refined white sugar, which is poison, so beware! The following are some of refined sugar's clever aliases:

Brown sugar—refined white sugar sprayed with molasses to give it a "natural" disguise.

Turbinado sugar—one step from refined white sugar and not any healthier. It is 95% sucrose.

High fructose corn syrup—do not be misled because the word "fructose" is in the name. It is about the same as refined white sugar both in form and how the body reacts to it.

Corn Syrup—this stuff is found in just about everything! It is shot into your blood like refined white sugar, and has other undesirable aspects as well: Because it is processed from corn starch, it frequently causes an allergic reaction in sensitive individuals. Also, the corn used in this product is commonly sprayed with pesticides. Triple threat!

The Good Guys

The Following are natural sweeteners that are not absorbed as quickly as refined sugars (and other natural sweeteners such as: Honey, maple syrup, unrefined cane juice, crystalline fructose, date sugar, concentrated fruit juice, and blackstrap molasses).

Brown Rice Syrup—because this is high in complex carbohydrates, it is absorbed more slowly into your bloodstream. The taste is more like butterscotch, and it is delicious in drinks and baked goods.

Barley Malt Syrup—like rice syrup, only the grain it originates from is barley. The flavor is like molasses, and can be used like brown rice syrup.

Stevia—this is an herb that is up to 400 times sweeter than white sugar, but has no calories! It is a healthy alternative, but the taste may require some adjustment.

Fruitsource—this is the brand name of a trademarked sweetener that combines grape juice concentrate with brown rice syrup.

Fruit Butters—try sweetening with the many kinds of fruit purees.

Unnatural—Unhealthy!

If it is too good to be true—it is! Many people choose their poison by color—pink or blue. There has been much published on how the pink one ravages the body, but have you read the studies on the blue one?

Aspartame (usually found in the market place as the trademarked NutraSweet) is the most popular sweetener today. It is in diet *everything*—found in over 1200 products! And the paradox is—studies show that people who use aspartame regularly gain weight, not lose it!

Aspartame is a *synthetic* additive—not a natural product made from benign amino acids like proponents would like you to believe. Although the ingredients themselves are found in nature alone—(phenylalanine, aspartic acid, and methyl alcohol) they are <u>never</u> found in this combination. And people consume tons of this stuff—about 10 pounds per person per year. Studies link large amounts of aspartame to cancer, brain and nervous system toxicity, and side effects such as: Headaches, dizziness, memory loss and confusion, decreased vision, depression, anxiety and irritability, drowsiness, seizures, nausea, insomnia, diarrhea, joint pain, and dehydration. (Dr. Gary tells us that many researchers feel it is one of the most toxic substances around.)

For aspartame to be eliminated, the body must first convert it to formaldehyde! If this doesn't sound toxic, I don't know what does! *They* (again, who are *they*?) used to tell us this stuff was safe. It now comes with an official warning! (Feeling like a laboratory rat again?)

CHAPTER IV

The Code You Came With

"I believed that no two people on the face of the earth were alike; no two people have the same fingerprints, lip prints, or voice prints. No two blades of grass or snowflakes are alike. Because I felt that all people were different from one another, I did not think it was logical that they should eat the same foods. It became clear to me that since each person was housed in a special body with different strengths, weaknesses, and nutritional requirements, the only way to maintain health or cure illness was to accommodate that particular patient's specific needs."

—James D'Adamo, N.D., in;
Eat Right For Your Type
Peter D'Adamo, N.D.

We are all unique; anatomically, physiologically, psychologically, emotionally, and spiritually—and we have unique combinations of how everything works together. Physically and biochemically we are each different. You need to determine what your key obstacles are to successful, long-term body fat reduction, muscle toning, and energy intensification.

GENETICS...THE ONE THING WE CAN'T CONTROL

According to a U.S. Public Health Service study, one out of three Americans is overfat.

Obesity has officially been declared an epidemic.

And this has all happened in the last century.

So what's up?

We can look at lifestyle, eating habits, and ethnic food preferences, but that still doesn't erase the fact that if you see an overfat child, you are not at all surprised when you meet his similarly overfat parent (the acorn didn't fall far from the tree, as they say).

Consider the fascinating experiments that scientists are doing with identical twins. They've studied twins who have been separated at birth and raised in different environments, and found that these twins grow up to be equally fat. Also, there was a research project done by Canadian doctors who deliberately overfed identical twins, compared them to other groups of identical twins who ate the same controlled amount of calories, and they found that the twins who were the genetic copies had exactly the same response to the food—but their response differed markedly from the other twins. These doctors did some math and figured out that about 65% of the difference between these people were a result of their genetics.

The theory that genetics play a significant role in obesity drove scientists into their laboratories. One of these scientists, Dr. Jeffrey Friedman, worked eight years on a project to identify and clone what is called "the obesity gene." This gene contains the information to make "leptin"...a protein that regulates metabolism and appetite, and when the gene is defective, the brain does not receive a message to "stop eating."

Another scientist, Dr. Alan Shuldiner, discovered a common mutation in another gene called "the thrifty gene." Early man frequently died of starvation, so our species evolved to compensate for this fact. Gene mutations developed that made it possible for our ancestors to survive periodic famines by making them have slower metabolisms. Of course, in this day and age, where there is an over-abundance of food in America, we can certainly do without this once-handy little mutation.

UNIQUE...AS A SNOWFLAKE

When you think "snowflake," what immediately comes into your mind? Right—a perfectly formed, beautiful creation that is like no other of its kind. Well, think of yourself the same way.

As I continue on my journey through this exciting new territory I am blessed with discovering brilliant minds and intriguing concepts. I never know where my path will lead me—one work turns me in the direction of another work, and so on. It has been quite an adventure. One name in particular seemed to keep coming up, and so I read his book. Jeffrey Bland,

Ph.D., is the author of *The 20-Day Rejuvenation Diet Program*, and he is a highly respected, frequently referenced and quoted doctor in what I will narrowly refer to as "The Nutrition World." The following are the Ten Principles of Dr. Bland's "Rejuvenation Program:" 1. Each person is biochemically unique. (Sunk in yet?) 2. The absence of disease does not guarantee the presence of health. 3. A personally tailored diet can help individuals overcome their unique health problems. 4. Plant foods and their constituents (phytonutrients) have health-giving properties. 5. Diet and lifestyle can help reverse the aging process. (I like that one so much that I think I'll repeat it.) Diet and lifestyle can help reverse the aging process. 6. Diet can help overcome living in a toxic world. 7. Oxidant stress can be prevented with diet and nutrients. 8. Many major diseases are diet-related—and diet modifiable. 9. Illness is related to problems of the digestive and liver detoxification systems and their influence on immune, nervous and endocrine function. 10. You are your own best health insurance provider.

In his book, Dr. Bland presents his program and how it addresses the following: Aging and Oxygen Radical Damage—Detoxification and Rejuvenation—Toxin Management—Powering Immunity and Preventing Fatigue—Balancing Hormones—Managing Pain and Inflammation—and Rejuvenating Your Brain Power. The diet plan has daily recipes and specific menus. There are screening questionnaires to evaluate your progress. There is so much information in this book, but being who I am and where I'm at, I will highlight what Dr. Bland says about aging: "After age 40, most people begin to lose strength, flexibility, cardiovascular function, hearing, eyesight, skin elasticity, kidney function, short term memory, reaction time and lung function. These are average changes for people whose lifestyle and diet are less than optimal. You may be living with a number of chronic health complaints you have associated with aging. I believe most of these complaints actually stem from the inadequate functioning of some of your body's systems, and <u>many of them can be corrected</u>.

You may have thought you were engaged in a race you must inevitably lose, against an unbeatable opponent called aging. I don't believe that's so. I believe there are ways to slow down the biological clock or turn it backward to achieve higher levels of function." (See, *Chronological Age Vs. Biological Age*)

"Why do I get sick so much?" "Why do I have so little energy?" "Why can't I lose weight?" "Why am I always depressed?" "Why am I so forgetful?" "Why does everything I eat turn to pain in my gut?" "Why am I so irritable?" "Why does it feel like I'm dragging myself through mud most of the time?"

"Why can't I get out of my own way???"

Do you ask yourself those questions? Positively maddening, isn't it?

BLOOD TYPE

As you may know by now, there are so many considerations in determining what your specific needs and issues are. Get ready—here is another one: Blood type. In his book, *Eat Right For Your Type*, Peter D'Adamo, N.D., talks about continuing his father's (James D'Adamo, N.D.) work in the field of blood type analysis. Dr. D'Adamo states: "Now we have begun to discover how to use the blood type as a cellular fingerprint that unravels many of the major mysteries surrounding our quest for good health. This work is an extension of the recent ground breaking findings concerning human DNA. Our understanding of blood type takes the science of genetics one step further by stating unequivocally that every human being is utterly unique. There is no right or wrong lifestyle or diet; there are only right or wrong choices to be made based on our individual genetic codes." Dr. D'Adamo breaks it down to: Four blood types—four diet and exercise programs. Each blood type is described regarding its unique history and identity, and advice is offered and recommendations given involving: Strengths, weaknesses, medical risks, diet profile, weight loss, supplements, and exercise. Dr. D'Adamo even factors ancestry into the equation.

According to the D'Adamos' literature, knowing our blood types allows us to "zero in" on vital health and fitness—nutrition and exercise information that corresponds to our exact biological profile. Dr. D'Adamo calls the specific food recommendations that are presented in *Eat Right For your Type*: "Clear, logical, scientifically researched and certified dietary blueprints based on your cellular profile." Eating the foods that "support" your blood type will help restore your body (*weight loss is one of the natural side effects of the body's restoration*) because these foods are tailored to the cellular composition of your body (*as opposed to being a generic, one-size-fits-all recommendation*). Certain foods will promote weight gain or weight loss for you, although they may have a different effect on a person of another blood type. For example, people are constantly asking about these "high protein diets," and why they seem to work so well. Dr. D'Adamo tells us his observation is that most of his patients who do well on a "high protein diet" are usually Type O's and Type B's. Type A's would not typically do well on such a diet because their systems are biologically unsuited to metabolize meat as efficiently as Type O's and Type B's. Type AB's would also fare poorly because they need a balance of appropriate foods for both Type A and Type B.

How did they arrive at this? Dr. D'Adamo explains:

"Nature has endowed our immune system very sophisticated methods to determine if a substance in the body is foreign or not. One method involves chemical markers called antigens, which are found on the cells of our bodies. Every life form, from the simplest virus to humans themselves, has unique antigens that form a part of its chemical fingerprint. <u>One of the most powerful antigens in the human body is the one that determines your blood type.</u>

The different blood type antigens are so sensitive that when they are operating effectively, they are the immune system's greatest security system. When your immune system sizes up a suspicious character, one of the first things it looks for is your blood type antigen to tell it whether the intruder is friend or foe.

Each blood type possesses a different antigen with its own special chemical structure. Your blood type is named for the blood type antigen you possess on your red blood cells."

Dr. D'Adamo further explains that it was found that many foods agglutinate (clump) the cells of certain blood types (not a good thing—it's like rejection). However, other foods, which produced similar results in other blood types, proved beneficial. He tells us that some doctors, scientists, and nutritionists explored these implications, and found that a part of our genetic inheritance is a chemical reaction that occurs between our blood and the foods we eat. Lectins (abundant and diverse proteins found in foods) have agglutinating properties that affect our blood. Dr. D'Adamo says: "When you eat a food containing protein lectins that are incompatible with your blood type antigen, the lectins target an organ or bodily system (kidneys, liver, brain, stomach, etc.) and begin to agglutinate blood cells in that area."

Stay with me now.

Incompatible lectin proteins do not get digested. Instead, they travel through the bloodstream and target an area, where they clump the cells (which makes them targeted for destruction by the immune system as if they were foreign invaders). This clumping can cause irritable bowel syndrome, or cirrhosis of the liver (among other things according to Dr. D'Adamo).

Dr. D'Adamo's work presenting that each blood type has specific reactions to certain foods has influenced how we present our nutrition plans in *Live It Or Diet Lifestyle Systems*. This association between blood typing and nutrition blends perfectly with our philosophy of "bioindividuality." When we look at the genetic characteristics of our ancestors (which still live in our blood today) we can see how adhering to a food plan that follows our code makes perfect sense:

Type O: The oldest and most basic blood type, the survivor at the top of the food chain—hunters who thrived on meat.

Type A: The first immigrants, forced by the necessity of migration to adapt to a more agrarian lifestyle.

Type B: The assimilator, adapting to new climates and the mingling of populations.

Type AB: The delicate offspring of a rare merger between Type A and Type B.

We had wonderful results when we field-tested *Live It Or Diet Lifestyle Systems* using blood type as our barometer for food recommendations. When "the foods to avoid" (according to Dr. D'Adamo's recommendations) were removed from an individual's diet, the individual became less bloated, had more energy, and lost some weight—<u>before</u> any further modifications were incorporated. Also, I found a very interesting correlation between food sensitivities and blood type avoidance foods. For example, I am Blood Type O. According to Dr. D'Adamo's book, I should do well on lean meats, and I should do poorly on certain grains, gluten and dairy. When I tested for food allergies (with blood testing, electronic testing, and kenesiology testing—see, *Allergy Testing*) I tested positive to sensitivities to wheat, gluten, and dairy, among other things. According to my blood type recommendations, most grains will make me feel sluggish, and lean animal protein (hormone-free, natural meats like the ones from Coleman—see, *Appendix G*) will vitalize me. Well, it's true. I have energy and a strong attitude when I eat animal protein (and my cholesterol level is low), gluten causes my body to bloat and completely disturbs my digestive system, and I get tired and foggy when I eat certain grains at certain times. Like, if I have a Cliff Bar as a snack in the afternoon, I need a nap afterward! (Cliff Bars are made from oats. Blood Type O's do not do well on oats according to Dr. D'Adamo. And I love them, too—dang it). Now, if I give a Cliff Bar to a client who is Blood Type A, they feel great—energized and happy! (Blood Type A's do well on most grains, but poorly on most meats.) I've compared "blood type avoidance foods" with food allergy testing on my *Live It Or Diet Lifestyle System* clients, and found that they correlated often enough to be more than a coincidence. Blood Typing is not a new concept. It has been around for many years. Dr. D'Adamo has taken it to another level, and it is exciting and innovative work that we embrace and practice. (We have included some general blood type recommendations in *Putting It All Together.*)

If you do not know your blood type, a personal blood-typing kit is available (see, *Appendix E*).

METABOLIC TYPE

Metabolic type is yet another marker of individual identification. Your body genetically has certain physical, mental, and emotional characteristics. As these characteristics are affected by different disturbances and imbalances, they change, reflecting the lack of harmony in the body.

In *Your Body Knows Best*, Ann Louise Gittleman defines "Metabolic Profiling" as: "A system of interpreting and understanding body language to determine an individual's genetically based nutritional requirements. The body gives us many clues to these needs, communicating them through physical, mental, emotional, and behavioral characteristics."

A paper entitled *Metabolic Profiling: A Breakthrough In Nutritional Science* by Mannatech, Inc., states the following regarding the *Nutritional Controversy* prevailing today: "Make no mistake about it, health is a hot issue and millions of Americans know it! Polls have shown that one out of every three people is on some kind of special diet. Over 20 million people take vitamin supplements every day. Unfortunately, however, confusion regarding nutrition pervades the entire health industry. Even physicians and nutritional authorities hold radically different opinions of what is "right!" As an example, Dr. Robert Atkins and the late Nathan Pritikin, noted American authorities on nutrition, each promoted a celebrated, yet diametrically opposed, dietary regimen. One was generally at the other's throat concerning the correctness of his personal program and the incorrectness of the other's. Atkins promoted a high-protein, low-carbohydrate, moderate-fat diet. Pritikin promoted a low-fat, low-protein, high-carbohydrate diet. While the numerous health proponents may be vastly different in their theories, they are all the same in one respect, and this is their collective critical flaw: They treat each of us as though we were exactly the same.

Roger J. Williams, Ph.D., D.Sc., the noted biochemical researcher from the University of Texas, cut right to the heart of that flaw. In one of his books on the subject of individualizing nutritional requirements he states, 'If we continue to try to solve nutritional problems on the basis of the average man, we will be continuously in a muddle. Such a man does not exist.'"

The idea of individualization based on metabolic profiling and oxidation is not new. Francis Pottenger, M.D., author of *Symptoms Of Visceral Disease* published in 1919, established the autonomic nervous system as a main consideration in "metabolic individuality," and described how different nutrients impact this system. Then, during the 1950's, two doctors—Dr. Melvin Page and Dr. Henry Bieler, separately worked on systems classifying "endocrine types" (thyroid, adrenal, and pituitary), with nutrient recommendations to support each type. The research done by Dr. George Watson on "oxidative rates" in the 50's and 60's and then published in his book, *Nutrition And Your Mind* in the 70's (see the section, *Oxidative Rates*) discussed the influence of macronutrient ratios on the oxidative system. Dr. Roger Williams, the discoverer of pantothenic acid (vitamin-B5), originated the *Genotrophic Theory,* describing the need for nutritional individuality. Dr. William Kelley (a dentist who became famous in the 80's for his work with terminal cancer patients) developed a system of metabolic profiling based on Dr. William's work. The Healthexel system (developed by William Wolcott and licensed to Mannatech, Inc.) incorporates the work of D'Adamo in blood typing, and Watson in oxidative rate. "The Power System" was developed in the 80's by Dr. Richard Power and Laura Power. They combined the work of Bieler and D'Adamo, and expanded the glandular types to seven. The Powers' found a close correlation between blood types and endocrine gland types. Dr. Power puts it this way: "The basic idea is to identify the dominant glands by clinical characteristics and blood type, supply the necessary nutrients for them, and support the corresponding recessive glands with proper diet and supplements—thus balancing natural strengths and weaknesses. Most people are not a pure prototype, but a combination. The blood type can be determined by a simple test, and the gland type can be determined by observing many secondary clinical signs, such as: Body shape, personality, skin texture, food cravings and allergies, etc."

There are many different approaches to metabolic typing. In her book, Ms. Gittleman describes The Healthexcel System of Metabolic Typing (developed by William Linz Wolcott), which is a four dimensional model adding Chinese medicine, (AyurVeda) to autonomic nervous system, oxidative system, and endocrine system considerations.

Mr. Wolcott was an associate of Dr. William Kelley's. Dr. Kelley's extensive and significant model of metabolic typing, The Kelly Program, is presented in the book, *Medicine's Missing Link*, by Tom and Carole Valentine. They write: "Dr. Kelley is the founder of metabolic typing as a science and a new medical paradigm. He developed a system for determining at least ten distinct metabolic types. Dr. Kelley's classifications and metabolic types are based on careful evaluations of physiological processes made over many years. Dr. Kelley reviewed the existing research on metabolism and individual uniqueness, then conducted intensive, long-term research of his own in order to develop a system for accurately classifying the various patterns into basic metabolic types."

(All right, if you need a break here, take it. I want you to absorb what I am saying about this subject, and it could get a bit confusing. Don't let it overwhelm you. When we build your *Live It Or Diet Lifestyle System*, we will evaluate all of this along with your other considerations. It will be exciting to see how it all comes into focus for you!)

Ready to continue?

Let's start with a question. What is the *autonomic nervous system*? Well, think "automatic" when you say "autonomic." It is our system of glands, organs, smooth muscles, nerves; all of the functions of the body that we do not have to think about. The two distinct components of the autonomic nervous system are the *sympathetic* and the *parasympathetic*. The sympathetic system is associated with *catabolism*, or *tearing down* (the stress response—fight or flight). The parasympathetic system is associated with *anabolism*, or *building up* (rest and repair). The Valentines continue: "The Kelley metabolic typing system first divides everyone into one of three general categories based entirely upon the autonomic nervous system in general. People, Kelley learned, may be sympathetic-dominant, parasympathetic-dominant, or balanced between the two."

I do not want to get so technical on you that I lose you. So, I will just tell you that from the three basic categories in Dr. Kelley's system, people are then divided into types based on other variables, including oxidative rate (see, *Oxidative Rate*). There are 3200 questions included in Dr. Kelley's evaluation procedure. It is clearly the model that has influenced metabolic typing today.

Dr. Carolyn L. Mein, in her book, *Different Bodies—Different Diets*, discusses how she expanded the aforementioned metabolic typing methods to include 25 metabolic types. She writes that she became frustrated when she observed that some people had the characteristics of more than one type.

Why does metabolic (or body) typing work? Dr. Mein writes: "The basic principle of body typing is that each individual body type needs a different set of 'rules to play by.' The reason people experience such contradictory results with diets is that not everyone reacts the same way to the same foods or food combinations. It is important to recognize which foods affect your individual body positively. All foods contain certain nutrients that support or stimulate specific glands, organs, and systems of the body. Diet can be as simple as eating the foods that support your body, and avoiding those that create unnecessary stress. By giving your body what it needs, food cravings disappear and your energy increases.

Since each type has its own characteristic shape, knowing your body type will lead to a more realistic expectation of your appearance. It is time we establish our own identity.

One of the first indications that your body is under excessive stress is an imbalance in your weight. From here on, 'diet' means: The consumption of foods chosen to support your body. When you begin to notice either weight gain or loss, your body is signaling you that it's time to restore its balance.

To identify your ideal diet, you need to determine your dominant gland. Your dominant gland is the strongest gland, and it has the greatest influence on your body. This gland is what determines your shape, appearance, and areas of weight gain. Losing weight is not simply about losing pounds, but losing them in the right places. 'Classic' diets cause the dieter to lose weight from the upper body and gain it in the lower body (see, *Cellulite*).

When the body is in crisis or over-stressed, it will crave the foods that provide the greatest relief in the quickest way possible by stimulating the dominant gland."

This is not what you want to do. It creates further imbalance, causing more weight gain. You must take the stress off your body, and give the dominant gland some rest. At this point, the focus needs to be on supporting the corresponding recessive glands.

Another individual who is actively practicing metabolic typing is nutritionist, Jay Cooper. I first read about Mr. Cooper's work in an article written by Laurie Tarkan, published in the June 1998 issue of *Fitness Magazine*. The article described how Mr. Cooper applied the published works of Dr. Henry Bieler and Dr. Elliot Abravanel on metabolic typing in his practice. The article said: "Some body types do not lose weight on low-fat diets because not everyone metabolizes food in the same way. Also, each body type craves particular foods that over-stimulate the dominant gland, which can lead to suppressed metabolic function." When Jay Cooper's book on metabolic typing, *The Body Code*, came out in 1999, I eagerly read it. In it Mr. Cooper writes the following:

"No one diet or exercise plan or lifestyle is ideal, or even reasonable, for all human types. Over countless generations, our physiologies have adjusted to our environments through natural adaptations and mutation. Governed by a survival mechanism, our gene pool has evolved to enable the perpetuation of our species by incorporating the many different threads of human history that have contributed to it. Each of the 100 trillion cells in each of our bodies is carrying this history. It is our history, the history of the human race, perpetuated through all generations of time into this living conglomeration that is today...you and me.

Since America is one big ethnic melting pot, and since most of us don't know our genealogy very well, we may not know exactly which threads from the strand of human history are predominant in our physiological makeup. That is why we must use the tools that we have to discover the lifestyle choices that are most harmonious for our own genetic type. Modern researchers have established that, for purposes of determining diet and exercise needs, the anatomical, glandular, and energy methods are the most useful.

Your glandular type affects your body's usage of basic macronutrients along with micronutrients that create the energy and building materials necessary for cellular regeneration. This process of converting raw materials into the building blocks of life is known as <u>metabolism</u>. Your dominant gland determines differences in body-chemistry balance, metabolic function, and energy usage. Your glandular type, like your anatomical type, is programmed by your genes.

To restore a healthy balance among your glandular secretions, you must cut back on foods that stimulate the subordinate glands. In this process, the key to health is <u>balance</u>—although one gland is always dominant, it should not be <u>too</u> dominant, or it will overpower the contributions of the other glands.

Your glandular type is determined by analyzing related characteristics such as physical shape, the size of your skeleton, the location of body-fat pads, your energy patterns, and how your body responds to proteins, fats, carbohydrates, and exercise."

Jay Cooper's glandular approach divides people into four body-chemistry types. They were outlined in Ms. Tarkan's *Fitness Magazine* article this way:

Adrenal

Personality: High-energy person who likes to have power and be in control. Typically workaholics and entrepreneurs, thriving on discipline and challenges.

Physical Characteristics: Straight torso, slightly-defined waist, low lower body fat compared to upper body—gains fat first in stomach, rib cage, and breasts or upper back, pelvis narrower than hips, flat butt.

Food Recommendations: Adrenals crave—and should avoid—saturated fats, alcohol, and meat. Eat a low-fat, high-fiber diet. Eat a light breakfast, light-to-medium lunch, and large dinner. Eat plenty of vegetables, fruits, and grains. Eat poultry and fish in moderation. If cravings strike, eat vegetables and fruit.

Exercise Recommendations: Since it is easy for adrenals to store fat, and hard to burn it off, do aerobic exercise in target heart rate zone for 45 -55 minutes, five to six days a week. Do weight training twice a week with light weights.

Thyroidal

Personality: Creative—likes to teach and communicate, tends to absorb and process information quickly, and then forget it. Overachiever and perfectionist.

Physical Characteristics: High, well-defined waist, medium breasts, semi swayback, long legs and arms, hourglass shape—gains weight first in upper legs and abdomen, teardrop shaped butt.

Food Recommendations: Thyroidals reach for sweets when energy levels fall, but should avoid them. Eat small meals every four hours that include low-fat protein, (egg whites, poultry, fish and tofu) and vegetables and beans. Eat grains in moderation. If cravings strike, eat protein.

Exercise Recommendations: Thyroidals have a naturally revved metabolism, so you can get away with less cardio, (30 minutes four times per week) and strength training two to three times per week.

Gonadal

Personality: Nurturer and mother of everyone—enjoys being social, gregarious and a caregiver.

Physical Characteristics: Small, low waist-line, small or medium breasts, very sway-backed, large, muscular legs—gains more body fat from the waist down, full, round, pro-truding butt, gains fat first in thighs and butt (saddlebags).

Food Recommendations: Gonadals should avoid high-fat spicy foods (which they often crave). These foods over-stimulate the ovaries, promoting fat storage in hips and butt. Eat a light breakfast, medium lunch, and large dinner. Eat fruits, vegetables, poultry and fish. Eat grains in moderation. When cravings strike, eat fruits and vegetables with high-water content.

Exercise Recommendations: Since Gonadals tend to gain weight easily, you should emphasize cardio—40 minutes in your target heart rate zone five days per week. Strength train twice a week with light weights—careful not to bulk up your lower body, which it will have a tendency to do.

Pituitary

Personality: Tend to be poets, artists, and composers—abstract thinkers who are analytical, and need time to themselves.

Physical Characteristics: Large head and eyes, narrow shoulders, slightly defined waist, small butt and feet—gains weight first in the abdomen and lower inner thighs, then equally all over body; bulges below navel.

Food Recommendations: Pituitaries are naturally thinner and have trouble building muscle. They should avoid trigger foods such as dairy, caffeine, and white flour, and eat high protein and starchy vegetables to stimulate the adrenal and gonadal functions. Eat primarily meat , poultry, and vegetables. Eat grains in moderation. When cravings strike, eat proteins like venison or turkey jerky, or a protein bar.

Exercise Recommendations: Since Pituitaries have little muscle definition, emphasize weight training. If you are over-weight, add cardio, two to three times per week. Do three strength-training sessions per week, using weights sufficient to build muscle. Pituitaries won't bulk up.

Interesting, huh? When I integrated metabolic typing into *Live It Or Diet Lifestyle Systems*, I was able to break through the frustrating "plateaus" that clients often experience. Metabolic typing wound up underscoring many of the recommendations from the other methods of identification we were already employing. Dr. Gary and I have studied the data on all of the systems that identify an individual's needs through observing body characteristics and behavior. There is an exciting correlation between metabolic typing, blood typing, and oxidative rate—along with the propensity towards certain food sensitivities and gut disorders, and impaired sugar regulation. On your *Live It Or Diet Lifestyle System*, we will add metabolic typing as a consideration in determining your game plan.

YOUR MISSION, SHOULD YOU CHOSE TO ACCEPT IT...

On a friend's refrigerator, the following saying is posted: "Nothing tastes as good as being thin feels." Well, add to that "nothing *feels* as good as *being healthy*," and you've got two profound little statements of fact. Because of them, I choose to never deviate from my seemingly rigid, narrow path. Companions glare at me with disdain when I order my "picky-picky-picky" meals in restaurants, or when I just have some vegetables when nothing else is suitable for me to eat in their homes. But I just go about my business, without being tempted (even if ridiculed) to "just this once—lighten up." I refuse to pay the price anymore. I don't just wear it, I *feel* it, and it's *not worth it*.

I have dedicated the past several years to getting to the core of my food issues so I can "take control" of them. Unfortunately, all of my research has taught me that there just is no one simple solution. Our answers are at the end of a maze...and each of us has to find the way out for ourselves. Just think of me as your scout.

CHAPTER V

TAKING CONTROL

Picture if you will...another diet.

And, it's going relatively well a far as you can tell. You are losing weight. So far the scale has been your friend, whispering sweet nothings each morning that carry you through the day on a magic carpet of success.

You have eliminated certain "enemies" from your daily food plan, and you are repeatedly eating only your safe, assigned "allies."

Then you find that you have begun craving certain things. Like sweets, or rich carbohydrates, or fats, or all of the above.

You have dutifully kept your enemies off your shopping list, so none of them currently reside in your kitchen. You can stand in front of your refrigerator peering in all night long, and all you'll catch is a cold. You have done your job well. Nothing that can harm your mission is lurking about in there.

But, the cravings become obsessions. You can think about nothing else. Every waking moment you are fighting the impulse to cheat. You are losing the battle. You're going nuts. "Can food really drive me nuts?" you ask yourself. You are losing control. You are back in the kitchen, going through cupboards, searching behind boxes, desperately looking for something, *anything*, to satiate the beast that has taken over your body.

It becomes a matter of survival. You get creative. Ketchup is sweet. Okay. What can I put it on? Nothing. "There is nothing to put it on! Why did I throw out those saltines?? Maybe I'll just eat it with a spoon."

Welcome to The Twilight Zone. Did you see the signposts?

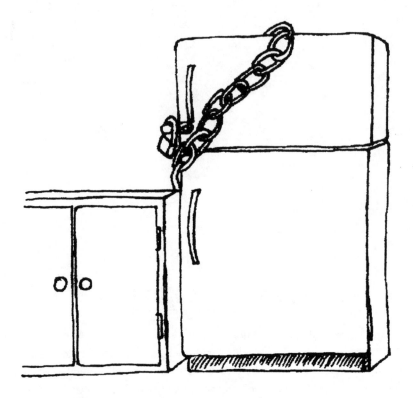

THE DEFINITION OF INSANITY

Do you know what the definition of insanity is? Some people answer by saying that it is "doing the same thing over and over again, but expecting different results."

I call that hope.

To me, the definition of insanity is "doing the same thing over and over again— knowing the results are going to be the same—*but doing it anyway.*"

Why do you think there are so many exercise/nutrition books, programs, diets— "solutions" out there? If the first one worked for everyone, would we have needed the others? If any one of these "revelations" worked for the masses, the subject would have been closed. Done. Let's solve another problem.

But we just keep trying them don't we? And when they fail, who do we blame? The authors? The doctors? The diet counselors? No. We blame ourselves. The program didn't fail. <u>We</u> failed.

The truth, my friend, is that there is no "off the rack" program that fits everyone.

ONE SIZE FITS ALL?...

No matter what your health and fitness goals are, *you cannot get there from here (and stay there) without understanding your bioindividuality.* Most people just blindly follow the Program Du Jour, with no awareness of the brutal fact that what works for one person may not work for another. Each one of us reacts differently to food, stress, exercise, etc. When you consider that there are more potential pitfalls in designing a perfect appearance enhancement program than in any other health care arena, you will understand the challenge of this chapter. I cannot ethically offer you another generic "program." I will not say "look at me...this worked for me and it will work for you, too." It might not. I don't know. But, what I will do here is teach you how to evaluate who *you* are. From there, based on your own *personal* evaluation, you will learn how to get into the best condition possible for *you.*

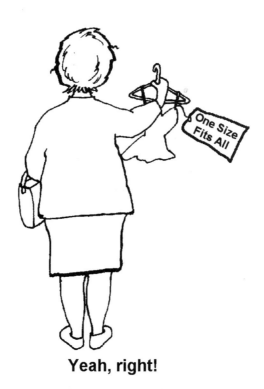

Yeah, right!

The following is a redundant statement, but *diets do not work.* Another redundant statement should be: *One-size fits all programs are irresponsible.* Both of these set you up for failure. Diets deprive. They either cut your calories to below maintenance (and your body's metabolism will slow down to compensate), or they cut out certain foods (which wipes out any nutrient balance you might have had). Yes, you will lose *scale weight* initially but, as we have discussed, some of that will be *muscle* and you now know that ultimately, your metabolism will slow down further as a result of that. Also, remember that fat is burned in your *muscle* (your body's furnace) and by decreasing the amount of your muscle you are decreasing your body's ability to burn fat. When you go on one of the gazillion plans that are out there, you will begin by losing weight on the scale. Yea! It's working! Then, you hit what your "diet person" calls a "plateau" and you are deprived further, but that's okay, and <u>you don't care</u> because the scale begins to move again. You reach your goal. You celebrate by dragging a wagon load of fat onto your TV tray, or you go on a shopping spree, or do whatever you do to officially recognize your victory. And then you go off your "diet." I do not need to tell any of you what happens next. You already know too well or you would not be reading these words. 95% of the people who go on these diets gain back all of the weight they lost and *more*. <u>We get fatter</u>.

If you have followed one of the more creative programs that simply eliminate a nutrient—like fat, or carbohydrate, or protein—well, you tell me, does this sound, well, *sound*? I mean nutritionally speaking, of course. Balance wise, you know what I mean? Will it supply your body with the nutrients that are essential to health? I'll put it to you this way, if you have children, would you allow them to eliminate a nutrient from their diet? No. You obsess over balanced meals and getting your kids to eat everything on the plate—including the vegetables. (How many daily servings of vegetables do you insist upon for yourself?) You worry about *their* health, but you are willing to sacrifice *yours* for a smaller number on the scale, on the dress tag, or on the measuring tape.

<u>This</u> approach and philosophy is based on creating <u>health</u> first and foremost, and then helping you achieve the most physically appealing manifestation of the healthiest possible body. Philosophically and ideologically this is what I believe to be the *right thing to do*...and, in my experience, is the *only* way to do it so that it is sustainable. Remember <u>my</u> story? I got the body of my dreams and destroyed my health in the process. You must create your optimal physique on a solid foundation of health. Forget..."It's not how you feel, it's how you look." I will not help you sacrifice your health for the sake of four hours in a New Year's Eve dress. It's not worth it, okay? I've been there. At 50 years of age I can tell you there is only one right way for you (as there is for me), and I spent years looking for it. Hopefully, the information in this book will end the search for *your* solution.

"WE INTERRUPT THIS BROADCAST"...

In the wake of the Surgeon General's warning that "lack of physical activity is hazardous to your health," an ever-increasing number of people will be seeking a way to commute this sentence with the least possible fuss. The reason I say this is because those who will be most affected by this dramatic message are the baby-boomers...38 to 55 year olds who typically—at this stage of our lives—are busy professionals/parents/community conscious—people who have serious agendas. At the same time, it is this population that will appreciate the implications of the Surgeon General's report and will look for effective, yet efficient ways of prolonging their lives and improving the quality of those extended years.

We are also old enough to remember the ominous warnings and dangers of yesteryear...the "cold war" years that found us digging fallout shelters and listening for the screech on the radio that signaled that we must run for our lives to our provision-filled cement tombs and await *the mushroom cloud.*

Kruschev was banging his shoes on podiums, Castro was razzing Kennedy, and cigarettes were quietly killing our loved ones.

Baby-boomers, for the most part, are in tune and, if not, they are in denial. But for most of us, the Surgeon General has put the last nail in our procrastination coffin. Members of "The Woodstock Generation" realize that this latest announcement is a landmark. We remember the Surgeon General's last official warning in the 60's about cigarette smoking and the reality of smoking-related deaths permeating our consciousness. We all know someone at this point who has died due to smoking...can we really get sick and die from lack of exercise?

Remember who we baby-boomers are. We are the generation of people who refused to accept everything that was put before us as "just the way it is." We confronted situations, questioned "authorities," and *rebelled.* We were activists! We didn't just passively give in. It would <u>not</u> be typical of us to passively accept changes in our bodies as a matter of age—*just the way it is*—and yet that is exactly what most of us are doing: "Well, what can I expect, after all I am 40, or I am 50." Horse manure. That's not the attitude you would have had in the 60's. Come on!

Consider this. A good many of these signs of age are a reaction to a lifetime of being bombarded with drugs (i.e.; birth control pills, antibiotics, etc.), pesticides, pollutants, inadequate and irrational eating habits—the list goes on, but you get the idea. We have been affected on a *cellular level* by all of these conditions, and our bodies react by deteriorating. *We have the power to stop this.*

Okay. So maybe we 78 million baby-boomers are ready to listen now as responsible health/fitness professionals deliver knowledge and instruction on how to get and stay fit. But, in order for these messages to be effective, you must access the information, learn how to evaluate what you need, and decide whether or not you need to seek counseling or help in a certain area. If you do, I offer referrals in *Appendix H*. Your fitness quest begins...or ends *here*. Your level of success depends on you, and how truthfully you will look at yourself, your behavior, and your willingness to adapt to the changes that will be necessary for survival.

I know, I know—such drama.

THE CAFETERIA OF LIFE

"If I'd have known that I was going to live this long, I would've taken better care of myself."

—George Burns

Life is like a cafeteria. (Here she goes again.)

You grab your tray at the start of the long stainless steel line that leads to a variety of choices. As you slide your tray across the shiny path, certain things appeal to you at that moment, and you place them on your tray. "I'll have some of that...more of this..lots of that...mmm, I'll take seconds of that..."and so on down the line. If you are anything like me in this "cafeteria of life," you have made some unfortunate choices. And, when you're young and "bullet-proof," you never consider that some day you will actually have to pay for all of this stuff.

Well, trust me, my friend—the time does come to pay for all of the garbage that we have heaped on our trays throughout our lives. I am 50 years old, and I've been at the cash register. "Wow, did all that junk really cost this much?"

$Too much sugar. $Too much fat. $Too much junk and fast food. $Too much meat. $Too much alcohol. $Too much protein. $Too many additives, preservatives, and processed foods. $Too many artificial sweeteners. $Too little exercise and physical activity. $Too much psychological and spiritual stress. $Too much exposure to electromagnetic radiation, toxins, fumes, pollutants, and pesticides. $Hormone imbalances. $Food and environmental allergies and sensitivities. $Upset pH (alkaline-acid imbalances). $Drugs that mask symptoms and exacerbate problems. $Drugs to lose weight. $Drugs to do drugs.

Ka ching $$$! It adds up, babe. The following is my case history. Take notes. Take inventory. Take care.

15 ROUNDS—MY CHAMPIONSHIP BOUT

"Float like a butterfly—sting like a bee."

(No Name Needed)

I want a cookie! I *need* a cookie! Cookie! Cookie!

My brain cried out like this after each meal. This can't be normal, can it?

Or, I would have to have wine with a meal. One glass, or two, or—sometimes I couldn't control myself. This began to worry me. Did I have an alcohol problem? "Situational alcoholism" someone called it. What the heck is that?

Oh, how I hate to lose control of *anything*, especially my body and its desires.

But I was. I did not feel good. I was tired. I was depressed. I was gaining weight. I had brain fog. I was losing my memory. I was losing more teeth. I was even losing my hair! ("I thought I had tile floors. Where did this carpet come from?")

Round one.

Okay, you have my attention.

And so, I began having tests.

The first was the food allergy testing with Dr. Gary (which gave me my first glimmer of hope). Testing positive to several foods, and then eliminating them, was the first step. I immediately dropped weight, and my bloating reduced.

Round two.

A *Biological Terrain Assessment* (blood, saliva and urine tests) illuminated some other probable issues, most noteworthy: An overall acidic condition, a depression of liver and kidney function, severe oxidative stress in the lymphatic system, impaired digestion, early signs of degenerative conditions and premature tissue aging, a depletion of available minerals, and a *biological age of 69!*

Oh, man.

Round three.

"I just can't wait for the next test, Doc.—hormones, right? Yea! What will we discover there, I wonder, if I am biologically 69 years old ???" I was beginning to feel that familiar, "This is more information than I needed to know" cop-out lurking in the shadows of my psyche. But, "What makes the 'hot n' tot' so hot?" queried the Lion.

Courage.

And so, once again I spit in a vile (every day for 28 days!) and sent them on their way. The results revealed (for the most part) normal hormone levels for a woman my age. "What does that mean? Normally *low*? They're low, right?" Oh, man.

Round four.

Feeling a little punch-drunk, Doc., but, okay—where do we go from here?

Blood tests with Immuno Labs to further test for food sensitivities and Candida (which their questionnaire indicated as a "red flag").

Oh joy, I'm allergic to more foods, *and* I have Candida. I can now eat two things, and I have to rotate *them*. (Candida Albicans is a strain of yeast that usually dwells in the gastrointestinal tract, among other places in the body. Even though it is considered "harmless," it will multiply rapidly when resistance and immune function are low. It feeds on sugars and carbohydrates, and releases many toxins into the bloodstream causing a myriad of disorders. It is a stress-related condition. When the body is severely out of balance, either from antibiotics, birth control pills, cortico-steroids, a nutritionally weak diet, a diet high in refined carbohydrates and alcohol, and too little rest, Candida has its shot. Judging from the above list, are you a candidate? (see, *Candida Albicans*)

Round five. (Am I bleeding?)

More viles. More saliva. This time for my adrenals (see, *The Endocrine System*).

Surprise. I have stressed out adrenals.

Round six.

I get to collect urine! All night! And...in the mail it goes. This will indicate any dysbiosis (see, *Your Food Must Become You*). Boy, did I have gut issues!

Round seven.

Basal temperature testing to indicate thyroid function. What thyroid function? The thermometer read 96 (and normal is between 97.8 and 98.2!)

Rounds eight through eleven.

Aggressive (is not even the word) homeopathic and supplemental regimen from Dr. Gary to address my low hormone levels and imbalances, dysbiosis, adrenal fatigue, and low thyroid function. Countless sublingual drops—precise combinations of nutrient formulas—dosing several times a day—I go nowhere without my bag of *stuff*.

Rounds twelve through fourteen.

Re-testing. Rotating in other remedies. Stabilizing. Holding ground. Regaining mental clarity. Losing weight. Circles under my eyes disappear. Basal temperature climbs to 97.3 (still not normal, but getting there). I don't need a nap anymore!

Round fifteen.

Victory! A little battle-scared, but *Live It Or Diet Lifestyle Systems* is conceived from the experience. And, that makes it all worth it to me.

THE "HERO JOURNEY" WITH NICK NOLTE

"Breaking out is following your bliss pattern—quitting the old place—starting your hero journey—following your bliss. You throw off yesterday as the snake sheds its skin. Follow your bliss. The heroic life is living the <u>individual</u> adventure. It is all about finding that still point in your mind where commitment drops away. It is by going down into the abyss that we recover the treasures of life. Where you stumble, there lies your treasure. You must return with the bliss and integrate it. 'As you go the way of life, you will see a great chasm. Jump. It is not as wide as you think.'"

—A Joseph Campbell Companion

Nick gave me the book that contained the above passage. He told me that I appeared to be on just such a journey. I know that <u>he</u> is.

Right there on the beautiful Atlantic Ocean in Fort Lauderdale is a very unique health club called The Zoo. That is where I met Nick. As I watched him—day in and day out—go through his routine of cardiovascular exercises, I waited for my opportunity to suggest integrating resistance exercise into his program. At the time I was the fitness director of The Zoo, so I considered it part of my job to enlighten people who are missing something—even if they do not ask for it. Ah, but how to approach a movie star with my gift?

Well, as fate would have it, we wound up at The Zoo's juice bar at the same time one day, and I seized the moment. Nick was preparing for his role in "The Thin Red Line"—a character that possessed a specific demeanor, posture, and movement that was the opposite of Nick's. We discussed how muscular "integrity" would create the body, thus the attitude of this man. Nick had already chosen a trainer at The Zoo, Tari Rose. Tari was a great choice, and so, we got to work. We tested Nick's body fat. I designed a series of exercises to target the muscle groups that would affect Nick's posture. Tari integrated them into a complete exercise program that addressed the total body, and Nick and Tari got to it. Tari's approach is fresh and fun. Some days they would work out on the beach, some days on the roof of The Zoo (where there is an outdoor gym overlooking the ocean), some days just concentrating on stretching in the aerobic studio. We addressed Nick's cardio more specifically, using a heart rate monitor and staying in the zone to burn just fat. Nick and I would do "Spinning" (a special stationary bike routine that has choreographed drills to music) on the roof of The Zoo, while we looked at the ocean (what a view!).

As far as the nutritional component, I started with the basics. I took Nick shopping at Wild Oats, and there we explored the wonderful organic, natural, and diverse alternatives to typical American foods. Then, we had a lesson in preparation (Nick likes to do his own cooking). But, now I am faced with my dilemma. *Who* is *Nick*, and what are *his* unique issues? I sent Nick to Dr. Gary to find out before I went any further with his diet.

Dr. Gary did a series of tests and "clearings" on Nick, and gave me my guidelines on what Nick should eat. When I originally analyzed Nick's diet, I knew that he needed to consume more protein than was his usual habit, especially since we had added the additional stress of the rigorous new exercise program. I learned from Dr. Gary that I needed to carefully design his food plan to be more "alkaline based," which meant I had to be mindful of the type and amount of protein in each meal (see, *Recipes From The Nolte Compound*). I received this information when I was at the "Nolte Compound" in Malibu where I was helping Nick redesign his gym.

The "Nolte Compound" is, as you would suspect, a beautiful place. But, it is also a special place. Nick has the most incredible gardens on his property. Along with the magnificent flora that is everywhere, there is an organic fruit and vegetable garden. This, I suspect, is what heaven on earth was like before we goofed. Each day we would pick raspberries, strawberries, and blackberries, and choose from the wide array of vine-ripened, nutrient packed vegetables and fragrant herbs from which I created the recipes you find in this book. It was glorious! If only all of us could just go into our backyards and pick our fresh, nutritious food on a daily basis!

Nick's commitment brought excellent results. He lost body fat and gained lean muscle tissue. Because he wanted to continue to work out on location, I trained him on a device that was invented by a friend of mine, Steve Kushner. It's called the T-2 (see, *Appendix D*). It's an awesome piece of equipment that is so small it travels *anywhere*, and so completely efficient and effective that its simplicity is positively brilliant.

Nick was intrigued and fully embraced the philosophy and approach Dr. Gary and I presented to him. He had already embarked on a journey—one in which he set his course in the direction of knowledge and self-discovery. He has a voracious appetite for informative books, and reads volumes of them passionately and relentlessly. He is open and warm and funny and fascinating—pure delight to be around.

It's interesting. When you see Nick on screen, you always say, "I like this guy." Now that I've gotten to know him, I understand why. The connection that we are making with him is to his "vital force." It is powerful.

METABOLISM

Right now, as you read this, you are burning calories, which is creating heat. Eating a certain way could help to increase the amount of heat you are generating, or "speed up" your metabolism.

Digestion is the absorption of food that you eat and conversion of that food into energy. During this process, each macronutrient has a different effect on metabolism.

In *The Body You Love*, a program developed by a friend of mine, Phil Kaplan (a renowned fitness professional who has a popular radio show in South Florida) shares with us what he has learned regarding the energy requirements of digesting the three macronutrients:

First, let's look at *Fat*.

It does not require a lot of work for your body to break down fat. Fats are "emulsified" into smaller molecules, and then either used for energy or transported for storage. For every 100 calories of fat that you consume, your body burns approximately five calories as energy to accomplish this process. In other words, you have a *five-percent metabolic boost* from ingesting fats.

With <u>Complex</u> *Carbohydrates* your body has to work a little harder. (Note that I am qualifying the type of carbohydrate here. What I am about to tell you does not apply to *refined carbohydrates*.) Complex, unrefined carbohydrates are long chains of sugars that your body must break down, and then release hormones to accomplish a variety of tasks such as transportation to cells, conversion to glycogen for storage as energy in muscles and liver, etc. Your body must work almost twice as hard to process complex carbohydrates as it does to process fat, so for every 100 calories of complex carbohydrate you eat, your body burns ten calories of energy in dealing with it. You have a *ten-percent metabolic boost* with unrefined complex carbohydrates.

Because digesting these carbohydrates makes your body work harder, it was observed that, calorie for calorie, by simply replacing fat with carbohydrate, people lost *weight*....and so the "Fat Free" craze was born. But, pay attention here...this does not mean the boxes and bags, and shelves-full and truck-loads and warehouse-stuffed processed and refined carbohydrates are going to accomplish this *thermic* effect you are looking for. *You will not get the metabolic boost from them* because machines used in the refinement process have done much of your body's work for you, and these products are quickly absorbed into your bloodstream. This all ties into the sections on *Insulin* and *Glycemic Index* in chapter 3, as well as *Food Allergies and Addictions*, so there are many issues we are addressing with this "refinement" subject. You will see that what keeps coming up in regards to carbohydrates in this book is: *Stay away from processed and refined foods.*

With *Proteins* your body has to do the most work of all. As I explained earlier in this chapter, proteins are long chains of amino acids, and they have to be broken apart, absorbed, and used for many jobs such as rebuilding tissue. This requires a lot of work, and your body uses about 20 to 25 calories of energy per 100 calories of protein ingested to do this work, or a *twenty-percent metabolic boost*. Now, I am referring, of course, to *lean* protein...otherwise you will have fat to work with in the "calorie for calorie" conversion, and you will not get the same effect. Therefore, because this phenomenon was observed on high protein diets, the "protein only" craze was born.

There are, of course, different opinions here as well. *In Live Longer, Live Better*, Dr. Barnard tells us that consuming <u>carbohydrates</u> elevates your metabolism by stimulating the production of thyroid hormone—and digesting this macronutrient provides the highest metabolic kickback. He says low-carbohydrate diets slow down metabolism.

Dr. T. Collin Cambell from Cornell University conducted a study in China, observing that the Chinese eat less protein than Americans do, and they are thinner. Dr. Cambell observed: "On a protein diet lower than what we have here (U.S.), it appears that the energy that is consumed is expended in the form of heat—a higher carbohydrate consumption allows the body to expend more energy as heat. A metabolic rate associated with loss of body heat tends to be increased. Therefore, it appears weight-loss can be achieved with a diet lower in animal protein, and overall protein as well."

Oh, boy.

Will we ever stop behaving like laboratory rats?

<u>Your body was made to process all of the macronutrients and do specific jobs with each one of them</u>...one of these jobs is the very one we are obsessing about at this moment: Liberating fat and using it for energy.

You must EAT to have energy, release energy, elevate your metabolism, and become less fat.

<u>A note on calories</u>...Both Protein and Carbohydrate contain four calories per gram. Alcohol contains seven calories per gram, and fat contains nine calories per gram. By limiting your fat intake, especially *saturated fats*, you will technically be able to eat more food to supply your body with its appropriate energy.

DIGESTION

"The ultimate truth out of all this is that it isn't the foods at all that are the problem. The real problem is with the digestive vitality of the person.

Think of the digestive system as resembling a flame. If you have a tiny flame, then you have to treat it with great care. The fuel must be pure and fine and added slowly, or the fire will flicker and possibly falter.

However, if you gradually build up that little flame so that it reaches bonfire pro-portions, then you can throw the occasional wet log or large chunk on it with only a little smoke being produced. However, many people are busily throwing wet logs on their digestive candles and wondering why their bodies are getting 'sooted up.'"

—John Matsen, N.D.

Eating Alive

Perhaps you've heard another analogy that addresses this same issue: Think of your digestive system as a large pail. You can fill it a little at a time, and allow the fluid to evaporate, or dump a whole lot in at once, eventually making it overflow. Digestion is very confusing because changing diet alone doesn't usually improve it. You can still remain highly sensitive to different foods. Dr. Matsen writes: "Sensitivities, or allergies to foods or external sub-stances like pollen or dust, decrease if the digestion is improved and the tox-ins eliminated. If a person can increase digestive vitality, the dietary range can also be increased."

This is when you can freely practice the "80-20" concept in your *Live It Or Diet Lifestyle System.* However, it is evident (by the prevalence of chronic physical, mental, and emotional disease in our society) that there are limits to what the body can take. It is not necessary that you become a vegetarian to be healthy, or that you need to eat meat, either. *What is important is that you digest quickly and efficiently whatever you eat. The result of digestive strength is dietary freedom.*

This is where food combining comes in. Some health-care practitioners advocate refraining from mixing carbohydrates and proteins to rebuild the digestive system. Eating these two macronutrients together results in the neutralization of the digestive juices, (alkaline for carbs, acid for protein) so the digestive process takes much longer. With the extension of the digestive process comes the increased chance of fermentation and putrification toxins being formed. Separating proteins and carbs speeds up digestion, and makes it more efficient. Improving the digestive function will decrease the need of food combining later on.

Dr. Matsen elaborates: "If digestion can be made so efficient that extra digestive energy is left over, that's what is sent out into the bloodstream to clean out the old accumulated toxins. Thus, it's surplus digestive energy that does the housecleaning in the body.

Since most of us have such overloaded digestive systems, we do little in the way of housecleaning over the years, which is equivalent to living in a house for many years without vacuuming it."

That is why it's good to get hungry. When you are hungry, your digestive energy goes out into the blood looking for fuel. The start of this process is beneficial, because it will digest some of the old "debris" lying around. (Don't be hungry for too long, though. Fasting is another topic, totally. It can help you detox and feel better emotionally, spiritually, and ultimately physically, but you can lose muscle, and have a "healing crisis." Some people are so toxic that their already over-loaded organs cannot handle the elimination. Thus, they feel <u>worse</u>.)

Also, the liver is the major organ involved in regulating blood-sugar levels. Most people have sluggish livers from years of "toxic accumulation" that do not do their jobs well. At this point, they are *functionally hypoglycemic* and get light headed, weak, and confused (brain fog!). Dr. Matsen says: "To cure hypoglycemia, the organs have to be detoxified to regain the proper regulation of blood sugar levels. It is therefore important to eat lightly in the morning in order to send surplus digestive juice into the bloodstream, but not so light so long that you actually get low blood-sugar symptoms. An hour or two of detoxification might allow the liver to slowly function a little better by the next day, week or month."

You can have the benefits of fasting *while you are still eating* if your digestion is efficient. According to Dr. Matsen: "The digestive system has highs and lows of energy, as do all the organs of the body. The digestive system is strongest between seven and eleven in the morning. The stomach "meridian's" peak is between seven and nine, and that of the pancreas (spleen "meridian") is between nine and eleven. This is the time to eat a big breakfast, like the nutritionists have been harping on us to do for such a long time. The problem with eating a big breakfast is that all the prime digestive juice is used up first thing in the morning, so it is virtually impossible to have any surplus digestive juice left for the rest of the day. No housecleaning will be done that day."

You can stimulate digestive juice in the morning with something light (that doesn't require a lot of digestion itself). You will notice on your *Live It Or Diet Lifestyle System* food plan that your day starts with water and fresh squeezed lemon. You can add to this a pinch of cayenne, and ginger to taste. These are all mild stomach stimulants, and they will stimulate the stomach to make more digestive juice. Grapefruit works great, too (and is good on a fat-loss plan).

So...a light breakfast (fruit, etc.), and mainly carbohydrates for lunch. Why? They are "clean-burning," and their wastes are easily eliminated. It is best to have mainly protein at night as they can be used as "building material," which is a better use for them rather than fuel (which has complex elimination). This might be a good regimen to follow (with individual considerations) in the beginning of your detox quest to "clean house."

Also, another consideration in the size of your early meals is your Oxidative Rate. According to Dr. George Watson in *Nutrition And Your Mind*, slow oxidizers are unable to burn sugar fast enough to also utilize a heavy fat-protein intake. He tells us that a *slow oxidizer* simply should not eat a heavy breakfast. If a *slow oxidizer* has had a substantial dinner the previous evening, he will think more clearly and feel much better if he eats something light in the morning. This, according to Dr. Watson, is not the case for the *fast oxidizer.*

In her book, *Different Bodies—Different Diets*, Dr. Carolyn Mein takes issue with "food combining." She writes: "In order for a food to be considered a food it has to contain fat, protein, and carbohydrates, even if the quantity is too small to appear on package labels. If any component is missing, the body doesn't register the substance as a food, and won't assimilate it. The assimilation of foods depends on the presence of all three components of fat, protein, and carbohydrates. Without the three elements, digestion and assimilation are incomplete, which, of course, leads to a system imbalance. Carbohydrates, which break down into sugar, are necessary for protein assimilation. Sugar enables protein to pass through a membrane between the bloodstream and the brain cells known as the blood/brain barrier. It also allows the same process to occur in other cells."

(For more debating on this subject, turn to *Alkaline-Acid Balance...*)

Do I advocate the principles of "food combining," or "food separation," as Dr. Dancey calls it, (see, *Cellulite*)? Well, I can tell you that when I incorporated it into the *Live It Or Diet Lifestyle Systems* of certain extremely challenged individuals, we had very positive results. It seemed that by simplifying the digestive process for them, it allowed their bodies to focus energy on healing and balance. Many uncomfortable and even debilitating symptoms subsided. I believe, like many of the principles presented in this book, food combining (food separation) has its place. Dr. Gary agrees—especially in the initial stages of balancing and healing—keep it simple!

THE "SET POINT THEORY"

Have you noticed that there always seems to be a struggle of "wills" between you and your body? You discipline yourself and deprive yourself and turn your back for one second and your ungrateful body has crept back up to its

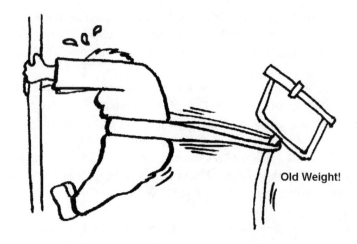

Old Weight!

comfortable (for it, not for you) old weight. Where it has slunk back to, stubborn wretch that it is, is its "set point;" the place where the metabolism stabilizes and "sets itself" as a result of habitual intake and expenditure of energy.

Dr. Ornish writes: "Your body resists change—both for better and for worse. Homeostasis, another word for equilibrium, is another evolutionary adaptation that makes dieting by traditional methods difficult. When you overeat, your fat cells grow larger. If you keep overeating, you begin forming new fat cells. You also gain weight. The size of your fat cells may decrease if you restrict food intake for a while, but the number does not. According to the set point theory, because of homeostasis your body tries to maintain your weight, even when you go on a calorie-restricted diet.

Recently, nutrition researchers at Cornell University published a study in the American Journal of Clinical Nutrition designed to disprove the set point theory, yet the results ended up confirming it. They wrote: 'First, it seems that some degree of weight loss can be achieved without the necessity of dieting. There is a great deal of evidence that conscious reduction in the amount of food consumed results in rapid losses of body weight, but almost invariably this lost weight is regained. Reductions in the fat content of the diet with no limitation on the amount of food consumed may lead to a more permanent weight loss than can be achieved through dieting.' According to the principal investigator, Dr. David Levitsky, your metabolic rate is related to the amount of carbohydrates you consume. 'Maybe the body can't detect a reduction in the amount of fat coming in, (if carbohydrates stay the same or increase) so the metabolism doesn't change.' When you increase consumption of carbohydrates, your metabolic rate may increase. Why? Your thyroid gland is a key regulator of your metabolism. Thyroid hormone increases your metabolic rate. Your thyroid gland makes a thyroid hormone called thyroxin, which can be converted to either an active or an inactive form. When you eat a diet high in carbohydrates and low in fat, then more thyroid hormone is converted to the active form."

There are those, of course, who disagree with Dr. Ornish. Their arguments (for higher protein, higher fat, whatever your blood type indicates, etc.) are presented in this book as well, along with more information on thyroid (see, FEMININITY, and *Thyroid Hormone*).

But, meanwhile—how do we change our set points? Well, you already know that caloric deprivation will not accomplish this. The more you restrict your calories, the faster your body will run home, back to its low metabolic set point and high body fat. Dr. Braly in *Food Allergy and Nutrition Revolution* states that: "We must change our diet and life-style and thus our metabolic set point, so that our body naturally stabilizes itself at a lower weight. In raising our set point—which is nothing more than the place where our metabolism has decided to park itself until further notice—we raise our ability to lose weight and keep it off permanently."

This sounds wonderfully simple. But I know that it's not. Theoretically, if we eat and exercise intelligently and often, we will maintain a higher metabolic set point. I know that by elevating lean muscle mass, engaging in appropriate aerobic activities, and eating nutritionally sound, frequent, small meals, our metabolisms are elevated. I do all of the above, but my body will still defy me at times. *Why* it would (and how it could) do this to me in the face of all I have done to insure that it *wouldn't* (and couldn't), sent me on yet another journey.

FOOD ALLERGIES AND ADDICTIONS

Have you ever considered yourself addicted to certain foods? Are there foods you crave? After you eat certain foods, do you find you are craving others? Do certain foods drive you to binge eating? Maybe it's time to pay attention to what "triggers" your actions and reactions in this area. Certain foods can be our "trigger foods"..foods that we are addicted to because we may actually be *allergic* to them.

Now, by allergies I do not mean the obvious ones, with the immediate reactions that you recognize, like hives, or vomiting, etc. I am speaking about the more insidious allergies, the ones that are called delayed onset. We may not even recognize the symptoms as *symptoms of a very serious problem*. We usually do not pay that much attention to every ingredient in every single thing we eat during the course of a day. Suddenly, we find ourselves driven to eat sugar, or bread. And somehow, we just cannot satisfy this desire. It controls us. We become bloated, depressed, tired, grumpy, foggy, and unrecognizable to ourselves. And we just think it's us. We are weak. We are not nice. We are not worthy of love. We are losers.

Consider this. There is a very strong probability that WE HAVE ALLERGIES TO CERTAIN FOODS. And these foods could be manipulating us in ways that we cannot defend. Imagine that! Food can be that powerful. The fact is, *food is the most powerful drug you will ever encounter*. It all gets translated to chemistry anyway, just like any other drug. I'll give you an example. We all acknowledge that heroin is an addictive drug. It ultimately controls an individual to the point of turning him or her into an addict. Okay, so where does heroin come from? Poppies. Something that grows in the earth. We take these pretty little flowers and process them and refine them and turn them into the drug, heroin. We have perverted something natural, transforming it into a chemical substance that we could not possibly react naturally to.

What else do we do that to? Nearly everything we eat? Think about it. What do we do to the foods that grow in the earth? Do we eat them as close to that state as possible, or do we process and refine them into something that is going to be as unnatural and addictive to our bodies as heroin?

No wonder we call ourselves addicts. No wonder we have eating disorders. I understand that many of our eating problems could be deeply rooted to emotional situations, but consider that with some of these issues, *eating the wrong foods may have preceded the emotional disorder*. We could actually be emotionally disturbed because of food.

We might have been born with certain allergies, or our food sensitivities could be adult onset, or they might be a matter of constantly introducing unnatural substances into our diets that throw us off balance. *Stop and consider some of the things you eat.* Do you know what is in that "mystery meat" that you just purchased at a fast-food drive through? When Hebrew National says, "We answer to a higher power," they mean for something to be certified "kosher" it must be more strictly regulated than most of the stuff we consume. That's why people today are turning to "organic" and "free range" and other more naturally grown livestock, produce, and grains.

Deprivation is another way to set yourself up for food allergies. Constantly eating just a few foods can cause your body to begin reacting badly to these foods. Couple this with the fact that a monotonous menu deprives your body of essential nutrients, and, before you know it, you are out of *balance*: You have now initiated numerous metabolic consequences that will wreak havoc with your behavior. You blame yourself when you simply can no longer resist that cookie; then that cookie leads to a whole box. You believe you lack discipline and you beat yourself up emotionally, which, of course, leads to more eating. And as you are stuffing and gaining and crying, you are completely unaware of the fact that this situation is in reality a built-in aspect of the program you are on. It is not you. You could not combat this if you had an army. Your body is missing something, or it has too much of something, or it is getting something it cannot handle, and, amazing machine that it is, it is reacting the only way it knows to survive. It will bypass your thoughts and desires and willpower totally. It will drive you against your will to a 7/11 at two a.m. to get something sweet long after the sane and controlled you has already thrown all that stuff out of your house. You are not in control anymore, and the only way you can *take control of your body* is to get off this ride completely and just *get still*. I say this because the best thing you can do when you do not know what to do is to be still so you can objectively filter knowledge through the computer between your ears. Being neurotic now will only lead to more harmful behavior.

I will use myself as an example here once again to illustrate this matter to you.

After I quit competitive bodybuilding, I underwent a year long holistic program (designed and supervised by Dr. Jiro Rodriguez—a chiropractor who specialized in biochemistry in New York) to get my body back in balance. The results of the tests that Dr. Jiro did showed *serious* nutrient imbalances, mineral deficiencies, and poor digestion; there was an entire spectrum of disorders that were causing my problems. I was suffering from severe gut pain, fatigue, that horrendous body acne (of course you know that it was the symptom that finally showed up on the outside that ultimately drove me to seek help), mental "fogginess," and other extremely disturbing problems. I had thrown my body into a virtual tempest of disease by the radical practices of competition. After adjusting and monitoring and modifying all conditions for a year, everything became stabilized, and I felt great—until my 40's.

Now, I am speculating here, but I have learned enough at this point to surmise that the return of my symptoms was caused by: Stress (I was practically working around the clock to build my business), sleep deprivation, imbalanced nutrition (I was subscribing to the fat-free, high carb "law" of the day), eating on the run, and the beginnings of arbitrary hormone behavior.

Along with the symptoms from my late 30's, the new, and even more disturbing symptom on the scene in my 40's was *weight gain*! Impossible, unacceptable, irritating bloat. My body was completely betraying me—ignoring my warrior workouts, my dedication to healthy food, my disciplined lifestyle.

Once again, I sought the natural, "alternative" route, and consulted with Dr. Gary (see *15 Rounds—My Championship Bout*). This is when I learned about food allergies and the accompanying syndromes. I had terrible abdominal pain again, with a whole series of gastrointestinal problems, but, of course, it was the terrifying bloat that initiated that first consultation. I was becoming unrecognizable to myself. No matter what I did—no doubt about it—-I was getting fatter. Now, I knew—from my experience and my education—that to resort to obsessive, radical behavior (like constantly doing cardio while engaging in calorie deprivation) would ultimately <u>backfire</u> on me, but I was (once again) desperate. When I discovered Dr. Gary and the connection between food allergies, poor digestion, and weight gain, I felt as if I had stepped out of my black and white tornado-tossed house into a Technicolor world. I tested positive to a wide variety of foods: Sugar, dairy, wheat, corn, and black pepper. I learned that when you are allergic to a certain food, you are unable to fully digest and absorb it. Partially digested food can enter the bloodstream, which could cause allergens to be deposited in tissue. In his book, *Food Allergy & Nutrition Revolution*, Dr. Braly states: "People who have a tendency to gain or lose more than a couple of pounds a day, or whose weight bounces around unpredictably, unassociated with the quantity of food eaten, should at least suspect food allergy. One of the ways in which the body can reduce the irritation of allergy is to hold on to a lot of water, in order to dilute the tissue-bound allergens—hence, edema (water retention). Because your body will not release these fluids as long as it is defending against allergic attacks, it is very hard to keep one's weight down until allergies are eliminated from your diet." Hello.

Rudy Rivera, M.D. And Roger Deutsch, authors of *Your Hidden Food Allergies Are Making You Fat*, tell us that the food allergies that we are referring to in this chapter—delayed onset food allergies—are actually food intolerances. They explain it this way: "Although a complex biological process, food intolerance is, simply stated, an individualized biochemical sensitivity to foods that are otherwise wholesome and harmless. This sensitivity causes the immune system to react as if it were protecting the body from an enemy such as a bacteria, virus, or parasite. This reaction to common foods causes intricate systems within the body to begin malfunctioning. One abnormal function triggers and impacts the next, like a series of dominos falling, until the slow dance of dysfunction surfaces in one form of ill health or another.

Food intolerances are often referred to as the "hidden" food allergy, since you usually have no apparent immediate reaction when you eat a food to which your body is sensitive. In fact, our body's reaction to offending foods usually occurs in small steps. Each step leads to the next until at some point, the body reaches a breaking point—the final straw. Our body then reacts by developing one or more of a wide range of symptoms and diseases such as obesity, arthritis, diabetes, gastrointestinal problems, sinus conditions, or migraines."

There are also many emotional, mental, and behavioral symptoms that Dr. Braly cites as possible indications of food allergies: Mental or physical fatigue, irritability, insomnia, mood swings, muscle and joint pain, and abnormal cravings (sometimes resulting in binge eating), among many others. This last symptom is linked to what is called the "allergy-addiction syndrome." It is believed that we "crave" foods we are allergic to because eating them prevents the "withdrawal symptoms" that we experience when we deny ourselves these foods. Dr. Braly says, "Simply put, allergic reactions may lead to an addiction to food that is bad for us, because eating the food temporarily relieves the discomfort it caused in the first place."

Is this what food addiction is all about? To examine this issue, I will first present what is stated in *Food Allergy & Nutrition Revolution*: "Addiction to food is biochemically and physiologically identical to the relationship between the alcoholic and liquor or a junkie and drugs. The body is an adaptive mechanism, always coping in physiological, biochemical ways with whatever demands you or your environment place on it. The body's natural reaction is to reject or throw off any substance it perceives as harmful or toxic—which is how it perceives any food or chemical that it is presented with too often and in excessive quantities. The addiction response is only one of the several actions your body takes to cope with allergic foods."

The body defends itself against the invasion of unfriendly foods in the digestive tract. It attempts to get this food past the absorption process, but this usually results in partially digested food finding its way into the bloodstream. The immune system retaliates by sending special antibodies, and the outcome of this battle is irritation and inflammation in the tissues where the enemy has deposited itself. Dr. Braly tells us that here is where the addiction comes in: "To cope with the resulting discomfort, the body sends out a rush of chemical mediators, including a group of narcotic-like substances called opiods. Thus, the very substance that is punishing your system seems to be giving you pleasure. You're unconsciously eating the allergic food in order to avoid the symptoms that would show up if you didn't eat it. You're bingeing on these foods; you're addicted to them."

Could this dilemma be an example of "the chicken or the egg?" For some of us, might addiction itself be the disease, an effect of genetics or unfortunate experiences?

Kay Sheppard, in her book, *Food Addiction, The Body Knows*, defines food addiction as "the compulsive pursuit of mood change by engaging repeatedly in episodes of binge eating despite adverse consequences." (Doesn't this sound very similar to the above arguments?) Ms. Sheppard further states that food addicts have a "metabolic, biochemical imbalance which results in the characteristic symptoms of addiction. The signs of addiction are obsession, compulsion, denial, tolerance, withdrawal syndrome and craving, plus distorted body image."

I briefly mentioned in my story how I hid my compulsive eating when I was younger. As far back as I can remember, I snuck food, ate in bathrooms and closets, stole bakery ingredients like chocolate chips from the pantry, kept candy (usually M&M's) in my pockets—I exhibited all of the classic behavior of someone who is powerless over their actions. I craved things like candy, cookies, bread—sweet, starchy foods. Eating these things *made me eat more of these things.* To this day, if I binge on sugar in one form, I cannot satiate the desire for more sugar in *any form.* Are my allergies to wheat and sugar a result of bingeing on these things in my youth? Or, did I always have a sensitivity to these foods, which caused the cravings, which caused the over-eating, which eventually caused my immune system to react?

In her book, Ms. Sheppard says that there is an addictive quality to certain foods, and the platform for programs that deal with food addictions is *total abstinence from refined and processed foods!* Most of the "trigger" foods that are cited in these programs include: Sugar, flour and wheat products, and foods with high fat content. Diets that do not take into account that these foods behave in our bodies like drugs, lock us in a pattern that can only result in a downward spiral; eventually, we must succumb to our cravings. The food plans for "food addict" and "eating disorder" programs are primarily lower carbohydrate events than most typical programs. They are not usually "low calorie" diets, because the metabolic inefficiency of such diets set the addict up to fail. They do, however, completely abolish all forms of sugar forever. These programs contend that sugar is to the food addict what alcohol is to the alcoholic. There has been much written on this subject. The book *Sugar Blues* is an entire volume dealing with the dangers of refined sugar. Also, an experiment done with rats implied that rats become addicted to sugar and could kill themselves eating it, even when good food was available to them. Along with complete avoidance of trigger foods, programs such as "Overeaters Anonymous" stress maintaining a balance between carbohydrate and protein, and eating a *variety of foods.* Eating one food too often may indicate that it is a binge food (which means an allergy or addiction), or that it might become a binge food.

Dr. Braly discusses the concept of "food rotation" in his book, and offers his *Food Rotation Diet.* There are five constituents to the food rotation concept. The first is that it helps prevent allergies (thus addictions) by limiting consumption of something to only once or twice a week. The second is that rotation of your foods promotes a more balanced diet and results in the presence of more nutrients. Third, it is almost impossible, as noted by Dr. Braly, "to continue to eat packaged, processed, and complicated foods on a rotation diet. Many packaged foods contain dozens of ingredients, which 'use up' foods that then cannot be eaten for ninety-six hours." (Dr. Braly's regimen allows you to eat a food no more frequently than once every four days for the first three months of the program.) Fourth, rotating your foods relieves stress to your digestive system, and fifth, it can lead to weight loss through clearing up food allergies.

Also, rotating foods (not repeating them for at least three to four days) could unmask allergies. If your reaction to a particular food, when it is reintroduced to your diet, is stronger than usual, it can be identified as a problem.

I mentioned that I underwent testing for food allergies, and when I eliminated these foods, I immediately dropped seven pounds, the pain and distention in my abdomen disappeared, and my cravings abated. I sailed through the following weeks like I was ecstatically reborn—and then, my symptoms returned—even though I stayed away from my trouble foods. Dr. Gary had warned me that this might happen, that we might be eliminating only one of the stressors causing my problems. Temporary relief ensued because my body had one less issue to deal with, but I was to discover that I—like many others—was battling other conditions as well (see, *15 Rounds..My Championship Bout*).

Food Allergy Testing

Isolating your sensitivity to particular foods is an important component of your *Live It Or Diet Lifestyle System*. There are many different testing methods used to determine which foods are sabotaging you. Dr. Ellen Cutler is a pioneer in this field. The following is an excerpt from her book, *Winning The War Against Asthma & Allergies*, which describes several allergy tests:

"Radioallergosorbent Test (RAST): This is an initial laboratory test administered to a patient's blood sample to measure the amount of IgE antibodies in the blood. The number of antibodies increases with the severity of the allergy. (For immediate-onset food allergies.)

Pulse Test: This measures the heart rate before and after exposure to a suspected allergen and is an effective method for determining allergic reactions to foods. Pulses can be felt at various points. The pulse generally deviates from normal in allergy patients. It usually becomes faster and more forceful, but can also become slower and weaker. Unfortunately, if one eats several foods at a time, it is hard to determine exactly which food is causing the allergic reaction.

Electronic Test: Electronic devices have been used for more than a century in the treatment and diagnosis of patients. Two German scientists, Voll and Werner, designed and built an instrument to chart and verify the relationship of acupuncture points to their corresponding organs and systems. Electronic devices work by reading the galvanic skin response, a measure of the flow of electromagnetic energy. Correlations with other test procedures have shown that the electroacupuncture device (EAV) test is accurate in detecting sensitivities to foods, chemicals, pesticides, herbicides, environmental irritants, dental irritants, fungi, bacteria, and viruses, as well as dysfunctions of organs and systems. This method causes little or no discomfort because there are no needles or puncturing of the skin. A low-level electric stimulus (not perceptible by the subject being tested) is passed through the body while the patient holds a brass handle in one hand and a metal probe is placed against acupressure points on the hands and feet.

Muscle Response Test: Also known as applied kinesiology, this test was developed in 1964 by Dr. George Goodheart, a chiropractor, to diagnose or read certain blockages in the body. Muscle response testing is also a method of using the relative strength of the muscles to uncover allergies, nutritional imbalances, and structural misalignments in the body. This method identifies blockages in the electromagnetic energy fields when one is exposed to an allergen. Muscle testing bypasses the conscious and subconscious minds. When a suspected allergen is held in the hand, a strong muscle will weaken if an allergy to the substance is present. The person to be tested generally lies down or sits up and extends an arm at a ninety-degree angle, thumb down, in front of the body. The facilitator pushes against the arm to establish the strength of the testing muscle (indicator muscle) while the subject resists. When the person holds a food or other substance to which he or she is allergic, the indicator muscle will immediately and markedly weaken. People can learn to perform this technique on others, and can teach others to test them. Muscle testing procedures can detect both hidden and active or acute allergies."

A state of the art IgG blood test called the Enzyme Linked Immuno-sorbant Assay (or ELISA for short), has been modified by Immuno Laboratories to be one of the most effective ways to detect delayed-onset food allergies. (Recent advances in finger-stick ELISA technology allows for home testing, and is part of our home test kit.)

Dr. Gary performed three food allergy testing methods on me: Immuno Lab's IgG ELISA test, electronic testing, and kinesiology (muscle response) testing. The comparisons between all three were amazingly similar.

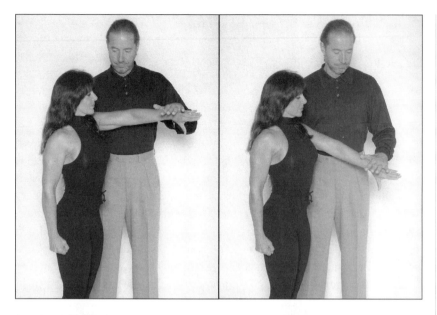

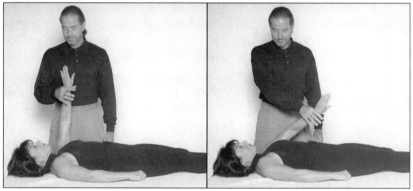

KINESIOLOGY (MUSCLE RESPONSE) TESTING.
(See page 162, *Muscle Response Testing For Food Allergies*—for instructions.)

Could You Have Food Allergies?

Muscle Response Testing For Food Allergies

You can test for food allergies (sensitivities) in your home. The following is how to proceed with Muscle Response Testing as described in *Say Goodbye To Illness* by Devi S. Nambudripad, D.C., L.Ac., R.N., Ph.D.:

"To perform standard muscle response testing, two people are required. The person who performs the test is called the tester, and the person on whom the test is performed is called the subject. The subject can be tested lying down, standing, or seated. (The lying down position is more convenient and gives more accurate results.) The subject lies on a firm surface, with one hand raised 90 degrees to his body, and his thumb pointing down toward his big toe (or his palm facing outward). The tester stands on the subject's side opposite the raised arm and gently rests one hand on the shoulder of the resting arm for balance. The tester, using his free arm, tries to push down the raised arm of the subject. The subject resists the push of the tester on his arm (the indicator muscle). The indicator muscle remains strong if the subject is well balanced at the time of the testing. If the subject is dehydrated, or out of balance in any other way, the raised arm is weak and gives way to pressure (we frequently find this test less accurate than it should be because many people tend to be dehydrated on a cellular level." (See, *Appendix F* for the *Live It Or Diet Hydration Formulation*—which can be used immediately to balance the subject.)

"The tester should not try to overpower the subject, and the subject shouldn't gather up all his strength from other muscles in the body to resist the tester with all his might. The tester needs to apply only about 5 pounds of pressure for about 3 to 5 seconds. If the indicator muscle remains strong with pressure, a suspected allergen can then be placed into the palm of the subject's resting hand. The sensory receptors in the palm side of the hand— at the tip of the fingers—are extremely sensitive to recognize the allergens. The fingertips have specialized sensory receptors that send messages to and from the brain. When the subject touches the allergen with his fingertips, the sensory receptors sense the charges of the allergen—and if they are incompatible to the subject's body—his indicator muscle will go weak with pressure. If they are compatible, the indicator muscle will remain strong."

You can use this test on any food you suspect might be causing you problems. I recommend that you test for some of the more common culprits: Wheat, dairy, sugar, corn, and yeast. Remember, I have compared my own muscle response testing with blood testing and electronic testing, and they all were in agreement. When done correctly, muscle response testing can be a very effective way of identifying your enemies.(See *page 161*)

Alternative Foods To Wheat And Dairy To Learn About And Love

(Wheat and dairy are two foods that come up most of the time in allergy testing.)

WHEAT: The average American diet is based upon the use of this grain. There are several other grains to choose from. Each grain has it's own taste, texture and smell. The whole grain can be cooked as is or it is ground into flour. From the flour comes breads, muffins, pancakes, pasta, crackers, cookies and quick breads. Some of the grains can be sprouted and made into breads.

The following grains are wheat alternatives:

- •AMARANTH: Available in whole grain and flour. There are recipes on the box.
- •BARLEY: Available in whole grain and flour. There are recipes on the bag.
- •BUCKWHEAT: Whole grain and flour, pasta (100% soba noodles), breakfast cereals, and hot cereal.
- •CORN: Flour (meal), pasta, breakfast cereals, polenta, tortillas, and corn chips.
- •KAMUT: Whole grain, flour (recipes on bag), pasta, breakfast cereals, bagels and bread.
- •MILLET: Whole grain, flour (recipes on bag), and breakfast cereal.
- •OAT: Whole grain, steel cut, rolled flakes, breakfast cereals and hot cereals.
- •QUINOA: Whole grain, flour (recipes on bag), pasta, breakfast cereals and flakes.
- •RICE: Whole grain, flour (recipes on bag), pasta, breakfast cereals, bread, crackers, cookies, chips, hot breakfast cereals, desserts and rice cakes.
- •RYE: Whole grain, flour (recipes on bag), bread, hot breakfast cereal, sprouted breads and crackers.
- •SPELT: Whole grain, flour (recipes on bag), bread, bagels, pasta and breakfast cereals.

See...no wheat...no sweat!!

All of the bags of flours have several recipes including cookies, biscuits, pancakes, muffins, waffles and quick breads. Your alternatives are all right there for you to choose from.

COW'S MILK (Lovingly Called "Dairy"): Another standard American diet staple. If you have an allergy to cow's milk you are not alone. The standard clichè is "Cow's milk is perfect—for baby cows!"

Here are some dairy alternatives:

- •MILK: How about trying *goat milk*? It is supposed to be the closest to human milk. If that doesn't interest you, try milks made from almonds, soy, rice, oat, and even from multigrains.
- •BUTTER: Margarine...is it a health food? How about one that is not hydrogenated? SPECTRUM NATURALS has a spread that is supposed to taste like real butter. There is always **goat butter**. And *rice butter*! Olive oil spread on toast tastes really good, too. Also, look for spreads made from soy.
- •CHEESE: Watch out for casein. The non-dairy cheeses have casein in them and it is dairy. The brand SOYMAGE is 100% casein free. It is available in mozzarella style and grated Parmesan cheese. They are primarily made from soy. Goat milk cheeses are available as well as sheep cheese (not cheap, this sheep cheese).
- •ICE CREAM: Some brand names that are dairy free are FARM FOODS Ice Bean, SWEET NOTHINGS, and IT'S SOY DELICIOUS. SHARON'S makes sorbet. You can always freeze a banana and blend it in your blender to make a frozen treat.
- •YOGURT: Available made from soy and goat milk.

HYPOGLYCEMIA

What is hypoglycemia? Most of us have an understanding that it is a condition that concerns blood sugar. We think of it as "low blood sugar" ("hypo" vs. "hyper"—high), but it is really more complex than that. In *The Do's And Don'ts Of Low Blood Sugar* by Roberta Ruggiero (the founder and president of The Hypoglycemia Support Foundation, Inc.), we read:

"In simple layman's language, hypoglycemia is the body's inability to properly handle the large amounts of sugar that the average American consumes today. It's an overload of sugar, alcohol, caffeine, tobacco and stress. In medical terms, hypoglycemia is defined in relation to its cause. Functional hypoglycemia is the oversecretion of insulin by the pancreas in response to a rapid rise in blood sugar or 'glucose.'

All carbohydrates (vegetables, fruits and grains, as well as simple table sugar) are broken down into simple sugars by the process of digestion. This sugar enters the blood stream as glucose and our level of blood sugar rises. The pancreas then secretes a hormone known as insulin into the blood in order to bring the glucose down to normal levels.

In hypoglycemia, the pancreas sends out too much insulin and the blood sugar plummets below the level necessary to maintain well being. Since all of the cells of the body, especially the brain cells, use glucose for fuel, a blood glucose level that is too low starves the cells of needed fuel, causing both physical and emotional symptoms."

(Dr. Gary tells us that hypoglycemia can also be complicated (or even triggered) by delayed onset allergy to sugar.)

The following are some of the symptoms of hypoglycemia: *Fatigue, insomnia, mental confusion, nervousness, mood swings, faintness, headaches, depression, phobias, heart palpitations, craving for sweets, cold hands and feet, forgetfulness, dizziness, blurred vision, inner trembling, outbursts of temper, sudden hunger, allergies and crying spells.*

If you have any of the above symptoms, you need to take a serious look at how you habitually eat and behave. Do you consume a lot of sugary, refined, and processed foods (cakes, donuts, breads, cookies, candy, etc.), sodas, caffeine, and alcohol? Are you under a great deal of stress? Do you smoke?

It is very important that you address this with some urgency if you believe that you have hypoglycemia. This is a serious condition that can lead to even more serious conditions if not attacked immediately, and your weapon is your <u>diet</u>.

We have discussed throughout this book the importance of individualizing diet and exercise programs. If you have hypoglycemia, it is vital that you take this approach. In *The Do's And Don'ts Of Blood Sugar*, Ms. Ruggiero says the following: "The key to a successful diet lies in its 'individualization.' Each one of us is different. Each one of us is biochemically unique. Therefore, every diet must be tailor-made to meet our individual nutritional requirements. Don't be afraid to listen to your body. It will send you signals when it cannot tolerate a food."

An extensive questionnaire to determine functional hypoglycemia is offered in your *Live It Or Diet Lifestyle System*.

(Additional testing options are listed in *Appendix E.*)

Could You Have Hypoglycemia?

If your *Live It Or Diet Lifestyle Systems* questionnaire results indicate probable hypoglycemia, you may need to take a *Glucose Tolerance Test*. Some doctors prefer using a "therapeutic diagnosis" (prescribing the appropriate diet and monitoring the response). Laboratory tests are not always conclusive, and if you have certain symptoms, they are an indication of a problem, even if test results are "borderline" or "negative."

If you do exhibit signs of hypoglycemia, the following recommendations are offered in *The Do's And Don'ts Of Low Blood Sugar:*

"•Keep a daily account of everything you eat, and your symptoms. A diet diary is your personal blueprint: A clear overall view of what you are eating, digesting and assimilating, and the first indicator that something is wrong.

•Start eliminating the 'biggies'—those foods, drinks and chemicals that cause the most problems: Sugar, white flour, alcohol, caffeine and tobacco.

•Be extremely careful when and how you eliminate the offending substances.

•Replace offending foods immediately with good, wholesome, nutritious food and snacks as close to their natural state as possible.

•Eat six meals a day or three meals with snacks in between. Do not overeat.

•Drink plenty of water

•Be aware that when you start on a hypoglycemia diet, you might experience migrating aches, pain in your muscles and/or joints, headaches or extreme fatigue. This is normal when eliminating refined foods. Call your physician if they persist.

•Be prepared to keep your blood sugar stabilized at all times, whether at home, office, school, or traveling.

•Rotate your foods. Eating the same foods over and over again for consecutive days can result in food sensitivities or allergies.

•Read labels. Avoid all sugars—dextrose, fructose, glucose, lactose, maltose, and sucrose. Read labels in health food stores, too. Just because you buy something in a health food store, does not necessarily mean you can tolerate the ingredients.

•Avoid artificial sweeteners, additives, preservatives and food coloring. MSG is a big problem for hypoglycemics—avoid it completely.

•Watch your fruit consumption. If you are in the early or severe stages of hypoglycemia, you may not be able to eat any fruit. Some can eat just a small amount. Avoid dried fruits completely.

•Be careful of the amount of 'natural' foods or drinks you consume. Even though juices are natural, they contain high amounts of sugar. Whether or not the sugar you consume is natural, your body doesn't know the difference. Sugar is sugar is sugar and your body will react to an excess of it.

•Dilute your juices, using about 2/3 juice to 1/3 water.

•Introduce new, unprocessed foods that have no preservatives, additives, or chemicals. Look especially for grains and vegetables.

- Broil, bake, or steam food.

- Understand the meaning of 'enriched.' It does not mean extra amounts of vitamins. It means a small amount of some of the vitamins that were processed out of the food have been replaced.

- Have your family stick to some of the basic principles of your diet. The big NO's for a hypoglycemic (sugar, white flour, alcohol, tobacco, and caffeine) are detrimental to anyone's health.

- Change your attitude about what constitutes a snack. We tend to think of snacks in terms of goodies or sweet treats. A good snack can be half of a baked potato with broccoli, half-stuffed tomato with tuna fish, some steamed zucchini and onions on a half cup of brown rice, a chicken leg or a slice of turkey.

- Store your food properly to avoid contamination and spoilage resulting from bacteria and molds.

- Wash your fruits and vegetables thoroughly to reduce or remove the amount of pesticide residue.

- Be aware that chemical sensitivities can aggravate Low Blood Sugar and induce reactions in vulnerable people.

- Know the seriousness of smoking cigarettes, especially for the hypoglycemic.

- Also realize that alcohol is extremely dangerous to the hypoglycemic."

Foods To Avoid For Hypoglycemia (based on the lists in *The Do's And Don'ts Of Low Blood Sugar* by Roberta Ruggiero)

DESSERTS: Anything containing white sugar (candy, cakes, pastries, custard, Jell-O, ice cream, sherbet, pudding, cookies, breakfast cereals, commercially baked breads). Avoid honey and other forms of sugar (brown, raw, turbinado, fructose).
GRAINS: Anything containing white flour (breakfast cereals, gravies, white rice, refined corn meal, white spaghetti, macaroni, noodles, refined bakery goods).
MEATS: Lunchmeats, bacon, sausage, processed meats (most contain corn sugar), meat or meat products with artificial colors, flavorings or preservatives.
BEVERAGES: Alcohol, caffeine, and all sugared soft drinks and fruit juices.
FRUITS: Dried fruits (figs, dates, raisins). Fruit juices can be tolerated at times if diluted. Avoid excessive amounts of fresh fruit.

Note: Tobacco should be avoided entirely.

Snack Ideas

Fresh vegetables (tomato wedges, sliced cucumbers, carrot and celery sticks, radish flowers, sliced summer squash and zucchini, cauliflower and broccoli flowerettes (steamed), mushrooms, pepper, fresh fruit—in moderation (apple wedges, orange slices, cantaloupe, watermelon, strawberries), cottage cheese, hard boiled egg, yogurt, nuts and seeds, popcorn, cold chicken, turkey, roast beef, cheese slices, whole grain bread or rice crackers with nut butter, whole wheat pretzels, applesauce (no sugar), baked potato (with steamed veggies).

CAN I GIVE MYSELF DIABETES?

78 million baby-boomers! Imagine. And, according to research, more than one-fifth of us (or nearly 15 million people) will develop diabetes. Why? We are the most educated generation in the history of mankind! We are a generation that paid attention, took control, and made a difference! And, we are also a generation that brought self-indulgence to a new level. We denied ourselves very little. Unfortunately, this includes the food and behavior that are coming back to haunt us.

Seven million Americans suffer from diabetes right now. There are two types of diabetes: *Diabetes Insipidus* (a rare, metabolic disorder) and *diabetes mellitus*. Did some of the people suffering from diabetes mellitus give themselves the disease?

What is diabetes mellitus? Neal Barnard, M.D., in his book *Food Is A Wonder Medicine*, explains: "Diabetes is, in essence, starvation. The cells of the body are starving for their normal food, which is a simple sugar called glucose. Normally, the cells use this sugar to run their microscopic machinery. The problem in diabetes is that sugar has trouble passing from the bloodstream into the cells where it can be used. It must be escorted into the muscle, liver, and fat cells by the hormone insulin, which can be thought of as a key that opens a door in the cell membrane for glucose to enter. When insulin is absent or not working properly, glucose simply waits in the bloodstream, unable to enter the cells."

Okay. This is very serious stuff. Diabetes can kill you. Dr. Barnard tells us: "Diabetics can develop aggressive atherosclerosis, leading to heart attacks and strokes. The poor circulation in legs, combined with trouble combating infections, means that a simple foot sore can progress to gangrene and amputation." Also, diabetes can lead to blindness and kidney failure.

How much responsibility can we take for all of this? In *Prescription For Nutritional Healing,* James Balch, M.D. writes: "Perhaps more than most diseases, diabetes mellitus is associated with diet. It is a chronic disorder of carbohydrate metabolism. Although genetics may make a person susceptible to diabetes,"..

ARE YOU PAYING ATTENTION?

"...a diet high in refined, processed foods and low in fiber and complex carbohydrates is believed to be behind most cases of the disease. Those who are overweight face the greatest risk of developing diabetes."

Wake up! I know this part is not fun, but this is important. Dr. Barnard tells us: "Diabetic treatments should always be individualized. The cornerstone of the diet is, first, to keep fats and oils to a minimum because they interfere with insulin. When I was a medical student, we did not appreciate the importance of this. We thought sugar was all there was to it. It is true that diabetics tend to develop high blood sugar levels in response to sugary foods. We used to chase our patients around the hospital to make sure they never bought candy in the gift shop, because we did not want their blood sugar to rise. But, all the while, the high-fat foods on the hospital trays were a much bigger problem because <u>fats interfere with the action of insulin</u>.

Although doctors used to believe that diabetics should steer clear of carbohydrates, we now know that just the opposite is true. Complex carbohydrates and fiber should be increased to allow a more gradual release of sugars into the blood. Many scientific studies have shown that blood sugar levels are under better control on diets that are high in fiber and carbohydrate and low in fat. A very low fat, high complex-carbohydrate diet also encourages weight loss, which improves insulin's action. Weight loss alone can make non-insulin-dependent diabetes disappear. The diet currently recommended by the American Diabetes Association could stand considerable improvement. Up to 30 percent of the calories in the ADA diet come from fat. Also, a recent report from the New England Journal of Medicine supports the suggestion that <u>cow's milk proteins stimulate the production of antibodies that destroy the insulin-producing pancreatic cells</u>. While this report was the first to bring the dairy-diabetes link to the lay public, researchers and clinicians have long suspected this possibility. It may well be that avoiding cow's milk would prevent the vast majority of cases of insulin-dependent diabetes."

Dr. Gary works with diabetes in his practice. He tells us that: "Many insulin-dependent (Type II diabetics) are allergic to sugar and insulin (insulin resistance). When properly desensitized, their clinical picture improves—sometimes dramatically. This work combined with proper diet and lifestyle modification could help eliminate this dreaded disease."

Also—<u>exercise</u>! Dr. Barnard writes: "Exercising muscles have a voracious appetite for sugar. They pull it out of the blood, even with very little insulin present. For this reason diabetics do well to maintain a regular program of aerobic physical activity. Caution is advised, however; a sudden increase in exercise can lower blood sugar too rapidly, and insulin doses will need to be adjusted by your doctor."

Okay. A quiz. If you do not (yet) have some form of diabetes, how can you decrease your odds of getting it?

Stop putting garbage in your body? Good answer.

SUGAR-SENSITIVITY
Could You Be "Sugar-Sensitive?"

Does this sound like you?

Sometimes I feel my confidence slipping away, and I am full of self-doubt and despair. I feel so crazy because one day I am at the top of my game—clear and focused, and the very next I am confused and desperate. It is as if I am entirely different people! I am moody and impulsive, and I cannot concentrate on any one thing. My attention frequently drifts, and I have low energy. I get tired easily, and I crave sugar and turn to sweets and snack foods to get myself going again. Sometimes I eat compulsively. I put on weight. I have no self-discipline, and I am frequently depressed and overwhelmed. I have tried Prozac and other drugs, but something is still wrong. My life is just not the way I want it, and I can't find the answer that works.

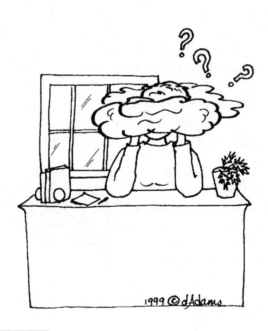

1999 © d Adams

Kathleen DesMaisons, Ph.D., addictive nutrition specialist and author of the book *Potatoes Not Prozac*, says if the above sounds like you, you may be "sugar- sensitive." She writes: "Sugar-sensitivity turns a person into Dr. Jekyll and Mr. Hyde. If you are sugar-sensitive your body chemistry may respond to sugars and certain carbohydrates (such as bread, crackers, cereal, and pasta) differently from other people. When you are biochemically sugar-sensitive, your body overreacts by releasing far more insulin than is needed." (Once again, they are playing <u>my</u> song.)

"If you are sugar-sensitive, there are three things in your body chemistry that contribute to the 'crazy' feelings: The level of sugar in your blood, the level of the chemical serotonin in your brain, the level of the chemical beta-endorphin in your brain. An imbalance in the level of any one of these bio-chemicals can bring about striking changes in the way you feel or act. When all three are out of balance, it is almost impossible to isolate which one is making you feel so bad."

Dr. DesMaisons' work in the field of addiction control led her to investigate and track the complex interactions, reactions, and delicate balance of brain chemicals and blood sugar. She recommends eating carbohydrates in their most complex form, to ensure slow absorption (see, *Evaluating The "Big Three" Macronutrients—Carbohydrate*). I especially love the way she broke her food categories into "White Things," "Brown Things," "Green Things," and Fruit. Basically, you want to stay away from any food that is a "White Thing," and Dr. DesMaisons tells us: Unless the first ingredient is whole wheat flour, think of it as a "White Thing."

Read labels. The more fiber, the less processed the food is. Refuse any product that has less than <u>two grams of fiber</u>, and certainly look for more. "Brown Things" include foods that are higher in fiber, like whole grains, seeds, and beans. They provide your body with solid nourishment and sustained energy, and will help you maintain a steady blood sugar level.

Vegetables ("Green Things") are complex carbohydrates that are loaded with fiber and slow to digest. Dr. DesMaisons recommends eating them at both lunch and dinner. Raw vegetables digest slower than cooked ones. Cooking vegetables breaks down the fiber, eliminating some of your body's work in digesting them.

As far as fruit is concerned, the higher the fiber content, the slower the absorption rate, making the fructose contained in certain fruits less of an issue.

Dr. DesMaisons goes into depth regarding brain chemicals. I urge you to read her book if you would like to know more about this subject. Briefly: "<u>Serotonin</u> is a brain chemical that is particularly important for sugar-sensitive people. It creates a sense of relaxation, 'mellows you out' and gives you a sense of being at peace with the world. Serotonin also influences your self-control, impulse control, and ability to plan ahead. When your serotonin level is low, you may feel depressed, act impulsively, and have intense cravings for alcohol, sweets, or carbohydrates." Dr. DesMaisons says that sugar-sensitive people naturally have low levels of serotonin. *Prozac* is frequently prescribed for people with the above symptoms because it raises serotonin levels. However, <u>you can raise serotonin levels through nutritional modifications.</u>

"<u>Beta-endorphin</u> is the brain chemical that's gotten the least attention in the diet, depression and addiction books. That's very strange because it is immensely powerful and can drive you inexorably toward deeper addiction—or raise your spirits to a level of health that you may never have known before. When your beta-endorphin is low, you feel depressed, impulsive and victimized. You may be touchy and tearful. Your self-esteem is low. <u>And you have a desperate craving for sugar.</u>"

Beta-endorphin is an "endogenous opioid," meaning that it is naturally occurring in the body, and has an "opium-like" effect like morphine and heroin (we've all heard of the "runner's high"—that feeling of euphoria and pain reduction that comes from a beta-endorphin release in response to a particular level of exertion). Dr. DesMaisons says that sugar-sensitive people naturally have low levels of beta-endorphin. (*Beta-endorphin levels are at their lowest in women just before menstruation.*)

Dr. DesMaisons recommends eating protein at every meal. Protein helps to slow down digestion (besides the other important reasons to consume adequate amounts of this nutrient—see, *Evaluating The "Big Three" Macronutrients—Protein*). Protein also affects your brain chemistry. <u>Tryptophan</u> is an amino acid found in protein, and it is used to make the brain chemical, serotonin. You want to eat foods higher in tryptophan (such as turkey, chicken, tuna, beef, and soy products). Eating <u>slow-absorbing</u> carbohydrates at certain times helps to get tryptophan to the brain. Dr. DesMaisons recommends a baked potato (with skin) as a snack before bed to raise the insulin level in your blood just enough to move the tryptophan to your brain. (Serotonin levels rise in the middle of the night.) You can accomplish the same effect with any <u>complex</u> carbohydrate, but she recommends a potato because of the research done measuring the "satiety index" of certain foods (putting potatoes at the top of the list).

Remember when we used to be able to buy L-tryptophan at the store? Well, that has changed, but there is something new out there that you can buy (until they change that too, of course). A natural compound called 5-HTP is available at most health food stores (isolated from an African plant called Griffonia simplicifolia and usually found in formulations including St. John's Wort). 5-HTP (5-Hydroxytryptophan) is made by the body from tryptophan. *It is used to synthesize serotonin.*

In his book, *5-HTP Boosts Serotonin Levels The Natural Way To Overcome Depression, Obesity, and Insomnia,* Michael T. Murray, N.D. says that there is "a massive amount of evidence to suggest that low serotonin levels are a common consequence of modern living," and he cites numerous clinical studies showing that 5-HTP is equal to (or better than) standard drug approaches to conditions linked to low serotonin levels. Dr. Murray recommends starting with 50 mg three times per day, and increasing to 100 mg in two weeks, if necessary. He says: "Because 5-HTP does not rely on the same transport vehicle as L-tryptophan, it can be taken with food. But, if you are taking 5-HTP for weight-loss, I recommend taking it 20 minutes before meals."

I loved the book *Potatoes Not Prozac.* So much made sense to me! The section on losing weight states: "A key element in weight loss is the separation of the physical and emotional components of compulsive eating. Compulsive eating, like nicotine use, is a multidimensional process, which demands real skill in knowing which factors are motivating you to 'use.'" Dr. DesMaisons tells us to keep a journal and record what we eat, and what we were feeling when we ate it. Then pay attention to how the food further manipulated your physical and emotional state. <u>Absolutely right on</u>!

As far as some of the popular diets out there—they will not help us (of course, we already know that, don't we?) Dr. DesMaisons emphatically describes how losing weight is not a matter of eliminating a nutrient (like carbohydrate), but "eating from what she calls the right side of the carbohydrate continuum—where the 'Brown' and 'Green Things' are." She tells us not to go on a high-protein diet (like the Atkins Diet). She says you do well on such a diet for a while because it eliminates most sugars, but it also inhibits the amount of tryptophan getting into the brain to make serotonin. *Less serotonin also means less impulse control.* Also, when we were field testing the *Live It Or Diet Lifestyle System,* we interviewed many people. Those who did well for a time on a high-protein diet were typically <u>Blood Type O</u>. According to the research, Type O's genetically fare better on higher protein than the other blood types. (This is an example of why we have put together many components to help you design a individualized game plan.) Dr. DesMaisons maintains that, contrary to what you may think you should do now, "it is essential that you maintain high levels of carbohydrates—but <u>very, very slow carbohydrates</u>. This means eating lots and lots of vegetables. Counting calories will not work for you. Eating more will. Eating more vegetables and protein will create an even balance in your brain, reduce the amount of insulin your body releases, and facilitate your losing weight."

What those of us who are sugar-sensitive must aim to do is *eliminate refined and processed sugars*. They are poison anyway, but especially to us. Dr. DesMaisons includes a questionnaire in her book (additional information on her program, *Radiant Recovery*, can be found in *Appendix H*). My friend, when I answered this questionnaire, it became a portrait of me. (Your *Live It Or Diet Lifestyle System* will include a questionnaire to determine your sugar regulation.) Many of the puzzle pieces that have been incorporated in this book (and thus *Live It Or Diet lifestyle Systems*) have been personal issues that have either developed with age, or have been lurking about forever—such as this one. From now on, when you reach for certain foods (such as candy, cookies, bread—any "white thing") think **crash**! That's what awaits you at the end of your roller-coaster ride.

Bet on it.

CANDIDA ALBICANS

Candida is not a disease. It is a strain of yeast commonly found in the gastrointestinal and genito-urinary areas of the body, which can cause a state of "inner imbalance." It is usually harmless until the immune system is compromised. Then it is unrestrained and able to multiply quickly, feeding on sugars in these tracts. As it does this, it releases numerous and damaging toxins into the blood. Candida is referred to as a "stress related condition." It occurs when the body is severely out of balance from antibiotics, birth control pills, a "junk food" diet high in refined and processed carbohydrates, alcohol, and too little rest.

There are numerous books on this condition. Among them are: *The Missing Diagnosis*, written by C. Orian Truss, M.D., in which he writes "...Candida albicans is in everyone..." and *The Yeast Connection: A Medical Breakthrough*, written by William G. Crook, M.D. The distinguished doctors who have pioneered this information and made it available to us have done so with much drama. The symptoms can be severe and all too recognizable to many of us. If you crave: Sugars, breads, alcoholic beverages—if you are fatigued, "drained," forgetful, "spaced-out," irritable—if you have chronic indigestion and bloating, upper respiratory issues, infections, etc...etc...you probably have a "yeast connected illness." According to most sources—you must not eat: Sugar (or sweeteners of any sort), breads and other baked goods containing gluten and yeast (or anything containing yeast such as vinegar and wine), dairy products (except certain yogurts), most fruits and juices, most nuts and nut butters, mushrooms and other "fungi," caffeinated

drinks, and carbonated drinks. Dr. Gary cautions that once again, "We must look at the big picture. Candida is a secondary condition (complication) to something else that has thrown off the immune system—challenging it so it can no longer focus on and control internal organisms (i.e., intestinal flora). As a secondary complicating factor, however, it could be major—increasing the overall immune toxic load. It is important to recognize that although some books may tell you that Candida is it (the cause of your woes), it is not just it. After treating people successfully with Candida for years, I realized that it was secondary to an overall condition that increases toxicity when the immune system is not in control. Everything starts stirring in the body, and that is when the body is more vulnerable to anything. The only way to truly get well is to look at the totality of that—toxicity, alergenicity, etc."
(See, *Your Food Must Become You*).

Your system will include a questionnaire that will effectively "red-flag" certain symptoms that can be abated by the elimination of specific foods from the diet.

OXIDATIVE RATE

The important thing to keep in mind with all the controversy in the nutrition arena is that your needs are *unique to you*. A critical factor in determining what your diet's ratio of carbohydrates, protein, and fat should be is what your oxidative rate is. According to the innovative work of George Watson, Ph.D. In the 60's, and published in his book *Nutrition And Your Mind* in 1972, there are "fast oxidizers," "slow oxidizers," and "normal oxidizers." When one extreme type followed a diet more "appropriate" to the opposite type, Dr. Watson observed a whole series of what he called "calamities."

Fast and slow oxidizers are metabolic opposites. Your oxidative rate is the speed at which your body breaks down sugar (a process called glycolysis). Fast oxidizers digest and break down food and convert it to energy too quickly. Conversely, slow oxidizers perform the same process too slowly. The objective here is to bring both extremes more into the "normal" range. There is an optimum range of oxidation where the body can function normally (all physiological functions are maintained). In this range oxidative rate is *balanced*. Above this range (fast) and below this range (slow) the body cannot function normally, and all mechanisms are thrown off, causing a domino effect in your system. Every action in the body is affected, including digestion, fat mobilization, sugar metabolism, energy production, etc. "Slow Oxidizers" need to stimulate complete oxidation of carbohydrates, while "Fast Oxidizers" burn through carbs too rapidly. In her book *Your Body Knows*

Best, Ann Louise Gittleman tells us that both "fast" and "slow" burners can have trouble with their weight. She writes: "The slow burner burns food too slowly, and therefore can feel lethargic and sluggish and gain weight easily. The fast burner burns food too quickly, especially carbohydrates, and so can feel hyped up, nervous, and easily stressed. Fast burners also burn out quickly, stripping them of the energy needed for exercising, the lack of which contributes to weight gain. The common denominator for both types of fuel burners is that they need protein to stabilize their blood sugar levels. The fast burner needs heavier <u>proteins</u> such as meat daily, and the slow burner (who does not handle fat well because it slows down the metabolism) needs to eat lean protein, such as chicken or turkey breast and fish."

Oz Garcia, a nutritionist whose book *The Balance* discusses oxidative and metabolic types, tells us the following: "Energy is produced by the neural (or nerve) and endocrine (or hormonal) systems of the body, specifically the sympathetic and parasympathetic nervous systems, the adrenal and thyroid glands, and the parathyroid glands and pancreas. Whether you are a fast or slow burner depends on which of these systems and hormone producers dominates your metabolism. Fast burners are dominated by the adrenal system and the thyroid gland (thus the sympathetic nervous system, which is associated with stimulatory hormones such as adrenaline and cortisol). Slow burners are dominated by the parathyroid gland and the pancreas (thus the parasympathetic nervous system which is associated with sedating hormones such as calcitonin)."

Live It Or Diet Lifestyle Systems addresses the needs of fast, slow, and balanced oxidizers. For example, slow oxidizers are dragged down by eating more food than they can metabolize. They do best by starting their day with a light meal (like fruit or a high-fiber cereal) than with a big breakfast. Fast oxidizers do best when they eat foods that take longer to digest. They feel great when they start their day with a hearty breakfast (like eggs, turkey or soy sausage, and whole grain toast with a little rice butter). Our system also incorporates methods to balance oxidative rate. We do this by adjusting the ratios of macronutrients, by emphasizing a particular type of exercise, and providing specific, natural metabolic formulas for each group.

The exercise component in the oxidative rate issue has not been thoroughly examined—until now. Recently Dr. Gary and I completed a research project studying the effects of exercise on oxidative rate. We put fast oxidizers on one exercise protocol, and slow oxidizers on another. We clinically tested oxidative rate at three intervals: Before they began their program, after one month of strict adherence to the prescribed protocol, and a month later after continuing on the same protocol—changing nothing. The results surprised and fascinated us!

The foundation of *Live It Or Diet Lifestyle Systems* is dietary and exercise individuality. In his book, *Nutrition And Your Mind*, Dr. Watson wrote the following:

"When planning either a reducing or a weight-controlling diet, perhaps the single most important thing to consider is that it is a serious mistake to think that all calories are alike and may be freely substituted for one another without taking into account the different rolls they play in the energy metabolism of the tissues.

It is generally agreed that it is impossible to specify an ideal diet, which applies to everyone, although the manner in which the body transforms food into energy does apply to everyone. But levels of energy expenditure differ, and hence what caloric reduction will be adequate for one will not be for another. In addition, individuals who are either slow of fast oxidizers will have to modify the types of foods allowed according to their own particular metabolic needs."

Live It Or Diet Lifestyle Systems incorporates a state of the art questionnaire that will tell you which oxidative type you are. Along with your blood type and metabolic type, this information is used to determine your dietary and exercise needs (as well as appropriate supplemental support). However, since questionnaires tend to be subjective, we prefer using a definitive method to discern oxidative rate—a test called *Biological Terrain Assessment*, or BTA (see, *Appendix E*), whenever possible. (Dr. Gary developed our questionnaire through research, working with his patients, and the study that we conducted in Fort Lauderdale using the BTA.)

THYROID HORMONE

Do you have low energy and are easily fatigued? Are you frequently cold when nearly everyone around you is hot? Are you forgetful, confused, depressed? Is it difficult for you to lose body fat, but you <u>are</u> losing your *hair*? You might be suffering from a sluggish thyroid, or *hypothyroidism*. Now, when a very young person complains of these symptoms, he or she is tested for a variety of things, among them low thyroid function. But, in an older person these symptoms are often dismissed as a sign of normal aging (again, my friends, what is *normal*—and what is *natural*?). Unfortunately, the belief that with aging comes an "inevitable downward spiral" still exists in some parts of the medical community. I hope that you are catching on that this does not have to be.

The thyroid is a butterfly shaped gland located in front of the throat below the Adam's apple. Thyroid hormones regulate basal metabolic rate (the rate of oxygen consumption while at rest). They stimulate cellular oxygen use (which makes the body's temperature rise), thus enabling it to deal with a cold environment. Thyroid hormones also regulate metabolism. Like our other hormones, thyroid hormone production declines as we age. In *The Superhormone Promise*, Dr. Regelson writes: "The usual age-related decline in the production of thyroid hormone is not considered to be true hypothyroidism. In order to be diagnosed as suffering from hypothyroidism, your thyroid hormone levels have to drop below what is regarded as normal <u>for your age</u>. The prevailing philosophy in the medical community is that the drop in thyroid hormone production is a normal part of aging and that restoring thyroid hormone to a youthful level is unnecessary for most people. I agree in part. If you do not have any of the symptoms of thyroid hormone deficiency and are perfectly strong and healthy, then despite your declined production of this superhormone, you are probably making enough thyroid hormone to satisfy your body's needs and you don't need more. On the other hand, many people have thyroid levels that are 'normal for their age' but are clearly suffering obvious symptoms of a thyroid hormone deficiency."

That would be me. Let me again relate to you my personal experience. It had become increasingly difficult for me to keep body fat off. I began needing a nap (a *nap* of all things!) in the afternoon. I was always cold. My memory was failing me. So, in the series of blood tests that I had taken I was tested for thyroid function. Now, blood tests can be very subjective. For example, in the case of thyroid function, three things are usually looked at; T3 (triiodothyrine), T4 (thyroxine) and TSH (a hormone produced in the pituitary gland that stimulates the thyroid gland to make thyroid hormone). If T3 and T4 are *below normal* and TSH levels are elevated (indicating that the pituitary gland has to work harder to stimulate the thyroid gland) this red-flags a thyroid problem. The difficulty in evaluating this issue with blood tests exists in the *range of normal* on the tests. T3 uptake is considered normal between 25-35%, T4 levels are considered normal between 4.5-13.0 ug/Gl, and TSH levels are considered normal between 0.4-6.0 u IU/mL. Those are pretty wide ranges, and if you fall anywhere in there, even if it is the <u>low</u> end (as I did), you fall between the cracks in this system. There is another method of testing for low thyroid function, however, and that is <u>taking your temperature</u>. In his book, *Hypothyroidism: The Unsuspected Illness*, Broda O. Barnes, M.D. says that *basal temperature testing*—taking your temperature under your armpit—is one of the most accurate methods of testing thyroid function. My temperature consistently read below normal. Add this result to my borderline blood test results and my symptoms, and you have a clear sign of an under-active thyroid gland. Normally so? I don't know. I (like most of us) do not have base-line levels taken at a young age to compare current levels to. So, what are the options?

Well, the first one would be to deal with it, because it is not extreme (or even *abnormal*). Obviously, not an option for me. The second option is, depending on the severity of the individual condition—hormone replacement therapy—and take a drug called Synthroid which contains synthetic T4, or a drug called Cytomel, which contains synthetic T3 (both will override and eventually shut down the thyroid). More doctors are now considering *desiccated thyroid*, an animal-based product that is more in keeping with the way the thyroid gland produces thyroid hormone. Dr. Regelson says, "I personally feel that a patient should use desiccated thyroid. I am convinced that it will not only be more effective, but will restore thyroid hormone in a more natural way."

 I opted once again to take completely natural homeopathic and supplemental products from Dr. Gary, which will support glandular function, not replace it. (Because my condition is not severe, this is an option for me. For some people, it may not be enough.) I routinely take my basal temperature to make sure my body continues to respond to the regime I am on. If basal temperature is not affected by supplemental and nutrient support to the thyroid, you may be a candidate for Armour Thyroid, a natural prescription (which is made from ground up or desiccated cow or pig thyroid—also called USP Thyroid) that Dr. Gary brings in when supplementation is not effective. Armour supplies both T3 and T4 in about the same ratio made by your human thyroid, and it does not have the side effects of synthetic drugs (after all, there are no synthetic receptor sites in the human body). Ask your doctor about this alternative to Synthroid.

There are many "thyroid support" formulas out there. *Live It Or Diet Lifestyle Systems* employs formulations containing the nutrients that are essential for proper thyroid function. Among these nutrients is the mineral iodine. Iodine deficiency was frequently observed in this country, and that is the reason that it was added to most table salts. But, if you have cut down or cut out your consumption of salt (as I and many others have) you might be deficient in iodine. (Some other sources of iodine are ocean fish, shellfish, spinach, and sea vegetables.)

It is important to be aware of "thyroid blockers;" the drugs and foods that block or decrease levels of one or both thyroid hormones. Dr. John Lee writes in his March 1999 medical newsletter: "The most common prescriptions (that block thyroid) include prednisone, barbiturates, oral contraceptives, cholesterol-lowering drugs, heparin, phenytoin (Dilantin), propranolol, and aspirin. Also, **soy** can block thyroid (it also interferes with Synthroid). Some women are eating soy products every day. This is overdoing it and leads not only to blocked thyroid function, but also blocked uptake of glucose in the brain, blocked absorption of minerals, and blocked absorption of protein. Like everything else, soy should be eaten in moderation. In addition, **cruciferous vegetables** such as broccoli, cauliflower, cabbage and Brussels sprouts can block thyroid function (if greatly over-consumed)."

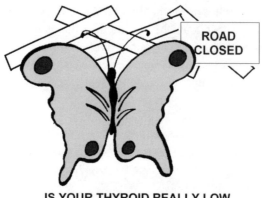

**IS YOUR THYROID REALLY LOW,
OR IS IT JUST BLOCKED?**

Thyroid is a key player in "The Hormonal Orchestra." Dr. Barnes writes in his book: "There is an old medical saying that just a few grams of thyroid hormone can make the difference between an idiot and an Einstein. It aptly characterizes the thyroid's role as a quickener of the tempo of life. When the thyroid gland is removed from an otherwise normal animal, all metabolic activity is reduced. Because commonly used tests for thyroid function are not accurate, particularly when it comes to mild and even some moderate forms of hypothyroidism, many, if not most of those with low thyroid function, remain undiscovered. I am convinced that as many as 40 percent of Americans are affected by some degree of hypothyroidism."

The following statement is from *The Superhormone Promise*: "It is heartening to note that as this book goes to press, an article appearing in "The Journal of the American Medical Association" (July 24, 1996) by researchers at Johns Hopkins University who urge physicians to include testing for an underactive thyroid gland as part of routine physicals for patients after age thirty-five. The article notes that low levels of thyroid hormone, which can lead to high cholesterol levels, as well as weight and depression problems, often go undiagnosed."

Dr. Gary agrees, but advises further: "More sensitive testing is needed (such as the basal temperature test). You want to establish the difference between a clinical problem and a functional problem. Several organs may be crying out for help functionally—but clinically not detected. For example, you may lose up to 60% kidney function before standard testing detects a problem. The biggest drawback with conventional testing is its lack of sensitivity. By the time a problem reaches a level where it is clinically detectable, it could have been functionally a problem for years. In the case of the thyroid, someone could manifest all the symptoms of hypothyroidism, but tests could indicate they are 'normal.' Our hormonal system is an amazingly intricate and complex messenger system. It is extremely sensitive and (in the female body especially) very easily thrown off. Women are more vulnerable hormonally."

•Note: Fatty acids are the transporters of our hormones. Vitamin E is a precursor to the female hormones. (A precursor "precedes" and is necessary to the formation of the next link in a "chain." The presence of Vitamin E is required in order for the manufacturing process of certain female hormones to be completed. Not enough vitamin E, we're in trouble.) And, chances are that if you are eating a diet high in refined and processed foods, *you are not getting adequate amounts of essential fatty acids.* Vitamin E is stomped out in the refinement process of grains. Women on their "fat free" diets are compromising their hormonal systems. It is imperative that we understand the interactive nature of all of this. But, again—just do not go out and buy a bunch of pills. Even though supplementation can be an effective tool in regulating your body's systems, let me remind you that nutrients function synergistically, and proper levels and ratios must be considered. An appropriate dose can be immuno-supportive, or too much can be immuno-suppressive (for example, Vitamin E and the mineral Zinc). More is not better. It is just more, and in some cases, dangerous. The big thing that people do not realize about supplements is that several grades of raw materials are available to make these products from. You want the highest grade possible, and this information is not listed on the label. Balance, quality of raw materials, processing—these are all keys to the bioavailablity (how well the nutrient is absorbed on a cell level) of a supplement. If it doesn't go to the cell, it doesn't do any good (and can even do harm, as in the case of calcium floating around—i.e., calcium deposits like bone spurs, kidney stones, etc.) That is why we have a series of nutritional products to offer with your system. We want to be assured that you were getting the best possible support.

Dr. Barnes' protocol for testing thyroid function is in *Putting It All Together.*

ALKALINE-ACID BALANCE...AND TOXIC WASTES IN YOUR BODY

An exciting series of tests that I underwent at The Clinical Nutrition Center was called *Biological Terrain Assessment* (a system developed by Dr. Rob Greenberg, M.S. D.C.). The following is how Dr. Gary clarified this procedure: "For the past one hundred years or so a battle has raged in medicine regarding the 'cause' of disease. While there are many complexities involved, simply put the debate centers around whether organisms or 'germs' (bacterial, viral, fungal) that invade the body's internal biological terrain 'cause' disease, or if it is the weakness and imbalance of the internal terrain, allowing the organisms to flourish, that is the 'cause.' Clearly the latter makes more sense and research has increasingly supported terrain not germs as the cause. In fact, Louis Pasteur, who discovered penicillin and was one of the most vocal advocates of the 'germ theory' finally admitted before his death 'it is the terrain.'"

Samples of my saliva, blood, and urine were analyzed to evaluate conditions not only on a serum level, but on a cellular level as well. Dr. Gary discovered that my body was dangerously out of pH balance, demineralized, and extremely toxic. What? When the body is in an extremely acid state (as mine tested to be), it can lead to acidosis which, when unchecked, can be lethal. I was handed a book called *Alkalize Or Die* (a rather dramatic title) by Theodore A. Baroody, N.D.,D.C.,Ph.D., and told to stay away from certain "acid producing" substances such as coffee and carbonated beverages. I needed to learn which foods were more "alkaline producing," and concentrate on adding more of them into my diet. It seems that, even though I eat extremely healthy, the foods I gravitate towards contain minerals that are acid binding (see, *Osteoporosis*). These are most proteins (including red meat, poultry, and some beans) and most grains. Most fresh vegetables and fruits contain minerals that are alkaline-binding. When you do not eat the appropriate balance of these foods, you tip the delicate pH balance in your body. This produces a "toxic" condition in the tissues, organs, and systems of your body that affect the way you look and feel.

In the book, *Reverse Aging*, by Sang Whang, we read further support of alkaline therapies. Mr. Whang is an engineer, a scientist, and an inventor. In his book he discusses the aging process, and the advantages alkalizing— specifically with "alkaline water." When toxic substances are introduced into the body, the body produces waste products. Mr. Whang writes: "Even if there were no toxic substances, the process of metabolism (the oxidation or burning of nutrients to get energy to function) creates residue waste products (acid) that the body has to get rid of. The waste products that we do not discard completely must be stored within the body somewhere. The process of aging, which starts from the very beginning of our life, is the accumulation of these non-disposed waste products. Cells deteriorate because waste products are being accumulated."

I would like to discuss this a little further, since pH balance is an important issue, which is often over-looked in health-fitness "programs." In order to sustain *homeostasis* (the balance and harmony of the body), the body must maintain a constant body temperature, and constant body fluid pH values. Optimum blood pH values fall within a narrow range, and there is a delicate balance because of all we are constantly dumping into our system. The body has to maintain this pH range in the blood to survive, so it deposits "acid wastes" from the blood to the body. The accumulation and storage of these wastes makes us feel (and look) awful. It is helpful to understand that what you habitually ingest might be extremely acid forming, and thereby harmful to you. For example: According to Mr. Whang, a glass of diet soda (or regular) is so acidic that it can change the pH of 10 gallons of alkaline water to acidic! Also, how do you handle stress? Whether it be mental or physical, *stress creates acid.* This is why stress speeds up aging.

In his book, Mr. Whang cites the work of several doctors and scientists. We do not want to get too technical here, but we want to share the following conclusions that these brilliant (and Nobel Prize winning) individuals agree upon: If the condition of the body, the extracellular fluids, *the environment for the cells* becomes too acidic, there is not enough oxygen for the cells to survive. This causes damage and disease.

Mr. Whang says we should drink *alkaline* water. Dr. Baroody says that we should combine starches, like rice and potatoes (which are acid-forming) with vegetables, like broccoli and carrots (which are alkaline-forming), and avoid eating two starchy foods in one meal. Dr. Baroody also says that it is not good to combine starches with heavy protein (like meat and potatoes). He says it is because "starch neutralizes hydrochloric acid, so protein digestion slows way down. The result is a process called 'putrefaction' (extremely acid-forming). This produces a climate for toxins and illness because starches and proteins are sitting in the stomach and intestines and not being properly digested." (Gas and bloating is the immediate obvious result.) He further recommends eating fruit 20 minutes before any other food—(other sources say at least 20 minutes before).

Is this beginning to sound like *Fit For Life*, a popular diet book from some years back that advocated a principle called "food combining?" This book told us not to mix carbs and proteins, and have fruit all by itself. Remember that one? Dr. Sears, in *The Zone*, of course, says that to actually be in "The Zone" you must eat carbohydrates with proteins. Listen, I am not advocating the *Fit For Life* diet, or Dr. Baroody's diet, or any other "diet" for that matter. The entire nutrition arena is filled with conflicting views, as we already have discussed. Just to get my feet back on "ground zero," I went to *Understanding Nutrition* (Whitney & Hamilton), which was the textbook given to students when I studied nutrition. The following is an excerpt from that book that addresses the "food combining" issue:

"Another common misconception about digestion is that people shouldn't eat certain food combinations (for example, fruit and meat) at the same meal, because the digestive system can't handle more than one task at a time. The art of 'food combining' is based on this idea, and it represents a gross underestimation of the body's capabilities. There is seldom interference between the absorption and utilization of one kind of nutrient and that of another. In fact, they often seem to enhance each other. For example, sugars taken at the same time as protein (within four hours) seem to promote better utilization of the protein. The sugars may slow down the digestive process so that it is more complete, or they may provide precursors for some nonessential amino acids so that whole proteins can be produced more readily and retained in the body. The interaction between the carbohydrate in one food and the protein in another is not unique; there are other interactions that have to do with the vitamins and minerals. For example, the vitamin C in one food enhances the absorption of iron from another."

Ground zero is right. What's up, Doc?

Once again, I asked Dr. Bach McComb to comment:

"If you eat a starch or fruit during or immediately after a high protein meal, you will interfere with the digestion of the protein. Protein needs to sit in the stomach for about two hours with a fair amount of hydrochloric acid for the large peptide bonds to break down. If it doesn't happen in the stomach as result of hydrochloric acid, it doesn't happen later on. If you have a big protein meal, and a lot of complex carbohydrates at the same time, it becomes a quantity dependent thing. They are going to conflict with each other, because complex carbohydrates do not really need to do much in the stomach. So, your stomach has this dilemma; is it going to be efficient enough to deal with this complex carbohydrate and let it go through a little early, and hold the protein back? Not likely. It's either going to dump it all a little early, which means you now have undigested protein, or hold the carbohydrate back in the acid media long enough to cause fermentation. Fermentation throws off the pH, and the signal for the food to leave the stomach to go into the small intestine is pH dependent. So, when the pH gets to a certain point (about 4.0, 4.5), the stomach says, 'Okay, the acid has done its job, protein is broken down, time to dump it.' But, it's the carbohydrates, as a result of fermenting in the acid media that brought the pH up. Now, in the small intestine, the protein has not been broken down small enough to be absorbed."

Elizabeth Dancey, M.D., author of *The Cellulite Solution*, writes the following about food combining: "Although medical research has yet to prove or disprove the facts, there is no doubt that many people have found a food-combining diet to be of enormous benefit in the treatment of a number of complaints ranging from digestive problems to chronic fatigue and cellulite (see, *Cellulite...Can You Really Knead, Rub...Punch It Out?*). In fact, the term 'food separation' is perhaps more accurate as the principle of this type of diet is that you separate proteins and starches so that they are never eaten together in the same meal. This enables the body's digestive system to function more efficiently. The reason for this is that proteins and starches require different sets of enzymes in order to be properly digested. Protein-digesting enzymes prefer to work in an acid environment, while starch-digesting enzymes prefer an alkaline environment. If the two are forced to work together, neither is working in its preferred environment and, consequently, neither is functioning at optimum efficiency.

The bulk of the diet should be made up of protein, carbohydrate (starches and sugars), and fruit and vegetables. Fruit should always be eaten separately from meals, with a gap of two hours in between. Protein may be eaten with vegetables (and beans,) but not with carbohydrates (starches or sugars). Carbohydrates may be eaten with vegetables and beans, but not with protein."

Dr. William Kelley, noted researcher and developer of a pivotal model of evaluating metabolic types (see, *Metabolic Type*), has an opinion on food combining. In the book, *Medicine's Missing Link*, the authors, Tom and Carole Valentine, write: "Kelley crossed the food-combining notions off his list of reliable sources of health information, for it is apparent from man's diverse nutritional history, around the world, that the digestive system is designed to cope with a wide spectrum of foods. Proper digestion handles all the combinations and variables."

I have a point to make about all of this. Can you guess what it is by now? That's right—*balance*. It all comes back to balancing the various aspects of life: Emotional, spiritual, physical, and <u>nutritional</u>. Remember the "puzzle" analogy? You may not be dealing with an acute acid condition in your body as I was, but I wanted you to know that such things do exist. The following is a list of symptoms associated with this condition: Acne, muscular pain, dizziness, low energy, joint pain, food allergies, agitation, PMS, bloating, heartburn, diarrhea, constipation, headaches, depression, swelling, insomnia, loss of memory, and many others that Dr. Baroody associates with beginning and advancing stages of acidosis. If you are suffering from some of the items on this list, you might consider having yourself tested. A urine pH of 6.4 is optimum for body function. An acid state exists between a pH of 0.5 (extremely acid) and 3.5 (mildly acid). An alkaline state exists between a pH of 7.5 (extremely alkaline) and 4.5 (mildly alkaline). 4.0 is a neutral state. Based on your results, you will probably need to adjust the ratios of foods that you eat. If you are like most Americans, there are not enough fresh, raw fruits and vegetables in your diet. Also, Dr. Baroody maintains that "refined, white sugar is one of the most damaging substances for consumption." (Sound like anything you've read recently?)

Another book that addresses this subject is *Your Health—Your Choice*, by M. Ted Morter, Jr., D.C., M.A. Throughout his book, Dr. Morter offers "Wellness Principles" and "Health Hints" such as: "pH indicates acidity or alkalinity <u>and</u> how healthy you are—the pH of the fluids in your body doesn't stay constant; it fluctuates according to what's going on. If it fluctuates too wildly or for too long, you encounter physical problems. Your body is an alkaline entity by design—it is important to understand that all of the body fluids, except those in the stomach, are alkaline. Your body is alkaline by design and acid producing by function—cells operate in an alkaline environment, yet acid is produced as they function. The second source of acid is from acid ash food. You need adequate amounts of vegetables and fruits to take care of the acid that is produced by meats, fish, poultry, dairy products, seeds, nuts, and grains." But what about all of the acids in fruits? "Fruits are acid entities that serve an alkalizing function. And—Negative Thoughts=Acid Thoughts=Disease."

Dr. Carolyn Mein discusses pH balance in her book, *Different Bodies— Different Diets*. She writes: "An easy way to determine your acid/alkaline balance is by using pH paper to check your saliva. You can get this paper at most drug stores. The best one to get registers a range of 6.0 to 8.0 in increments of .2 to .4. To use, tear off a strip, put one end of the paper in your mouth, and get it thoroughly wet with saliva. Then check the resulting color against the graph on the dispenser. The ideal result is a pH between 6.8 and 7.0. If you find that your level is less than 6.8, your system is too acidic. Eating more vegetables and acid fruits like lemon, limes, and oranges will usually increase your alkalinity. (This is a typical example of two acids producing alkalinity.) If your reading is greater than 7.0, your system is too alkaline, and you'll need more acid-forming foods. These would include high protein foods like meats and grains.

The most common imbalance is acidity. If you're getting enough fruits and vegetables and you're still too acidic, it could be caused by one of several factors. Generally it means your immune system is stressed, like when you're fighting a cold, chronic illness, or toxic condition."

Get Rid Of the Stuff!

Toxins. Toxic. Detoxification. Huge issue? Apparently so, since it has been brought up in most of the works I have recently read, not to mention my own radical encounter with it (see, *15 Rounds—My Championship Bout*). And so, my friend, I cannot *not* address it.

I will begin by giving you the definition of "detoxification" as presented in the book *Detoxification & Healing* by Sidney MacDonald Baker, M.D.: "Detoxification is what your body's chemistry does to rid itself of unwanted chemicals, whether the chemicals are left over from your own metabolism or enter your system from the air you breathe, the food and water you consume, substances you rub onto your skin or use to treat your hair, or the toxins and allergens produced by the germs that inhabit your intestine. The word 'detoxification' is also used to describe a treatment intended to improve or assist this process."

Okay, that's how most of us understand this word. We associate it with alcohol and drug programs, and certain "cleansing" products and treatments. Some of us (at one time or another)—misguided and desperate—might have even abused the process. This is not really what is being referred to here, although an appropriate regimen might be prescribed if indicated. I am talking about the *biological process of detoxification*—the body's own natural mechanism that, for some of us, may be seriously impaired. When this vital function and its team of organs is "down," imbalance is the result. Dr. Baker writes; "Imbalance is the precursor of disease."

Therefore, another determination you must make (puzzle piece you must fit) is whether or not your body's detoxification system is working. If it is not, it must be addressed. I will give you an example. One of the places the body stores toxins is in its fat (see, *Cellulite...*). When fat in the fat cell is liberated, it goes into your body's system, <u>along with all the toxins that might be stored in it.</u> This could make you feel quite awful, and it certainly is not healthy for your body. That is why, along with a fat-loss program, you might need to consider some sort of detox. Doctor Gary cautions that this is a sensitive procedure: "It is not a good idea to just run out and buy detoxificants and colon cleansers and such. Your body has to be ready for such an event, and it should be supervised. I strongly recommend that you speak to your health-care practitioner about the appropriate way for you to proceed."

Remember, I thought I was healthy. I certainly appeared to be. Oh, but my friend, it is not how you *look*—it is how you *feel*, and you know how *I* felt. Why was my system so *distressed*? Looking in the mirror gave me positively no satisfaction (even on a low water-retention, good-hair day). I had to get to the bottom of this!

A popular notion trotting around this time was (and in some circles still is); "You cannot have too much protein." Several "credible" and powerful sources espoused this concept. I, figuring that I needed more protein because of all of the stress I was placing my body under (never realizing that I was not digesting the protein I was eating), significantly increased my protein intake. Earlier in this book you read how overdosing on protein could lead to calcium-leaching in the body, and I would like to expound a bit on this here because it is so important for us to know it. In the book, *Healing With Whole Foods* by Paul Pitchford, it says; "An excess of any kind of high-protein food causes the body to become saturated with uric acid, which significantly weakens all of its functions, especially that of the kidneys." Remember—I have already mentioned that most protein sources are "acidic." Mr. Pitchford also writes; "Cravings (for sweets) can be caused by hyper-acidity, which often results from lack of exercise, eating too quickly, and too much, or an excess of meats and refined foods."

However, an indomitable sweet tooth was not my only issue, as you know. What was the big picture—my complete jigsaw puzzle?

In reading Dr. Jeffrey Bland's book, *The 20-Day Rejuvination Diet Program*, the following anecdote jumped out at me, so I want to share it with you:

"Some time ago I woke early on a rare Saturday morning when the weather was fine and I had no commitments. I was full of energy and health, and I decided to go for a long bike ride. When I got back, I ate breakfast and proceeded to take care of some fairly heavy yard chores. Just as I was completing those jobs, my 21-year-old son appeared and suggested we go water-skiing. We spent the next couple of hours out in the boat, taking turns skiing and running the boat. The activity didn't stop there. In the afternoon we decided to work out with weights and do some strength and flexibility conditioning. At the end of an hour of this activity, I suddenly felt overwhelmingly fatigued. I realized I had, in the course of a single day, gone from being an unusually healthy and vital individual in the morning to feeling very ill. By evening I had sore muscles, a headache, low energy, and a set of symptoms which felt very much like a low-grade flu. I knew this was a classic example of becoming 'toxic' by having exceeded my metabolic threshold, or the reserves of function in my vital organs.

I chastised myself for pushing my healthy body so hard. I had made myself temporarily sick, but at the same time I realized that many people have this feeling of unwellness, not just once in a while, but every day. They wake up each morning not having metabolized the toxins their bodies built up the previous day. Each day they add more toxins, until eventually they develop significant symptoms."

Do you think this is all some sort of mumbo-jumbo? Well, I can tell you that I felt terrible before I adopted these principles, and then felt much better after I began to pay attention to the macronutrient and pH ratios (along with the variety) of my meals. In fact, I began to wonder if the incredible, overpowering cravings for something sweet that always followed one of my high-protein meals wasn't simply a case of my body crying out to be in pH balance. After every meal, I <u>had</u> to have something sweet. (Does this happen to you?) Now, this made no sense to me. No one ate healthier than I, was my belief. Could it be that it was asking for something alkaline to neutralize the acid that I had just consumed? Think about *when* you experience your cravings. Write down whenever they happen, and see if there is not some correlation to either consumption of refined carbohydrates (see, *Sugar-Sensitivity*) or imbalanced meals. (A Home Tesing Kit will be available with your *Live It Or Diet Lifestyle System*. See, *Appendix E*.)

YOUR FOOD MUST BECOME YOU!

In order to effectively build an individual's weight-management system on a foundation of health, we must first look at the functioning of the digestive system. Who do you know that hasn't had a digestive complaint (including yourself)? There is always some irritant: Gas, bloating, constipation, fatigue, etc., that accompanies us on our daily tasks. We overlook these hitch-hikers, or attempt to rid ourselves of them through anti-acids, caffeine, and other junk that seems to make them go away, but in reality only suppresses the problem (thus complicating it).

Finally, there is a growing awareness that the digestive system plays an important role in total body health. It greatly affects our immune system, acting as a barrier that provides our first line of defense against invaders. However, when the health of the digestive system becomes compromised, all manner of dis-ease and dis-comfort can result. *Leaky Gut Syndrome, Dysbiosis*, and other digestive disorders lead to inefficient cell nourishment, toxicity, pH imbalance, and a whole series of aggravations and conditions.

Leaky Gut Syndrome

Elizabeth Lipski, M.S., C.C.N., and author of *Leaky Gut Syndrome* (a Keats Good Health Guide), tells us: "'Leaky gut syndrome' is really a nickname for the more formal term, increased intestinal permeability, which underlies an enormous variety of illnesses and symptoms. It is not a disease or an illness itself. Rather, it manifests itself in an enormous variety of ways depending on your genes and your personal ecology.

Common clinical conditions associated with increased intestinal permeability are: Acne, aging, AIDS, alcoholism, allergies, arthritis, autism, food sensitivities, inflammatory bowel disease, intestinal infections, irritable bowel syndrome, liver dysfunction, malabsorption, malnutrition, chemical sensitivities, pancreatic insufficiency, psoriasis, schizophrenia, ulcerative colitis, among others.

Common symptoms are: Abdominal pain, aggressive behavior, anxiety, asthma, bloating, chronic joint and muscle pain, confusion, constipation, diarrhea, fatigue, fuzzy thinking, gas, indigestion, mood swings, nervousness, poor exercise tolerance, poor immunity, poor memory, recurrent bladder and vaginal infections, shortness of breath, skin rashes, toxic feelings.

Our digestive system provides us with our most intimate contact with our environment. It is a 25 to 35 foot hose that runs from mouth to anus, and provides a barrier between the outside world and what actually gets absorbed into us, becoming our bodies. Seventy percent of our immune system is located in or around the digestive system. Specialized cells called Peyer's patches in the intestinal lining sample foreign substances and send them to the intestinal mucosa to be gobbled up." Leaky gut syndrome develops when the mucus layer is weakened. Bacteria and fungi can then pass through into the bloodstream, and throughout the body. Some of the most common causes of leaky gut syndrome are: Prolonged use of anti-inflammatory drugs, stress, food sensitivities, immune overload, alcohol abuse, chronic infections, and Dysbiosis.

Dysbiosis

Dysbiosis is the imbalance between "friendly" gut flora, and harmful gut flora (*Candida* is a type of dysbiosis). Antibiotics, birth control pills, and other prescription and over-the-counter drugs instigate dysbiosis. These medications kill not only bad guys, but good guys—changing the delicate balance of the flora, and allowing opportunistic conditions to thrive in the mouth, digestive system, vagina, and on the skin (see the section on *Candida Albicans*).

The Liver

Leaky gut syndrome also taxes the liver because it allows toxins and particles from incomplete digestion to circulate and cause irritations. The liver is responsible for filtering and converting toxins into byproducts that can be safely excreted. When the liver is overwhelmed, it cannot do its job efficiently, so it begins storing fat-soluble toxins in fat cells (see section on *Cellulite*) hoping to deal with them later, but in reality never catching up. Today (more than ever) our livers are so besieged by enemies like: Alcohol, environmental pollutants, pesticides, food additives, along with the byproducts of our own metabolism, that they cannot function efficiently. When the liver is overloaded there is an increased risk of free-radical damage in every cell of our bodies. Mood fluctuations, depression, and irritability are indicative of liver problems (in eastern philosophies the liver is considered not only the center of health, but also *the seat of emotion*). Remember that the objective is to create homeostasis (harmony and balance in the body) and to do that we must also address the toxicity and functional capacity of the liver. *Live It Or Diet Lifestyle Systems* takes the holistic approach and considers the interactions of all the organs (see the section on *Acid-Alkaline Balance and Toxic Wastes*).

Parasites

Research shows that between 85 to 95% of Americans are unknowingly harboring one or more parasites (there are over one thousand species). Larry Clapp, Ph.D., J.D., author of *Prostate Health In 90 Days*, writes: "Parasites that can live in the human body range from 30-foot-long tapeworms down to microscopic organisms that burrow into body tissue or attach themselves to individual cells. Some parasites literally eat us, sucking their nutrition out of our cells or cutting into the body tissue in search of food. Others satisfy themselves by snatching nutrients away from the food we've eaten before we've had a chance to use the nutrients ourselves. For example, some people who crave sugar do so because parasites are robbing them of it." (•Note: Because of the proximity of the prostate (and other considerations), prostate problems can be exacerbated by leaky gut syndrome, dysbiosis, and other digestive disorders. I strongly recommend that you guys read Dr. Clapp's book, *Prostrate Health In 90 Days*.)

The way parasites rob us can be very harmful. For example, calcium-leaching parasites burrow into our joints and can cause arthritis. Other parasites eat the proteins that protect our nerves, causing nervous system disorders.

Worms eat away at intestinal walls, and "liquefy" colon tissue. They all drain our energy, compromise our immune systems, and cause a myriad of diseases. And, they are easy to get! They enter our bodies through food, handshakes, bare feet, utensils, polluted water, when pets lick us, and even through inhaling air that contains them (how's your air-conditioning system?).

Elizabeth Lipski lists common symptoms of parasites as: "Abdominal pain, allergies, anemia, bloating, bloody stools, chronic fatigue, constipation, coughing, diarrhea, gas, irritable bowel syndrome, itching, joint and muscle aches, nervousness, pain, poor immune response, rashes, sleep disturbances, teeth grinding, unexplained fever, and unexplained weight loss."

You can have trouble losing weight and have parasites as well. Actually, anyone can have parasites. One of my *Live It Or Diet Lifestyle System* clients eliminated a foot and a half long worm after one month on her system! This parasite had been starved to death by forced abstinence from offending foods—along with the client's detoxification, hydration, and an entire reconstruction of eating patterns that are symbiotic to the individual (not the parasite). Parasite screening is incorporated in *Live It Or Diet Lifestyle Systems'* clinical programs.

A Systematic Approach

Once we begin to restore homeostasis, fat can be liberated, bloating subsides, energy is increased, etc. The process starts with healing the gut. We must deal with food sensitivities, treat dysbiosis, replenish gut flora, reduce oxidative damage with antioxidants, and so on. Then we can begin a detoxification program that will remove toxins and eliminate parasites. There are many homeopathic remedies that we employ in *Live It Or Diet Lifestyle Systems* to assist our efforts. There are also various cleanses and fasts that can be used (careful, though—remember that after 24 hours of fasting, muscle wasting begins).

THE ENDOCRINE SYSTEM

The glands of the endocrine system perform a complex and interactive series of actions and reactions that control many of the major functions in the body. Picture this system as a huge telephone network where each gland is a generator, and they are all connected by wires (your blood stream). When one generator (gland) outputs too much or too little juice (hormone), there is a breakdown in communication throughout the network. Messages are not being delivered effectively through the blood stream, and hormone balance is disturbed. This has a cascading, domino effect, and in order to stop it, the malfunctioning generator (gland) must be pinpointed. For example, a hypothyroid condition must be evaluated by also looking at the generator (pituitary gland) that sends messages to the thyroid (TSH-thyroid stimulating hormone) to make thyroid hormone, as well as looking at the thyroid itself.

Now, the hypothalamus gland communicates with the pituitary gland, which is also responsible for the release of growth hormone (as well as other hormones that communicate with the reproductive system). If there is a short-circuit in the communication between the hypothalamus and pituitary glands, this will affect the release of growth hormone. (The hypothalamus secretes GRH-growth releasing hormone, which is a message to the pituitary to release growth hormone.)

The adrenal glands respond to messages via the sympathetic nervous system, and will initiate the "fight or flight" response as a reaction to: Fear, anxiety, pain, trauma, hemorrhage, exercise, extreme cold or heat, hypoglycemia, and hypertension. The adrenals also produce vital precursors to our endogenous sex hormones—beginning with cholesterol, which is converted to pregnenolone. The adrenals then make DHEA, which is a hormone that travels through the bloodstream into our cells, where it is converted to male hormones (androgens) or female hormones (estrogen). So, when there is a sex hormone imbalance in an individual, the function of the adrenals must also be examined. Constant stress (and other factors) fatigues the adrenals, causing them to work inefficiently.

And on and on it goes.

Whether the endocrine system relays messages efficiently or inefficiently will greatly influence the metabolism of carbohydrates, proteins, fat, minerals, and water. The messages (secretions) of the glands of this system also significantly influence what passes through a cell, and oxidative, as well as other phases of cell activity. Therefore, when evaluating many of the issues that accompany weight management, the endocrine system cannot be overlooked. In *Live It Or Diet Lifestyle Systems*, we troubleshoot a breakdown in the endocrine network through questionnaires and clinical testing.

WHAT ABOUT STRESS???

How often do you declare that you are *stressed-out!!!*? Do you know what that *stress!!!* is doing to you? Not many of us do. It's not just a matter of blowing your cork and not being able to cope. There are extreme physical consequences to the pressure cooker that your life has become.

Stress depletes our bodies and compromises them in countless ways. It exac-

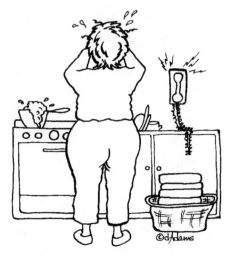

erbates (intensifies) already existing conditions, and creates new health problems that seem to come from "nowhere" (our inner intelligence shutting us
down to rest, regroup, and chill out, perhaps?). In her book, *Your Body Knows
Best*, Ann Louise Gittlemen, M.S., tells us: "In addition to burdening the heart,
blood vessels, and immune system, stress also adversely affects our adrenal
glands (which regulate the body's minerals, as well as work with the thyroid
gland to produce and maintain the body's energy levels)." When a "stress alarm"
sounds, the adrenals respond by revving up and producing extra hormones. If
this stress continues, the adrenals "adapt by increasing in size and function—
drawing nutrients from the body's reserves until the body weakens due to lack
of nutrients and energy. Adrenal insufficiency happens when the body's reserves
of both energy and nutrients are exhausted. The body can take only so much
abuse."

Ms. Gittleman continues by saying: "If you think emotional stress is the
only form of stress we subject our adrenal glands to, think again. Physical
stress, including physical injury, overwork, and lack of sleep (see, *Sleeping
Beauty—Don't Wake Me Up Before 8*) affects the adrenals as well. Any chemical
substance (whether from environmental pollutants or diets high in refined and
over-processed foods) must be detoxified by our bodies (see, *Get Rid Of The
Stuff!*) and this, too, puts stress on the adrenal glands. In addition, job stress,
lack of or excessive exercise, and the use of stimulants such as coffee, sugar,
and 'recreational' drugs, all contribute to adrenal burnout. Early warning signs
of adrenal insufficiency include: Chronic low blood pressure, fatigue, low sta-
mina, sensitivity to cold, and addictions to either sweet or salty foods."

Dr. John Lee, in his new book, *What Your Doctor May Not Tell You About
<u>Pre</u>menopause* (co-authored by Dr. Jesse Hanley and Virginia Hopkins),

explains how stress can contribute to osteoporosis (see, *Osteoporosis*). He writes that: "If you are experiencing chronic stress, your adrenal glands are pumping out cortisol. Chronic stress creates a chronic demand for cortisol, which competes with progesterone in the bone. Cortisol and progesterone give opposing messages: Progesterone tells bone cells to build, while cortisol tells bone cells to stop building." **Did you read that?** If you spaced-out for a second—go back and read it again! We are at an age when we need to pay closer attention to this stuff, my friend.

Also, Dr. Lee warns us about the unfortunate combination of estrogen dominance (see, *Hormone Replacement Therapy And The Great Dilemma*) and stress. He says: "This creates a self-perpetuating cycle where stress causes estrogen dominance, which then causes insomnia and anxiety, which pulls on the adrenal glands, which then creates more estrogen dominance. A woman who has been caught in this type of cycle for a few years will find herself in a constant state of 'wired but tired,' which will eventually result in dysfunctional adrenal glands, blood sugar imbalances, and debilitating fatigue that may be diagnosed as chronic fatigue syndrome."

Are you tired when you wake up, and spend the rest of your day trying to compensate with shots of caffeine (in one form or another), along with sugar, and nicotine? Well, as a result of this behavior, your artificially over-stimulated adrenals will keep you up at night. And so the cycle continues—until you are felled. Adrenal exhaustion is not a joke. It's yet another case of us charging through life, not paying attention to the signals from this precious vehicle we are charging <u>in</u>.

What Can We Do About It?

Stress management.

Don't you hate that term? "I DON'T HAVE TIME FOR STRESS MANAGE-MENT!!!! Trying to manage my stress is stressing me out even more! Can I make the time to read that book on 'stress management,' or escape to that yoga class, or meditate, or pray? NO! I CAN'T! There's always <u>something</u> being demanded of me from <u>someone</u>!" Believe me, my friend, I understand (see, *The Crash Of '92*). But, we just cannot ignore the red flags our bodies are putting up all over the place. My advice is just to start by turning your life-volume down to a low roar. I did it by taking little bits of time here and there—not big chunks of time requiring scheduling in my stupid appointment book. The following is how I succeed at becoming less of a "Tasmanian Devil:" First thing in the morning I spend time with God. I pray, read a few passages from the Bible, and try to become more centered and focused. (I truly did not believe I had the time for this until I tried it!) Throughout the day, I take moments here and there to speak to Him (He is very good at calming me down). I say a short prayer before I eat instead of just shoving food down my throat like I used to (see, *Upon This Rock I Build My Church*). At night I spend a little more time with my Bible, and I pray. I no longer exercise like a obsessed maniac, I take deep breaths and think before I respond like a possessed lunatic, and in general I try to have more balance in my life.

There are measures that we can take nutritionally to combat stress (your *Live It Or Diet Lifestyle System* will plug this component in). In fact, nutrition is one of our more powerful weapons against the ravages of stress. Our nutritional needs dramatically increase when we are under any kind of stress. Ms. Gittleman states: "We need to fortify our bodies with the extra reinforcement they need so that our reserves are not depleted during stressful periods. Adequate protein is one of the key remedies of a stressed-out body, (see, *Protein—The Under-Rated Nutrient*) as are a number of vitamins and minerals that can support and enhance adrenal function during this time. Magnesium, calcium, zinc, potassium, sodium, and copper are all depleted from the body tissues as a direct result of stress. Surprisingly, the very best food sources of naturally balanced minerals come from the sea (see, *Acid-Alkaline Balance*). Sea vegetables, sold in capsules or in dried form in the health-food stores (see, *Get In Touch With The World And Your Food*), provide high amounts of magnesium, potassium, phosphorus, iodine, and other key trace minerals like manganese, chromium, selenium, and zinc. B-complex vitamins, known as anti-stress vitamins, are crucial to take during stressful times." Eat plenty of fresh fruits and vegetables, legumes, and eggs and lean meats to stockpile depleted nutrients. Listen to beautiful music, like Vivaldi's "Four Seasons" (that's what I am listening to as I am writing this. Positively glorious!)

And pay attention to your body when it tries to speak to you.

EAT TO *LIVE*

This section nearly didn't make it into this book. I hadn't considered heart disease a major issue in the over-all theme of a book that targets baby-boomer health and fitness. After all, if you follow the eating guidelines within these pages, you would automatically have a "heart healthy" diet. However, a recent event in my life compelled me to call Evan Reynolds, our publisher, and ask him if I could insert this chapter. I am so grateful to him for "stopping the presses." I need for you to read this story. It could save your life.

We generally judge a book by its cover. We design a cover to entice you to explore the book's contents—where the real value is. Sometimes you do, sometimes you don't—that is the way of it. In our society, appearances are everything. Beneath the Surface (nearly the name of this book) is what counts. I could talk on and on about "weight management," but what if heart disease is quietly killing you?

I was in the Midwest a few weeks ago doing just that—lecturing on "weight management," when I received the news. I had made my routine daily phone call to my parents, and got my weeping father on the other end. "Mom's had a heart attack," he was barely able to say. I cut my trip short and flew to West Palm to be with my family. My sisters, brother and I all converged on the hospital where my mom was in intensive care. She survived the heart attack, but had to undergo bypass surgery.

Cardiovascular Disease

The staggering, debilitating fear that descends upon you when you are faced with the possibility of losing a loved one is something I cannot describe. We went through it with my dad, first with prostate cancer, and then with bypass surgery. We couldn't believe that Daddy had heart disease. He was so healthy and fit. At nearly eighty years old he was full of energy and vitality. Meanwhile, heart disease was slowly claiming his cardiovascular system. Thankfully, he flunked his stress test. The cover of his book was completely misleading!

When Daddy had his bypass surgery his surgeon, Dr. Downing, was upbeat and optimistic. (Dr. T. Peter Downing is one of the best cardiovascular surgeons in the country. He was also my mom's surgeon.) My dad pulled through like a champ. In just a few days he was up joking and laughing and flirting with the nurses. He can still jitterbug anyone of any age under the table (of course, while wearing his heart-rate monitor—Daddy's learned to listen to his body's signals).

It was not the case with my mother.

My mom has always been the rock, the strength, and glue that holds the family together—fiercely protecting, quietly nurturing, strong-willed—and hard-headed. No one ever believed she could be so vulnerable—except me. I've learned too much. She was over-weight. She had high blood pressure. She was a smoker for years. She had shortness of breath. She was easily stressed. And, she lived to prepare the sumptuous Italian meals that were the foundation of all family gatherings.

Mom had to undergo bypass surgery on her carotid artery about two years ago, but she didn't make any changes. I warned her. I begged her. I remember I was on my knees in a parking lot one afternoon, crying and pleading with her to listen to me. Dr. Gary had made it very clear to me that if she had a blockage in her neck it was not an isolated event—they would be elsewhere—around her heart. She had to allow us to design a program for her. This is what we do!

Well, she had the heart attack we predicted. Hadn't her doctors warned her? Didn't they tell her she would have a stroke or a heart attack if she didn't make lifestyle changes??? What's wrong with them? Do they think their job is just to ride up on their white chargers and save a life in the nick of time—all drama and glory? What about <u>prevention</u>!?

We almost lost her. During the surgery they encountered more damage and blockages and calcification than they had anticipated. After the surgery she went into cardiac arrest. They had to shock her. She developed a potentially fatal arrhythmia. They had to take her back into surgery. Dr. Downing came out and told us it wasn't good. He was going to stay close. If he blinked his eyes, she could die, he said. He wasn't upbeat and optimistic like he had been with my dad. Eyes like saucers, white-knuckled and crying, we all surrounded him, near hysteria...what does this mean??? She could die??? My father announced, "If she dies, I die. I cannot live without your mother." We would lose them both.

No one took a breath that day. We were paralyzed with fear, praying and begging and bargaining with The Lord...please, just a bit more time...please. We paced the hospital corridors—unable to comprehend life without Mom—for what seemed like an eternity.

It was touch and go for nearly a week. There was one crisis after another, all handled by The Lord. I am so grateful to Him. I am not ready to face the passing of my parents.

Dr. Downing told us that he could not "fix" all of Mom's damage. She needs to take great care. I did the intervention I should have done years ago. I cleaned out her house, her refrigerator, her cabinets. I got rid of the food that almost killed her, the high fat stuff, the high sugar stuff, the refined and processed garbage that filled her shelves. Done. History.

There are no options for my mom. She must learn to "eat to live," not live to eat. I filled mom's house with healthy, high fiber, saturated fat-free, cholesterol-free, low-fat, whole, natural foods. I consulted with Dr. Gary and designed a Live It Or Diet Heart Healthy system for her. I am determined to show her that eating healthy is the opposite of deprivation!

Yes, food can make you fat. Food can make you miserable. Food can rob your energy and affect your moods. Food can also kill you.

Why did I want to paint this vivid and depressing picture for you, my friend? Because I want to save you from a disaster like the one invited in by my mother. Heart disease doesn't just "happen." It is a condition that develops slowly over decades. It is not just a disease for "old people." It could be building in you right now. Baby-boomers are not exempt. We are not just a bunch of granola-eating health nuts. We are also incredibly self-indulgent experts on denial. And, by the way, bypass surgery, despite what they will have you think, is anything but "routine." It is an extremely dangerous operation that takes a tremendous toll on the body. Julian Whitaker, M.D., in his book, *Is Heart Disease Necessary?*, writes: "Bypass surgery must be done rapidly. For the duration of the operation, a patient is on a heart-lung machine, which takes over the function of oxygenating and pumping the blood. Once on this machine, the patient literally begins to die. The machine starts inflicting damage to the brain and to all other organs the minute it is turned on. Even a short stay on the machine under the most skillful hands will cause some brain damage." And, even when bypass surgery "works," it is only a stopgap measure. It doesn't correct anything, and should never be considered as the remedy for eating badly.

In *Prescription For Nutritional Healing*, Dr. James Balch writes: "Unfortunately, despite remarkable new technology for both diagnosis and treatment of heart conditions, the first sign of cardiovascular disease may be a life-threatening calamity. Disorders of the cardiovascular system are often far advanced before they become symptomatic. Every minute—someone in the United States dies of a heart attack." Dr. Gary says: "And about half of those people did not even know they had it! Their first symptom was death."

The Good News

In his book, *Is Heart Surgery Necessary?*, Dr. Whitaker explains why he "gave up being a surgeon to become a healer:" "Heart disease is the number one killer in this country. Half of all Americans who die this year will die from heart disease and related cardiovascular illnesses. The causes of these ailments are known, and there are proven treatments that can prevent or reverse the condition. These treatments are painless and noninvasive. But the disease continues to kill more than a million people every year. When someone dies of heart disease, it is listed as a 'natural cause.' Yet dying of clogged arteries is no more natural than being run over by a truck."

So, cardiovascular disease is not an inevitable by-product of the aging process. There are many things you can do to prevent heart disease. And, according to Dr. Dean Ornish in his book, *Dr. Dean Ornish's Program For Reversing Heart Disease*, (as well as Dr. Whitaker in his book) if you do have it, it can be stopped, or even reversed. (Dr. Gary has witnessed the same results clinically.) The research on these heart-disease reversal protocols have been extensive and dramatic. It is reported that patients began feeling better—and blood flow to the heart was found to improve—within weeks. Within one year, severely blocked arteries began to clear. On the average, the progression of heart disease stopped or began to reverse after four to five years. Arteries became less blocked, and quality of life improved.

Also, Dr. Gary recalls that diet and exercise had been documented back in the 70's by Nathan Pritikin to reverse up to 80% occlusion of coronary artery disease.

The Bad News
We must take responsibility for embracing a lifestyle that will keep us healthy and alive. Why is this the bad news? The most difficult thing that I've had to do in the 20 years that I have been in this field is to get people to make lifestyle changes—even if it meant that they could die if they didn't! Dr. Ornish warns: "Even a single meal that is high in fat and cholesterol may cause your arteries to constrict and your blood to clot more quickly." That's not good. Why would someone who is already at high risk for a heart attack opt to have that potentially dangerous meal? But they do. You do! Dr. Whitaker writes: "I have found that even patients aware of alternatives to invasive cardiac procedures often don't have enough strength or support to seek them out. Changing one's lifestyle is not easy. Taking responsibility for your own health can be a lot harder than just giving in to the man with the knife who promises to solve all your problems while you are asleep on the table."

Coronary Artery Disease

The blockages in coronary arteries and reduced blood flow to the heart is the end product of a chain of events that occurred over a lifetime. High fat, saturated fat, cholesterol, refined and processed baked goods, weight-gain, smoking, inactivity, and emotional stress all contribute to this condition. Everything boils down to choice, and it is the choices that we make on a daily basis regarding what we eat and drink, how much we exercise, and how we react to stressful situations, that can lead to heart disease.

How Are Blockages Formed?

Blockages aren't formed over-night. They develop slowly and chronically over decades. I used to think that coronary blockages were cases of our arteries just being plugged up by the sludge that we eat. But, the sludge that we eat accumulates in the area of the artery where the lining has been damaged. This damage to the arterial wall can be caused by: Excessive amounts of cholesterol and saturated fat in the diet, high blood cholesterol, high blood pressure, and smoking. Once an artery has sustained an injury, our bodies try to fix it by applying a "Band-Aid" over it. This Band-Aid is comprised of cholesterol and other stuff. Year after year these Band-Aids become thicker and thicker if the damage is chronic. After a while, you have a blocked artery.

Isn't It Just In My Genes?

We love to write things off to genetics, but the truth is the extent of this disease is life-style related. Dr. Ornish writes: "There is a genetic variability in how efficiently (or inefficiently) a person metabolizes dietary saturated fat and cholesterol. Drs. Michael Brown and Joseph Goldstein won the Nobel Prize in Medicine in 1985 for their discovery of LDL-cholesterol receptors. These receptors are located primarily in liver cells, and they bind and remove cholesterol from the bloodstream. The more cholesterol receptors you have, the more efficiently you can metabolize and remove cholesterol from your blood. The fewer cholesterol receptors you have, the more your blood cholesterol level will increase when you eat saturated fat and cholesterol." Your lifestyle influences the number of cholesterol receptor sites as well. A diet high in saturated fat and cholesterol produces "double trouble." The dietary fat and cholesterol not only saturate the receptors, they also decrease the number of receptors—a bad combination. Your body makes all the cholesterol it needs. It is the excessive amount of cholesterol and saturated fat in our diet that leads to coronary heart disease.

This is where genetics comes in. The number of these cholesterol receptors is (in part) genetically determined. This will give you a pre-disposition for heart disease. But it doesn't mean you have to get it! Dr. Gary tells us that if in fact you do have a familial tendency to high cholesterol, you need to take a more aggressively preventive stance to neutralize that. He says: "The body manufactures approximately 80% of blood cholesterol (whether you consume it or not), primarily in the liver, and cholesterol is essential to many bodily functions. Dietary saturated fat and sugar are the primary culprits here, not dietary cholesterol. Unfortunately, both cholesterol and saturated fat are usually contained in the same foods."

So, dietary cholesterol is not necessarily a bad guy, unless the liver is not converting excess cholesterol into bile and releasing it through the gallbladder. This process is obstructed by excessive saturated fat in the diet (which congests the liver) by liver toxicity, by lack of exercise, and lack of vitamin C (which helps transport excessive cholesterol back to the liver). Other antioxidants, like selenium, Beta-carotene, vitamin E, and Co-Q10 help to block the free radical damage contributing to the elevation of LDL ("bad" cholesterol).

· Regarding the importance of specific supplementation in the fight against heart disease, Dr. Whitaker writes the following: "Another aspect of cholesterol research that has not received the attention it deserves concerns the relationship between cholesterol and vitamin C. Low-density lipoprotein(a) is an offshoot of the LDL ('bad') cholesterol particle, with a small strand of protein. This protein makes the lipoprotein(a) sticky, which allows it to adhere to and protect damaged or cut arterial walls. Without vitamin C, which enables tissue to heal properly, lipoprotein(a) steps in and acts as a bandage. The problem, however, is that when vitamin C levels are low, lipoprotein(a) begins to build up on artery walls and thickens into plaque. Obviously, vitamin C levels should be kept reasonably high." Dr. Whitaker is an advocate of supplementation, and recommends specific vitamins, minerals, and amino acids (that he calls heart helpers to lower your blood pressure, clear out cholesterol, prevent heart attacks, reverse disease, and give your heart rhythm) when treating heart disease. Dr. Gary recommended mineral support (especially magnesium, which helps to regulate calcium balance, corrects heart irregularities, controls blood pressure, and can even prevent heart attacks) for my mom, among other supplements.

High Blood Pressure

Hypertension, or high blood pressure, also damages the lining of arteries because the blood hits the lining harder. Dr. Whitaker writes: "The increased pressure on the inner walls of the arteries makes them much more vulnerable to the buildup of fatty deposits. High blood pressure also causes the heart to work harder, which means it needs more oxygen." Dr. Whitaker tells us that most of the factors that contribute to high blood pressure are controllable. These factors are: High salt intake, high sugar intake, fat imbalance, lack of nutrients, and lifestyle conditions such as stress, excessive caffeine and alcohol, lack of exercise, and smoking.

Smoking

By now we all know that cigarette smoking is not benign. All of the poisons and toxins in tobacco are absorbed into your blood. This damages the linings of arteries as it circulates. When you smoke, it also causes your arteries to constrict, and exacerbates the risk of blood clot formation.

Heart Attack

"Heart attacks usually happen when a small blood clot lodges in an artery that is already significantly blocked with cholesterol and other deposits—so the blood clot is the final blow in a person who already has significant coronary atherosclerosis," writes Dr. Ornish. "Aspirin interferes with blood clot formation, so the risk of heart attack decreases when you take it. For the same reasons, though, the risk of bleeding in your stomach or brain or heart increases." Dr. Gary notes that cold water fish oils (EPA/DHA in supplement form) similarly reduce platelet aggregation, without the bleeding side effect.

Irregular Heart Beat

I mentioned that my mom had what was described as a "potentially fatal arrhythmia." The same lifestyle conditions that can lead to heart attacks can also cause irregular heartbeats, or arrhythmia. Dr. Gary has found that there are usually mineral deficiencies present when there is an irregular heart beat. There are irregular heartbeats that are not life threatening, and there are those (called ventricular fibrillation) that are. Ventricular fibrillation is caused by reduced blood flow to the heart. Using caffeine or other stimulants can put you at higher risk for both types of irregular heartbeats.

How To Reverse Cardiovascular Disease

Exercise
A sedentary lifestyle will contribute to the development of heart disease. Although it is necessary to move, if you already have heart disease, an exercise program must be introduced that does not increase your risk of heart attack. Moderate exercise such as walking or biking will be beneficial when combined with your other lifestyle changes. Consult your physician. Do not add exercise as another stressor if you continue to eat poorly, and if you do not learn how to manage your stress. Remember, being sedentary contributes to obesity, and this will put a strain on your heart that it might not be able to handle. So, not doing some form of exercise is really not an option. Your *Live It Or Diet Lifestyle System* will include exercises that are best suited for you. You must learn how to move, how to eat, and how to stay calm.

Manage Emotional Stress
How does emotional stress lead to coronary heart disease? I mention elsewhere in this book that there is a direct connection between your heart and

your mind. I was not just speaking philosophically. Nerves (called the sympathetic nervous system) responding to an order from the brain, stimulate receptors in the heart that make it beat faster and harder and can cause the coronary arteries to constrict (the fight or flight response). As a response to stress, the brain causes other organs, such as the adrenal glands, to release hormones that cause a series of physiological reactions such as constriction of arteries and quicker blood clotting. This mechanism is there to protect us in times of crisis. Unfortunately, we chronically activate it in our stressful lives, and what was put there to save us, can also kill us. It can cause a heart attack in a person with advanced heart disease.

Also, according to research, when a diet is higher in fat and cholesterol, the chance of stress contributing to blocked arteries is magnified 30 times! Caffeine and other stimulants exacerbate the stress response. They make your fuse shorter. If anything, we all need much longer fuses. *We must learn how to manage stress.*

Limit Fats

Your body stores fat in the form of a substance called triglycerides, described by Dr. Ornish as: "Ugly yellow fat globules that appear in your bloodstream about an hour after you eat a high-fat meal. High triglycerides increase the risk of coronary heart disease." Partially hydrogenated fats should be avoided. They are higher in saturated fat—on purpose! Hydrogenation extends the shelf life of the products containing it. That's why this process is employed. There is, however, absolutely no regard for the length of your life in this scenario.

Also, be careful of products advertising "cholesterol free." They often have saturated fat and (as Dr. Gary has already told us) eating saturated fat will raise your blood cholesterol level even more than eating cholesterol!

All oils are 100 percent fat! One gram of fat supplies 9 calories, while protein and carbohydrates supply 4. So, fat is more than twice as calorically expensive as the other macronutrients. If you reduce the oil in your food and cut down on fat, even the "good" fat, you can eat more food and not get fat. Also, all oils contain <u>some</u> saturated fat.

Eliminate Sugar And Other Refined And Processed Foods

These can be poison to you for several reasons—but primarily if you already have impaired sugar regulation. If you have hypoglycemia, insulin resistance, or adult-onset diabetes (which are usually lifestyle induced), they can be lifestyle reversed. Diabetes increases the risk of heart disease (see, *Can I Give Myself Diabetes?*).

Eating refined products causes your blood sugar level to rise rapidly. In response, your pancreas releases insulin, causing your blood sugar to drop. This mechanism has been compromised in you if you have blood-sugar issues. Also, this roller-coaster effect causes mood-swings, fatigue, cravings, and can lead to obesity. Remember that insulin is a storage hormone (see, *Insulin And Glucagon*). Along with allowing sugar to enter your cells, it stores food as fat. Your prime directive here needs to be mobilizing fat from your fat stores, not increasing the size of those stores. Therefore, you must reduce these dramatic insulin episodes—not only to lose weight, but to reverse diabetes and other blood sugar disorders. All refined and processed carbohydrates can contribute to weight gain.

According to Robert Pritikin in his book, *The Pritikin Weight Loss Breakthrough*: "If you discipline yourself to eat a high-carbohydrate diet, but do not exercise enough, the excess carbohydrates you eat can be converted to triglycerides, or fats, in your liver, and then flood your bloodstream with tiny globules of fat. Elevated triglycerides can lower high-density lipoproteins or HDL's, the 'good' cholesterol that reduces your risk of heart disease."

Consume Enough Fiber

The importance of fiber cannot be overstated. Research shows that we need between 20 and 50 grams of fiber daily for disease protection. As I discussed earlier in this book, the typical American diet supplies 0 fiber on an average day! Refined and processed foods such as most conventional muffins, bagels, breads, cookies, crackers, pastas and white rice contain 0 fiber! Start thinking of these products as poison. Among other benefits, fiber slows down the absorption rate of carbohydrates and cholesterol into the blood stream.

Fiber is the nondigestible part of plants, comprised mostly of complex carbohydrates. Fiber is found in all whole grains, legumes, fruits, and vegetables. Refining foods removes fiber (along with other important nutrients). Dietary fiber consists of soluble and insoluble forms. *Your Live It Or Diet Lifestyle System* will be high in both.

How The Typical Cardiovascular Drugs Can Deplete Your Body

Chances are, if you have been diagnosed with some form of heart disease, you are taking several medications. They all deplete certain vital nutrients from your body. These nutrients must be replaced to insure optimal health and functioning of your body. The following are some of the most-often-prescribed drugs and their negative effects on your body:

Ferosemide (a diuretic) depletes: *B-12*, which can lead to anemia, improper digestion and metabolism of starches and fats, nerve damage, fatigue, digestive disorders, memory loss, eye problems, and an uneven walk—*Magnesium*, which can weaken muscles, nerves, and bones, and cause depression, high blood pressure, and heart disease—*B-6*, which can cause fatigue, water retention, irritability, allergies, arthritis, and a compromised immune system—*Potassium*, which can lead to irregular heart beat, elevated blood pressure, muscle twitches, and fluid alterations in the body—*Zinc*, which can slow wound healing and compromise your immune system.

Zocor (a cholesterol-lowering drug), **Lopressor** (a beta-blocker), **Glyburide** (an anti-diabetic drug), along with many other medications, all deplete *Coenzyme Q10*. This can lead to more cell damage from free radicals, compromised immune system, accelerated aging process, increased fatigue, respiratory disease, diabetes, and increased risk for heart disease.

Along with your eating modifications, you would need to take a multi-vitamin to replace lost vitamins and minerals and Co-Q10. Your Co-Q10 supplement will be one of the most important weapons in your arsenal to fight heart disease. Co-Q10 increases oxygenation of the heart and aids circulation. Research shows that it can prevent reoccurrence in individuals who have had a heart attack. Also, a 6-year study demonstrated that people being treated for congestive heart failure had a 75% chance of survival with the addition of Co-Q10, compared with a 25% chance for those who did not use Co-Q10. *In Prescription For Nutritional Healing*, Dr. Balch tells us the following about this important substance: "Coenzyme Q10's actions resemble those of vitamin E, but it may be an even more powerful antioxidant. It plays a critical role in the production of energy in every cell of the body. Deficiencies of Co-Q10 have been linked to periodontal disease, diabetes, and muscular dystrophy. Research has revealed that supplemental Co-Q10 has the ability to counter histamine, and therefore is beneficial for people with allergies, asthma, or respiratory disease. It is used by many health care professionals to treat anomalies of mental function such as those associated with schizophrenia and Alzheimer's disease. It is also beneficial in fighting obesity, candidiasis, multiple sclerosis, and diabetes. Co-Q10 also appears to be a giant step forward in the treatment and prevention of cardiovascular disease. In Japan, more than 12 million people are reportedly taking it at the direction of their physicians for the treatment of heart disease (it strengthens the heart muscle) and high blood pressure, and also to enhance the immune system."

•*The amount of Coenzyme Q10 present in the body declines with age, so it should be supplemented in the diet—especially by people who are over 50.*

Many studies have been published demonstrating the effectiveness of

Coenzyme Q10. Among them are: *A Six-Year Clinical Study of Therapy of Cardiomyopathy with Coenzyme Q10, Usefulness of Coenzyme Q10 in Clinical Cardiology: a Long Term Study, Effect of Coenzyme Q10 Therapy in Patients with Congestive Heart Failure,* and *Perspectives on Therapy of Cardiovascular Disease with Coenzyme Q10.* You can pull these and many other studies off the Web.

Another strong advocate of Co-Q10 is Stephen T. Sinatra, M.D. Dr. Sinatra is a board-certified cardiologist and a fellow of the American College of Cardiology, as well as the author of several publications on Coenzyme Q10. In a recent interview, Dr. Sinatra discussed how the conventional medical community is finally responding to the findings on Co-Q10. He said: "Being a board-certified cardiologist and a director of medical education helps me get the message across. It's ironic that a lot of doctors haven't been comfortable with nutritional supports, yet they're comfortable with potentially harmful drugs. A lot of drugs are thrown on the market with very little study. That's the conventional medical model (to ignore what a drug is going to take away in the long term in exchange for short-term results). In alternative medicine we nurture the body to heal itself to prevent future illness. That's where a paradigm shift in medicine is occurring this century. You've got 78 million aging baby-boomers, many of whom are fed up with managed care. They're reclaiming responsibility for their health, as well as their medical care. And that means taking supplements, exercising, eating healthier diets and being tended by alternative methods.

If I had a heart attack, I'd want the best conventional doctor around. Let him patrol the case; do an angioplasty if he has to. I just want to survive. Get me through the crisis. I applaud and embrace conventional medicine for its ability to handle crisis. But after they're done, get me to an N.D., a naturopathic doctor. When that paradigm shift blows through in 2000, many people are going to want to see an N.D. More than an M.D."

Dr. Whitaker, Dr. Ornish and the other distinguished individuals who have created programs for reversing heart disease have provided us with sound, well-researched guidelines on diet, exercise, and supplement recommendations. But, the problem is that it is all still one size fits all. *Your Live It Or Diet Lifestyle System* will incorporate these sound principles in an individualized format. If heart disease is one of your issues, it will be factored into your system, along with your other unique considerations.

It is important that you recognize that this chapter may have been written for you. God has a way of sending us messages. Sometimes He has to do something dramatic to get our attention (like He did with my mom). Or, sometimes, it could be just a voice in our head, a verse in the Bible...or a chapter in a book.

OVERALL GLANDULAR FUNCTION

Your glands work in concert with one another in the "interactive dance" that is the function of your body. When glandular function breaks down anywhere in your body, the harmony turns to cacophony (see, *The Endocrine System*).

Live It Or Diet Lifestyle Systems incorporates specific formulations that will support glandular function. If our questionnaire indicates that there is an issue present for you, we can plug the appropriate supplementation into your daily regimen to help bring your systems back into balance.

(It is also advisable that you consult your health-care practitioner.)

Who Ya' Gonna Call?

"The doctor of the future will give no medicine, but will interest his patients in the care of the human frame."

—Thomas Edison

Today we are becoming increasingly aware of the many options available to us for treating our ailments. Once upon a time we all ran to our family doctor for everything, and we got patched up—one way or another. But, as you may have already noticed in this book, I am not a fan of patches anymore. I want it fixed, whatever it is. The days of, "let's just silence it now, and deal with it later" are over for me. "Later" has arrived. Basically, Dr. Gary is my health-care practitioner now, but I have been consulting chiropractors for years. I learned quite a few years ago of the relationship between my musculoskeletal system and the organ and glandular functions of my body. As a competitive bodybuilder, I stressed my spine and my joints pretty good. Although I still continue to strength-train, I no longer use very heavy weights, and I have cut back from seven days of training to five. But, once upon a time, I was a maniac. And I had the back problems, the joint problems, and a long list of ailments and conditions to prove it. By addressing the condition of my structure, I also found relief from the discomfort of some of my body's imbalances.

I believe that God has put at our disposal many forms of healing arts: D.C. (doctor of chiropractic), N.D. (naturopathic doctor), O.M.D. (oriental medical doctor/acupuncturist), M.D. (medical doctor), D.O. (doctor of osteopathy). Sometimes you absolutely need an M.D. or D.O. Accidents happen, and emergency medicine in this country is second to none. Also, we let ourselves get so far gone in this society that we run out of time to help our body heal itself. But, that is what chiropractic and other natural healing arts are about.

According to the Association of Chiropractic Colleges: "Chiropractic is a health care discipline, which emphasizes the inherent recuperative power of the body to heal itself without the use of drugs or surgery. The practice of chiropractic focuses on the relationship between structure (primarily the spine) and function (as coordinated by the nervous system) and how that relationship affects the preservation and restoration of health. In addition, doctors of chiropractic recognize the value and responsibility of working in cooperation with other health-care practitioners when in the best interest of the patient."

But remember, if you have a chiropractic problem, nothing else will correct it. Also, many chiropractors have special training and certification in nutrition, homeopathy, acupuncture, and other areas of natural health. The chiropractors employing *Live It Or Diet Lifestyle Systems* fall into this category.

The best way to find any doctor is through a referral from a friend. Chester A. Wilk, D.C., in his book, *Chiropractic Speaks Out*, advises us on how not to choose a chiropractor (or any other doctor). He writes: "Doctors that rely on flamboyant advertising should be avoided since they are in violation of their professional code of ethics."

More and more people are seeking "alternative" forms of medicine. A good chiropractor can treat you for everything from strains, sprains, and other injuries to gastrointestinal disorders, headaches, and colds. Spinal adjustments (and other energy balancing techniques) relieve pressure on nerves that travel to various organs and glands in the body. When the nerve is no longer stressed, the message (or flow of energy) to the corresponding part of the body is restored. This will relieve imbalances that can cause fatigue, weakened immune function, and in general affect the homeostasis (harmony) of the body. In *Appendix H* you will find our *Information Hotline Number* for referrals.

For now, don't forget the following considerations: Are you eating meals that are balanced and nourishing for your body's organs and systems? (See, *Eating For Health, Healing, and Harmony*.) Is your liver overworked and therefore toxic? (See, *Your Food Must Become You*.) Do you have issues with your gut, such as Leaky Gut Syndrome or Dysbiosis? (See, *Your Food Must Become You*.)

And...what about your hormones???

Please...continue.

"I dont know why they call this 'alternative.' It's the 'original.'"

—Pat Surface
My Husband

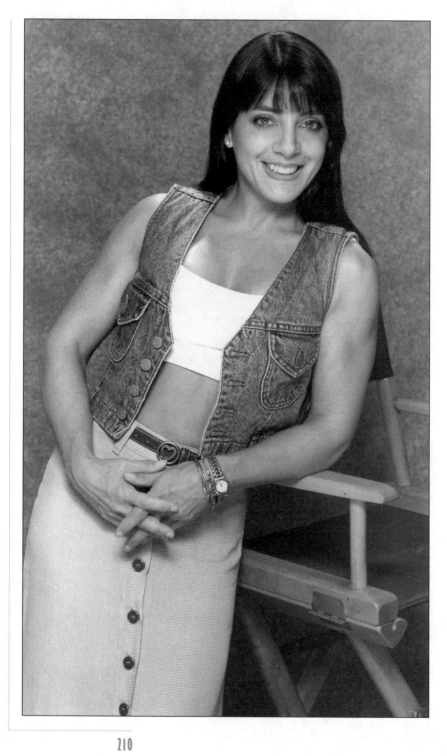

CHAPTER VI

FEMININITY

THE JOURNEY WITHIN (THE ONE THAT REALLY COUNTS)

"I am tired of all this nonsense about beauty being only skin-deep...what do you want—an adorable pancreas?"

—Jean Kerr

I remember waking up when I was fat, hoping that the condition of my body was just a bad dream. When I realized that it wasn't, I would spend the rest of my day depressed. Hating yourself from the jump really sets the tone of the day, don't you think? It's hard to expect anything good to come out of a day that you are moving through without confidence or self-love. Even at those rare times when you are somehow able to convince yourself that you are "a creature unlike any other," a brutally honest remark can cut into that fantasy like a machete.

I once had a boyfriend who confided to a friend of mine that there was one thing about me that bothered him—the cellulite on my thighs. Imagine having that graphic little image burned in your brain? Talk about having a bad day.

Or, later in life—after an extremely intimate moment—another boyfriend "shared" with me that my age "frightened" him. "Exactly what do you mean?" I asked, sorry that I posed the question the second it came out of my mouth. Well, my number—one that was so close to fifty—was a constant unpalatable reminder to him that I was "middle-aged" (and thus about to decay at any moment, I suppose).

YOU ARE MORE THAN YOUR NUMBER

"I have everything now I had 20 years ago—except now its all lower."
—Gypsy Rose Lee

It's all so remarkably tedious, isn't it? When will we finally discover that we are not a number—a dress size, or an age?

I prefer to subscribe to the baby-boomer attitude of "no more middle-age." In a recent magazine article, Lynn Snowden writes: "Now just because we are chronologically qualified (to be middle-aged) doesn't mean we have to look or act it. Middle-aged used to be the description of the point in life when, if we doubled our present age and consulted a life-expectancy chart, we could see that we were halfway to being dead. To be "middle-aged" is to have had the good, open-minded, adventurous person in you replaced by a pod person, a middle-aged pod person who takes seven minutes to put on makeup no matter what, and it shows. In other words, to be middle-aged is to be past it. Unhip. Uncool. Old."

When we baby-boomers were young, people in their 40's and 50's (like our parents) seemed old to us. Now that we have arrived at this age, we have done so without getting "old." Look at us. We are every bit as sexy and compelling as we used to be. *More.* More, I say! We have added "interesting" to the list. We have stories, history, experiences—*colorful* pasts. We banned bras, burned draft cards, marched (and sometimes "tripped") our way to adulthood. We were different then, and we are different now. Our role models are stunning, accomplished creatures (can you believe that Goldie Hawn is 53 and Lauren Hutton is 55?). They certainly make "50" a less frightening number for me.

Victor Hugo wrote: "The forties are the old age of youth, while the fifties are the youth of old age." Any way you view it, this time is another transitional period for us, just as adolescence was. Like it or not, we are going through another series of "changes."

THE PASSAGE DECADE.."THE OLD AGE OF YOUTH?"

"Nature gives you the face you have at 20; it is up to you to merit the face you have at 50."
—Coco Chanel

Recently I was having a discussion with a male friend on the obsession in this country with youth—specifically the youth of women.

Why do I do this to myself?

Anyway, this guy is forty-ish (great looking—pretty body) and his preference leans towards younger women—sometimes much younger. However, he does admit to an "appreciation" of me. How did I get so lucky?

"Well," he said, "guys like you because you have a young body."

He elaborated.

"Women's bodies begin losing firmness" (from his experience, I suppose) "in their early thirties. They just do not look and feel the same as women in their twenties. You are different, and so we like you."

Now I am nauseous.

What about my sense of humor, my wide variety of interests, my life experiences...my *mind*?

Now, as I see it, this is the problem with America. We celebrate our youth when we should be baby-sitting them—and celebrating our mature adults. European men idolize their older women, who are put on pedestals and worshipped.

I'm moving.

I have this image of American men going through life endlessly fondling the fruit in supermarket produce sections—rejecting the ones whose flesh does not spring back with the "zing" of youth. Someone ought to remind them that riper is sweeter.

Okay, so being the glutton for punishment that I am, I brought this topic to another male friend. He listened politely, and replied, "What's your point?"

Is it me?

I'm about to conduct a survey on the Internet.

Yes, I am appreciated for my body, but I work for it. Please appreciate the work. Appreciate the commitment—the dedication—the *person* behind the "behind."

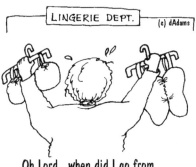

**Oh Lord...when did I go from
a 36 D to a 36 Long???**

There are countless women in this country who are making themselves sick trying to be in shape—to recapture the firmness of youth. I alternate between being thrilled when a man says, "You are the ultimate—a mature woman in a young woman's body"—and being horrified. It horrifies me because someday I will be a mature woman in a mature woman's body. In her book, *On Women Turning 50*, Cathleen Rountree profoundly writes: "As I reject the inevitable process of aging, my fundamental fear and anxiety continues to consume me."

I do not want to drown in an obsession to stay young. Instead, I want to celebrate my maturity. I advertise it. I'm proud of it. But I am also proud of the fact that women are beginning to give the "fourth decade" a new image.

AGE REVERSAL...A QUESTION OF SCIENCE OR ATTITUDE?

"Age is a very high price to pay for maturity." —Tom Stoppard

Menopause. What a horrid word. When we think of that word, images of crinkly skin, sagging breasts, fatter hips, dried up vaginas, mood swings, and night sweats flash into our minds with the fury of the hot flashes that we have no doubt begun to experience, but are totally in denial of—"Who turned up the heat?"

The Change. What does this mean? Changing from what to what? From a young woman to an old hag? No wonder we are constantly in the mirror—looking for signs of changing. "There they are! Oh no! *I'm...CHANGING!!! AHHHH...*"

Sounds like some awful science fiction movie, doesn't it? Too bad it's not. This is what society has done to women. And, 20 million of us—the unconventional, revolutionary, rebellious *baby-boomer women*—are on the brink of this change. Like it or not. Accept it, or not. Here we are.

Menopause. "Get out of Dodge—find a young one—this one's done." No wonder I hear that my age "frightens" men. It is what our culture associates with this time of a woman's life. Men do not have such a clear signal of the passage of time. Their markers are subtle, small bumps in the road (a little libido trouble, dear?)—mere annoyances. Not huge, brightly lit neon signs that are as easy to spot as the ones that announce the approach of Las Vegas. In his book, *What Your Doctor May Not Tell You About Menopause*, Dr. John Lee writes, "In native cultures menopause tends to be a cause for quiet celebration, a time when a woman has completed her childbearing years and is moving into a deeper level of self-discovery and spiritual awareness. In these cultures menopausal women are looked up to and revered. They are sought out for advice and their opinions are heavily weighed in the decision-making process of the community. How strange that sounds to us! We know menopause as a death knell, the end of a woman's sexuality, a descent into a dried-up and painful old age of arthritis and osteoporosis."

Forget Europe. I'm moving to New Guinea.

OSTEOPOROSIS

Quite frankly, I never thought much about it. Osteoporosis was for little old ladies who didn't get around much, not for a woman who pumped iron—like me! Then, I started losing teeth, and was told of the tremendous bone loss in my mouth. "Osteoporosis can start in the jaw," Dr. Gary told me. "Your body is losing calcium, and that is osteoporosis." How could I have osteoporosis? (The answers to that question, my friend, are throughout this book.)

Dr. Lee discusses osteoporosis in his book. He writes: "Osteoporosis is the disease American women are most likely to develop as they age. It is the most common metabolic bone disease in the United States. Over 45 percent of white women age 50 or more have bone mineral density over two standard deviations below the mean of normal young women. The lifetime risk of fracturing a hip, spine or forearm is 40 percent for white women in the United States (twenty percent of the women who fracture their hip die within a year)." Dr. Christiane Northrup in her book *Women's Bodies, Women's Wisdom*, tells us that as much as 50 percent of a woman's bone loss occurs before menopause! Dr. Lee tells us that osteoporosis can begin anywhere from five to 20 years prior to menopause while estrogen levels are still high (debunking the myth that it is a menopausal disease). Why is this happening?

Have you ever said to yourself, "Grandma seems to be shrinking?" Well,

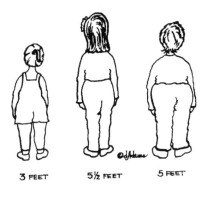

3 FEET   5½ FEET   5 FEET

you are not imagining things. She probably is. And you might be too. When bone withers, so do we.

Dr. Lee defines osteoporosis "as a progressive disease with many factors contributing to its cause. It is a disease of excessive bone loss and decreased bone density. More bone is being resorbed than is being made." Women in their early or mid-thirties have the highest bone mass, and then it starts to decline until menopause, when the bone loss accelerates. This indicates a relationship between declining sex hormones and loss of bone mass. Dr. Lee writes: "It is now generally agreed that estrogen therapy temporarily retards osteoporosis progression, but it does not truly prevent it or reverse it (and it is not without risk)." (See, *Hormone Replacement Therapy And The Great Dilemma.*)

Dr. Lee continues regarding the role <u>Progesterone</u> plays in all of this: "In preventing bone loss, we have to look as far back as a woman's early thirties. Dr. Jerilynn Prior at the University of British Columbia in Vancouver, British Columbia, Canada, measured estrogen and progesterone levels in female marathon runners who were developing osteoporosis. She found that they had stopped ovulating, a common syndrome in female athletes, and their progesterone levels had fallen. It was the lack of progesterone that brought on the osteoporosis. <u>These women were estrogen dominant and progesterone deficient!</u> Since it is clear that estrogen can retard, but not reverse, osteoporosis and estrogen cannot protect against osteoporosis when progesterone is absent, the addition of natural progesterone should be used in preventing or treating postmenopausal osteoporosis. Further, since some estrogen is produced by fat cells (see, *It's Not Fair!—Our Stubborn Baby Boomer Fat Cells*) muscle cells, and skin in postmenopausal women, it is possible that progesterone alone is sufficient to prevent and/or reverse osteoporosis."

Dr. Northrup agrees that natural progesterone (along with estrogen replacement, dietary adjustments, and exercise) can be effective in reversing bone loss. She also says: "It is clear that progressive bone loss in women is due to factors more complex than simply estrogen or calcium deficiency. Women need to realize that taking calcium is only one part of building strong bones. Magnesium, boron, vitamin D, vitamin C, and trace minerals are important. And while dairy products are pushed as a panacea to prevent osteoporosis, <u>it's entirely possible to create and maintain health bones without eating dairy.</u>" She recommends that we: Switch to a nutrient-rich <u>whole foods</u> diet, do weight-bearing exercise such as weight training and walking, cut back on alcohol and caffeine, and quit smoking. Dr. Lee explains that "the lack of exercise diminishes the stimuli that promote bone strength. (The exercise should be against resistance, such as bicycle riding, tennis, and weight lifting.) This, along with nutritional deficiencies, is probably the primary reason for the decrease in bone mineralization now evident."

Regarding the kinds of foods to eat, Dr. Lee tells us the following: "Other factors being equal, vegetarians uniformly have better mineralized bone than people who include meat in their diet. This isn't just because vegetarians are getting lots of high-quality calcium in their diet. Meat is high in protein, and too much protein in the diet creates an excess of acidity in the body (see, *Alkaline-Acid Balance*). If one eats more protein than required for nutritional purposes, it is not stored by the body (*other books say that it can be stored as fat*) but it must be excreted. The kidneys need to buffer the acidic protein waste products before they can be excreted in the urine. This buffering is accomplished with calcium, and if there's not enough in the bloodstream to buffer the acidic protein waste products, it will be pulled from the bone. This excessive loss of calcium creates a negative calcium balance."

Dr. Gary tells us that there is a urine test to measure calcium lost in the body. It is often found that a strict vegetarian on a 70 to 80 percent alkaline diet loses 200 to 300 mg of calcium daily. On a highly acidic diet (typical of today's fast food/junk food average American diet) up to 2500 mg of calcium can be lost daily. Considering you can only absorb a few hundred milligrams of calcium daily, it doesn't take long to do the math.

In the book, *Prescription For Nutritional Healing* by James Balch, M.D. and Phyllis Balch, C.N.C., the following are some recommendations for osteoporosis prevention that are listed:

"•Eat plenty of foods that are high in calcium and vitamin D such as broccoli, chestnuts, clams, dandelion greens, most dark leafy vegetables, flounder, hazelnuts, kale, kelp, molasses, oats, oysters, salmon, sardines (with the bones), sea vegetables, sesame seeds, shrimp, soybeans, tahini, tofu, turnip greens, and wheat germ.

•Consume whole grains and calcium foods at different times. Whole grains contain a substance that binds with calcium and prevents its uptake.

•Take calcium (at least 1500 mg daily) at bedtime when it is best absorbed and also aids in sleeping. (The most absorbable form is calcium citrate according to many sources. Dr. Gary likes calcium citrate in a mixture with several other forms.)

•Include onions and garlic in diet (as well as eggs if your cholesterol level is not too high) as they contain sulfur, which is needed for healthy bones.

•Limit your intake of almonds, asparagus, beet greens, cashews, chard, rhubarb, and spinach, as they are high in oxalic acid, which inhibits calcium absorption.

• Avoid phosphate-containing drinks and foods such as soft drinks, high protein animal foods, and alcohol. Avoid smoking, sugar, and salt. Limit your consumption of citrus fruits and tomatoes; these foods may inhibit calcium uptake.

• Avoid yeast products. Yeast is high in phosphorus, which competes with calcium for absorption by the body.

• If you take thyroid hormone or an anticoagulant drug, increase the amount of calcium you take by 25 to 50 percent."

Calcium needs to have other things present to be absorbed into bone, such as enzymes. These enzymes require magnesium and vitamin B6 to assist them. Other essential players are: Zinc, vitamin D, vitamin A, vitamin C, and boron.

Listen...this is important. There is something more to consider regarding calcium depletion. Drugs. The following is a list of prescription and over-the-counter drugs that deplete calcium and its coworkers (among other nutrients):

• Antacids containing aluminum such as Tums (that's right—what does that commercial say about supplying calcium???), Rolaids, Maalox, and Mylanta deplete calcium.

• Sodium Bicarbonate antacids such as Alka-Seltzer and baking soda deplete magnesium.

• Antibiotics such as Neomycin deplete calcium. Tetracyclines deplete magnesium.

• Anticonvulsants such as Phenobarbital, barbiturates, Phenytoin, and Dilantin deplete calcium.

• Anti-inflammatory agents (Corticosteroids) such as Prednisone deplete calcium and vitamin D.

• Cardiovascular medications such as Digoxin and Lanoxin deplete calcium and magnesium.

• Cholesterol-lowering drugs such as Cholestyramine, Clofibrate, Colestid, and Questran deplete vitamins A, D and K.

• Diuretics (blood pressure regulators) deplete calcium, vitamin B6 and magnesium.

• HRT drugs such as Estrace, Premarin, and Prempro deplete vitamin B6 and magnesium.

• Oral contraceptives deplete vitamin B6, vitamin C, zinc, and magnesium.

• Laxatives deplete calcium, and vitamins A and D.

• Ulcer medications deplete calcium and vitamin D.

One last note regarding a drug developed to treat osteoporosis—*Fosamax.*

In Dr. Lee's July, 1998 medical newsletter, he wrote an article entitled "Throw Away Your Fosamax." The following is an excerpt:

Fosamax is billed as the only non-hormonal drug approved to treat osteoporosis, but studies of this drug were cleverly stopped at four to six years. This is just the point at which the fracture rate for women taking similar drugs such as Didronel began to rise. The problem is that these types of drugs temporarily create denser-looking bones in bone density tests because they block the resorption of old bone. But old bone is constantly resorbed and replaced because it's weak and needs to be replaced, and it can't be replaced if it isn't resorbed. **In people who take Fosamax, the old bone remains in place and over time begins to crumble, and eventually this is likely to cause the fracture rate to sharply increase.**

Fosamax also causes deficiencies of calcium, magnesium, and vitamin D.

IT'S NOT FAIR!
Our Stubborn Baby Boomer Fat Cells

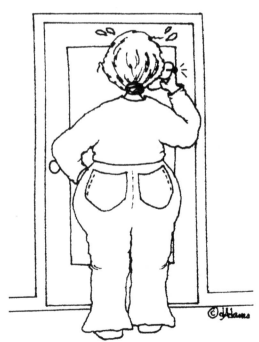

Yes, I KNOW they're back in style, but now the bottom is wider than the bells, so forget it!

I began writing this book at 45 years of age. Why? What could possibly compel me to sit at a computer for five years—translating clinical data into a form that someone could (and would) read? What possessed me to spend 1800 nights struggling and sifting through material and 1800 days writing about it—focused and driven and determined. What set me on such a noble course? My butt.

Yep. It was...growing. "Oh man. There it goes again. I haven't changed anything. I am eating the same, training the same, doing the same amount of cardio. The same routine! Totally! What's going on???"

45. That's what was going on. At 45 it seems to become a whole new ball game. So, we better learn the rules if we want to win.

I suppose you can figure out by now that hormones are calling the shots in this game. What can we do about that? Well, some of the books I have read say that we must learn to accept our new larger bodies, and embrace them and love them and...

This is not for me.

Listen. I'm not saying that we'll all look 20 again (thank the Lord, I was a blob at 20). But at 50, I __am__ determined to be in the best shape of my life. Now, that takes in a lot of factors. (I may not be as lean as I was at 37 years old, but I was destroying my health to be that way then.) I am talking about _really_ feeling good about ourselves. But I am not going to do that by adopting some mantra that will help me chant my way to self-love. I am going to put an honest effort into being the best I can be.

So what about our baby boomer fat? What do we need to address to keep it under control?

Outsmarting The Female Fat Cell (published in 1993) is a book written by registered dietitian, Debra Waterhouse. In it we read about our 30 billion fat cells and how female fat cells are larger, more active, and more resistant to dieting than male fat cells. Debra showed us how to "outsmart" our fat cells through exercise and nutrition, and at the end of the book, she warned us that once we all reached peremenopause, we would have to "outsmart" them again.

In 1998, _Outsmarting The Mid-life Fat Cell_ was published, and Debra was at it again—only this time regarding the fat gained during the "transition." When our hormones begin to decline, this signals the body to call other resources into action. Debra writes: "As soon as your fat cells detect a slightly lower estrogen level, they come to your aid to produce estrogen for you (it's one of their highly evolved functions). They know that eventually your ovaries will stop producing estrogen, so they start preparing to take over the ovaries' job."

Debra tells us that at this time of our lives, our fat cells grow in size and ability to store fat. Have you noticed that your waist is growing? Well, Debra says it is because the fat cells in our mid-section are better equipped to produce estrogen, and the larger they become, the more benefits we will receive.

Thank you very much.

So, what is happening is our fat cells are activating more fat-storing enzymes, de-activating fat-releasing enzymes, and growing by 20%! And, don't try to diet to fight this. Debra writes: "The harder you try to lose weight by dieting, the more powerful your menopausal fat cells will become, and the more weight you will gain. Diets don't work for most women regardless of age, but for menopausal women, diets have close to a 100 percent failure rate. Even on an 800-calorie diet, your fat cells will refuse to shrink and will fight back by growing even larger. Fat cells have an important mission of manufacturing estrogen and balancing your body during the transition—and they will do everything possible to make sure that they don't let you down. Most women who are in mid-life today started dieting in their teens and have been on at least fifteen diets, losing and regaining the same ten, twenty, or fifty pounds. Each time we dieted, our estrogen levels dropped and our cortisol levels (one of the stress hormones) rose. After years of yo-yo dieting and yo-yoing hormones, our systems eventually wore out. The result: A longer transition, a more severe experience, and more weight gain.

In summary, fat cells become more efficient at storage during the transition to menopause, but dieting makes them super-efficient by doubling the fat-storage enzymes and cutting the fat-releasing enzymes in half. Everything you've been concerned about during mid-life, from memory loss to hair loss, and from osteoporosis to insomnia, may be partially caused by dieting and is definitely exacerbated by dieting.

You can't force your fat cells to shrink during mid-life; they have to grow to produce estrogen."

What???

Okay. Wait a minute. If our estrogen levels are low, and our fat cells are staying fat to make estrogen for us, what if we started using some natural hormone replacement (see, *Hormone Replacement Therapy And The Great Dilemma*) to just chill those fat cells out a bit. In his book, *Natural Hormone Replacement*, Jonathan Wright, M.D. tells us about the natural alternatives to synthetic hormones, and how to alleviate some of the symptoms of menopause. By *using transdermal-penetrating creams* that can be rubbed into "hormone sensitive areas," we can raise our levels of estrogen and progesterone. We can also affect our estrogen (and testosterone) levels by taking DHEA. (Remember, you <u>must</u> be tested to know how low your hormone levels are and how much is required to do the job.)

Now, will that be enough to send our fat cells on a vacation so we can empty them while they are not looking?

Debra Waterhouse says we need to make the following adjustments to lose any fat at all: "Because menopausal women are highly efficient fat storers, it's imperative that we modify our eating behavior to match our new mid-life metabolism. Your metabolism decreases during the transition, so your caloric needs decrease as well. This does not mean that you have to choose lower-calorie foods; it means that you have to choose <u>less of any food</u>."

Debra tells us to: Eat less at night, eat smaller, more frequent meals, give up dieting, be aware of the fact that we will eventually need to decrease our daily calories by 400, and <u>exercise four to five times a week</u>.

Excuse me?

That's correct. She writes: "Now is the time to take action. You need to move during your mid-life years more than you have ever needed to before. Your menopausal body is depending on you to exercise to: fight fatigue, recharge your metabolism, reduce mental sluggishness, sleep soundly, stabilize your moods, diminish food cravings, reduce hot flashes, achieve greater mobility, strengthen your bones, reduce your risk of breast cancer, reduce your risk of heart disease, stabilize your blood sugar, and live a longer life.

If you want to do everything you possibly can to deter menopausal weight gain and combat mid-life fat—EXERCISE."

Debra offers research demonstrating that women who stay fit throughout their mid-life years are leaner, stronger, and healthier. They carry at least 13% less body fat, weigh almost 30 pounds less, and have about 5 pounds more lean muscle mass.

"When you become fit, your fat cells automatically become smaller. Each of your 30 billion fat cells learns that there is another existence. They don't have to function solely as fat-storage receptacles—they can also manufacture fat-releasing enzymes and shrink in size."

A combination of aerobic exercise *(to manufacture the fat-releasing enzymes that trigger the emptying of fat into your blood stream)* and strength training *(which will speed up your metabolism and condition your muscles to burn up that released fat)* is what is needed. (See, *Under Construction* for more on aerobic conditioning and strength training.)

Debra continues: "Exercise also encourages fat release in another way. It helps your body produce another source of estrogen so that your fat cells can willingly shrink without compromising your health. A recent discovery is that exercise stimulates your muscle cells to manufacture 25 percent of the estrogen your menopausal body needs. The more fit your muscles are, the more estrogen they'll produce, the less work your fat cells have to do, and the more cooperative they'll become in releasing fat. It's a win-win situation!"

Okay. I <u>was</u> exercising. But my body fat had still become more stubborn than it ever was before. It's all in the timing, Debra says. "Because our mid-life fat cells take longer to release the fat, exercising (aerobically) for a full 60 minutes will give them the time they need to release fat and direct it to the muscle to be burned."

Don't forget to integrate strength training into all of this. If you don't, you will continue to lose a half-pound of muscle a year. With strength training, *this can be 100 percent prevented* according to Debra Waterhouse and other sources.

And that sounds good to me.

MY JOURNEY THROUGH THE LOOKING GLASS

Whooo are youuu???
The Caterpillar, in

Through The Looking Glass
—Louis Carroll

If what you have read so far has triggered a desire to enter a brave new world and conquer your dragons—bravo! But, before you go any further into the information I have to offer you, allow a brief pause here to read about my experience.

The 40's for me were a wild ride. There were extreme highs—and extreme lows (see, *THE CRASH OF '92*). As I enter a new decade, I feel that I am more prepared for what life has to offer a woman who is maturing. I needed to learn about all of the options open to us, and then I wanted to explore them personally so that I could share my experience with you.

Science Or Nature?

We have to admit that the science in this arena these days is very compelling. Anti-aging doctors and clinics are offering us youth in a syringe. A growing number of people are taking this "Super Hormone Cocktail" in hopes of reversing the signs and symptoms of advancing age. Some dramatic results have been reported. Provocative studies have been conducted—mostly on men and rats ("...Sure, if you want to know how something works for a woman, just test it in rats first..." Dr. Christiane Northrup).

Although I'm told there is significant data to support how super-hormone replacement therapy could work for a woman in her late 40's, I couldn't find as much as I would have liked. So I conducted my own six-month study—on myself. I went to Dr. Lord-Lee Benner, an anti-aging doctor who gets wonderful results with his patients, and who probably has a portrait of himself somewhere decaying to dust (the man looks 20 years younger than he is!).

I took my savings (super-hormone therapy is not cheap) and began my journey. First—hormone tests—full spectrum: Estrogen, progesterone, testosterone, DHEA, pregnenolone, growth hormone—for $1200 you get the works! My levels were all "normally low" for a woman my age. The mission? To raise serum levels of my hormones to the levels of a 25 year old woman.

Then—the prescriptions.

Oh my. A prescription for syringes. (Scary.) Vials of synthetic Human Growth Hormone. Plus: Testosterone, DHEA, Pregnenolone, Melatonin, Premarin and Provera.

I injected myself twice a day, and took some pills. I did this for six months, and then I stopped. The results?

Oh boy was I disappointed!

Before I began my therapy I had a menstrual cycle that was starting to act screwy, terrible night-sweats, debilitating cramps, radical mood swings, alarmingly heavy bleeding, and relentless bloating. After six months on my super-hormone therapy, I had all the same complaints—but worse!

Every day I would wake up and say, "This will be the day the magic hits!" I would look in the mirror expecting to somehow appear "younger." I would pull my skin looking for the reported increase in elasticity and youthful "thickness." I would examine my body for the promised reduction in body fat.

And another day of needle sticking and pill popping would end without a miracle. Finally, my six-month deadline arrived, and I ended the siege on my body. (Please remember that this was my experience. After much more research, I understood that my negative reactions were probably due to the Premarin and Provera. Perhaps combining closely regulated super-hormone therapy with natural estrogen and progesterone would provide a more favorable outcome. Dr. Lee-Benner and other anti-aging doctors do get some great results with patients. Everyone is different. And, don't forget, miracles only come from One source.)

I gave my body some time to stabilize, and went back to Dr. Gary.

More testing: *Female Hormone Panel*, (this time not blood for serum levels, but saliva for cellular levels. I had to spit in vials for 28 days!) *Adrenal Stress Index*, (more saliva) and *Dysbiosis Urine Test* (well, you know).

(See, *15 Rounds—My Championship Bout*.)

My regimen ever since has been: Natural progesterone creme (which doubles my estrogenic hormonal receptor sites), a natural formulation containing (among other things) Black Cohosh Rt., Scullcap Rt. (and other ingredients proven to be beneficial for women), natural hormonal sprays, and a diet that rotates in soy foods such as tofu.

I have never felt better! I have a normal menstrual cycle. The cramping and bloating and bleeding are less. My bed is dry. I will never be pure joy to live with, but my mood swings inscribe a much smaller arc. And I am not about "Better Living Through Chemistry," which allows me to stay true to my beliefs and have peace.

Once again, this is my journey. There is so much that is available to us now. But, like most things, as they are with us for a while, our current "miracles" have begun to show some fallibility. Experience has begun to show us that (although there have been some dramatic studies and encouraging results) super-hormone therapy is not for everyone. Dr. Gary says: "It all comes back to everyone being unique. Although some have experienced a degree of success (and even drama) on super-hormone replacement therapy, it has virtually failed others. We are discovering now that the levels of these "cocktails" are too high for many people. Natural hormonal sprays and patches secrete minute amounts of hormones that will activate what was meant to be. It is important to be tested and then we can administer low, safe levels of the support indicated."

The moral? Before you step through the looking glass—know yourself very well so when things are not what they seem, you are not trapped in a world that is *bizarre*.

HORMONE REPLACEMENT THERAPY— AND THE GREAT DILEMMA
Estrogen and Progesterone

What is menopause, exactly? Dr. Lee says, "strictly speaking, menopause is the cessation of menses, the end of menstrual cycles." Now, to a lot of us, this does not necessarily sound like a bad thing. In *On Women Turning Fifty*, Cathleen Rountree writes, "During her middle years, when a woman is no longer a sexual object, she begins to experience herself as a truly sexual being. In our late forties and early fifties, with the onset of menopause, we enter a season in which we no longer need concern ourselves with unwanted pregnancy and birth control. We become more concerned with female production than reproduction."

Still, we do not want the usual physical consequences associated with this "gift." So, what are our options? Well, once again, the answers are unclear, conflicting, and controversial. And, once again, we women are allowing ourselves to be treated as laboratory rats. First, it was "Estrogen is the answer!"— and the birth of Estrogen Replacement Therapy in the late 1950s. By 1965, numerous magazine articles had been published heralding "The End Of Menopause!" Then, in late 1965, a book entitled, *Now! The Pills To Keep Women Young! ERT The First Complete Account Of The Miracle Hormone Treatment That May Revolutionize The Lives Of Millions Of Women!* by Ann

Walsh hit the scene. Women were dancing in the streets. In 1975, the dancing stopped. Women on ERT were developing uterine cancer four to eight times more often than those women who did not opt for it. Researchers confirmed this fact.

Just a temporary setback for the medical community. They rallied and found that cancer occurred because the estrogen that was being prescribed was "unopposed." And so, ERT was replaced by HRT (Hormone Replacement Therapy) and estrogen was prescribed with the addition of *progestins* (synthetic progesterone).

I do not know how many of you have already been prescribed Premarin (a form of estrogen derived from a *pregnant mare's urine*) and Provera (synthetic progesterone), but this "dynamic duo" was prescribed as part of my H.R.T. Why? I was experiencing certain symptoms that I suspected to be connected to premenopause (waking in the middle of the night in a sweat-soaked bed might have been a clue—see, *My Journey Through The Looking Glass*). When my symptoms did not abate, I was advised to increase the dosage of Premarin, suggesting that I actually needed to further elevate my estrogen levels. The *ratio* of estrogen to progesterone in my body was not considered.

Dr. Lee says, "A woman's hormone balance can begin to shift at anywhere from her mid-thirties to her late forties, depending on a variety of factors such as heredity, environment, how early or late she began menstruating, whether she had children and if so, at what age and how many, and her lifestyle. Hormone balance is intimately connected to stress levels, nutrition, and the environmental toxins encountered daily." Dr. Lee believes that the American woman's experience of menopause is "a combination of poor diet, unhealthy lifestyle, environmental pollutants, cultural attitudes, the incorrect use of synthetic hormones, and advertising." He further states that the symptoms that many of us experience as we approach menopause are actually a result of estrogen *dominance*, not estrogen *deficiency*, and to prescribe estrogen at all is a mistake. As we enter premenopause, ovulation is at best an erratic event. And if we aren't ovulating, we aren't producing progesterone. Dr. Lee elaborates that, "Menstrual cycles can continue even without progesterone, so women aren't aware that the lack of progesterone is causing their symptoms. This is known as peremenopause, or premenopause. During this time, the ovaries continue to produce estrogen sufficient for regular or irregular shedding, creating what I term 'estrogen dominance.' When estrogen surges, women may notice breast swelling and tenderness, mood swings, sleep disturbance, water retention, and a tendency to put on weight. These may be symptoms of estrogen dominance caused mainly by lack of ovulation and thereby lack of progesterone while estrogen levels are still in the 'normal' range. The fall of progesterone levels at menopause is proportionately much greater than the fall of estrogen."

In an article published in *Time Magazine* on June 26, 1995 entitled "The Estrogen Dilemma," Claudia Wallis comments that, "Estrogen is indeed the closest thing in modern medicine to an elixir of youth—a drug that slows the ravages of time for women. It is already the No. 1 prescription drug in America, and it is about to hit the demographic sweet spot: the millions of baby boomers now experiencing their first hot flashes. The risk of uterine cancer can be virtually eliminated, experts say, by adding synthetic progesterone. Estrogen, it seems, can prevent or slow many of the ravages of aging."

We know that estrogen is powerful stuff. It is the hormone responsible for the changes that occur at puberty for girls, such as; breasts, body hair, and a revved-up ability to store body fat. It figures that it is also responsible for the changes that occur later on in a woman's life (increased body fat, more hair in strange places). Also, Dr. Lee states in his book that, "When women consume considerably more calories than needed, estrogen production increases proportionately to supernormal levels and may set the stage for estrogen dominance syndrome and exaggerated estrogen decline at menopause." (Make no mistake; estrogen and body fat are linked—see, *It's Not Fair!—Our Baby Boomer Fat Cells*.) We credit estrogen with the many wonderful, youthful qualities of our earlier years when, in fact, Dr. Lee says the credit belongs to <u>progesterone</u>. The following are the effects of progesterone as listed in *What Your Doctor May Not Tell You About Menopause*: "Maintains secretory endometrium, protects against fibrocystic breasts, helps use fat for energy, natural diuretic, natural antidepressant, facilitates thyroid hormone action, normalizes blood clotting, restores sex drive, normalizes blood sugar levels, normalizes zinc and copper levels, restores proper cell oxygen levels, prevents endometrial cancer, helps prevent breast cancer, stimulates bone building, restores normal vascular tone, necessary for the survival of embryo, and precursor of corticosteroids." The following is a list of symptoms that can be caused or made worse by <u>estrogen dominance</u> (also listed by Dr. Lee in his book): "Acceleration of the aging process, allergies, breast tenderness, decreased sex drive, depression, fatigue, fibocystic breasts, foggy thinking, headaches, hypoglycemia, increased blood clotting, infertility, irritability, memory loss, miscarriage, osteoporosis, premenopausal bone loss, PMS, thyroid function mimicking hypothyroidism, uterine cancer, uterine fibroids, water retention and bloating, fat gain (especially around the abdomen, hips, and thighs), gallbladder disease, and autoimmune disorders (such as lupus), mood swings, heavy or irregular menses, and craving for sweets." Nice list. I don't know about you, but I sure recognized many of the symptoms on that list. This is the exact <u>opposite</u> picture from the one that was painted by Dr. Robert A. Wilson in his book, *Feminine Forever*. In <u>his</u> book, Dr. Wilson wrote, "For the first time in history women may share the promise of tomorrow as biological equals of men. Thanks to hormone replacement therapy, they may look forward to prolonged well-being and extended youth."

Dr. Lee maintains that "we have a progesterone deficiency in premenopausal and menopausal women in Western societies." He associates this phenomenon with a diet that is dominated by <u>refined and processed foods</u>. (Are you getting the message here?) Dr. Lee says, "In nonindustrialized cultures whose diets are rich in fresh vegetables (thus consuming the over 5000 known plants that have progestogenic effects), progesterone deficiency is rare."

What About Soy?

Regarding natural sources of estrogen (dietary phytoestrogen), I would like to quote from an article in "The Soy Connection" called *The Phytoestrogen Paradox*, written by David T. Zava, Ph.D., that I found really interesting. Dr. Zava developed the *saliva hormone assay testing procedure* at Aeron Lifecycles. Basically, what he stated in his article is that studies have shown that Asian women consuming traditional high-soy diets have few menopausal symptoms and lower rates of osteoporosis than women in western countries. Dr. Zava reports: "Soyfoods posses many unique properties that protect against cancer, as well as cardiovascular disease, osteoporosis, and menopausal symptoms. One of the most distinctive features of soyfoods is their exceptionally high content of isoflavonoids such as genistein and daidzein (weak phytoestrogens with about 1/1000th the activity of estradiol). In Asian countries where much larger amounts of soyfoods are consumed, blood levels of these phytoestrogens are 100 to 1000-fold higher than in western countries. The circulating levels of genistein in individuals eating a traditional soy-laced Asian diet is up to 1000-fold higher than the highest levels of endogenous estradiol in premenopausal Asian and Western women. Declining endogenous estrogens associated with ovarian failure during menopause is closely associated with an increase in menopausal symptoms, as well as a marked increase in the risk of developing cardiovascular disease and osteoporosis. However, despite the low endogenous estrogen levels in post-menopausal women from Asian and Western countries, Asian women consuming a traditional high-soy diet have far fewer menopausal symptoms and fewer hip fractures (osteoporosis), hallmarks of estrogen deficiency. In fact, hot flashes in Japanese women are so rare there is no word to describe them. Soyfood consumption may be responsible to some extent for this freedom from symptoms." The article goes on to state that more research is needed, but that there is data to support the view that in post-menopausal Asian women who typically consume a low-fat/high-soy diet, genistein acts as a surrogate estrogen agonist, without the harmful side effects of promoting the growth of "estrogen-sensitive" tumors. Once again, a lot of our problems seem to come back to one place—diet.

There are products available in health food stores such as "Genistein," which is a supplement containing substances derived from soy. Products such as this are offered as natural alternatives to Premarin. Dr. Zava now cautions us that genistein is an anti-nutrient (toxin), and since the above article was printed, his "jury" is back out. Dr. Zava told Dr. Lee in an interview in Dr. Lee's medical newsletter dated May, 1998: "When I first began to study soy's anti-cancer properties, I thought genistein was the answer. As I read on in the scientific literature I became less convinced that genistein was beneficial." Both Dr. Zava and Dr. Lee recommend that we eat the _food_ that has been fermented and cooked, not take the supplements. He also tells us that, although the phytoestrogens in soy products such as miso, tofu, and tempeh are known to inhibit the growth of cancer, and the Japanese _do_ tend to have lower rates of breast and prostate cancer, they also have one of the highest rates of stomach cancer in the world.

Too Much Of A Good Thing?

Dr. Lee explains that the Japanese stomach cancer could be caused by many factors, but there are some reasons to be cautious about eating too much soy. One is that soy is a protease inhibitor—it inhibits the enzyme protease, which is responsible for breaking down protein in the digestive tract. This, however, is not the only issue. Dr. Zava continues in his interview with Dr. Lee:

"People do fine with average soy consumption, eating it here and there, but the way Americans are jumping into it, we are going to have problems. I reviewed the literature on soy very carefully, and what I found is that there are an enormous number of toxins (antinutrients) in unfermented soy. These are plant chemicals produced naturally in the soybean that, if not removed first by soaking, slow cooking, and fermentation can cause serious health problems if you eat too much of them. (Over thousands of years of experimentation, the Asians learned how to remove the toxins from soybeans and reap the remarkably rich nutrients from the bean.) There are five types of plant chemicals in the soybean that can be toxic to humans: Allergens, phytates, protease inhibitors, genistein, and goitrogens. The allergens (in soybeans) probably account for some 10 to 20 percent of allergic reactions in Western population. The phytates can be a problem because they tightly bind up essential minerals (particularly zinc, which is needed for over 50 enzyme reactions in the body, including many of those necessary for brain function), preventing them from being absorbed by the body.

Soy foods can be important as one part of a balanced nutrition and lifestyle approach to menopausal symptoms, but they aren't a solution by themselves. With natural progesterone and/or estrogen replacement therapy, women often get complete relief of menopausal symptoms."

Dr. Lee's interview with Dr. Zava regarding "the dark side of soy" caused quite a reaction from many people—and one was Dr. Earl Mindell, author of many books on nutrition and health, including *The Vitamin Bible*. Dr. Mindell stated that most Americans do not even know what soy products are, and that eating too much is not an issue. Dr. Lee responded by saying: "Dr. Mindell is right—most Americans don't eat enough soy. Eaten in moderation, and in fermented forms such as tofu and miso in which the anti-nutrients have been reduced or removed, soy is an important part of a balanced diet. Dr. Zava emphasizes that the soy products we need to be wary of are those that aren't fermented, such as soy milk and soy powders. He has done laboratory studies of soy powders and found that they tend to have very high concentrations of anti-nutrients." (*Live It Or Diet Lifestyle System's* protein powder is <u>rice protein</u> based, which is tolerated by most individuals.)

Soy can also block thyroid. One of the anitnutrients in soy, goitrogen, prevents iodine from being absorbed into the body. Iodine is needed to make thyroid hormone. It is important to eat soy in moderation for many reasons, but especially if you have low thyroid function—and best to eliminate it if you are taking Synthroid. (See, *Thyroid Hormone* for other thyroid blockers.) Dr. Lee concludes by saying: "Soy is a food that is a medicine in moderation and a potential poison in excess."

Oh, my. Take heart if you are an advocate of soy (which I am). There is new technology on the horizon that involves sprouting soy and eliminating the toxic properties. Dr. Gary and Dr. Hinze, along with the rest of Live It Or Diet's product development team, are researching a process developed by Zane Baranowski that will potentially provide the benefits of soy without the side effects. In *The Living Soy Superfood*, Mr. Baranowski, along with Tonita d'Raye, tell us: "Raw soybeans contain trypsin inhibitors, which are chemicals that disrupt digestive enzymes. For this reason, soy foods must be heat-processed or chemically extracted to neutralize these enzyme inhibitors in order to be consumed safely. Consuming soy foods such as tofu, miso, soymilk, powdered soy protein, and many of the isoflavone soy supplements are beneficial. However, many health-promoting benefits of nutrients in soy products are devalued by heat processing to deactivate trypsin inhibitors in order to make products more digestible. <u>Many soy supplements on the market boast of very concentrated isoflavone content but are not 'alive.'</u> Therefore, while the quantity may be impressive, they lack biologically active quality. Now there is a new technology for processing soybeans that does not involve heat processing. This technology eliminates the problem with trypsin inhibitors. Now we have a highly concentrated soy complex that is 'fully alive,' biologically active and bioavailable, and can be powdered, encapsulated, and used as a dietary supplement. Furthermore, the highly concentrated live complex retains soy's vital phytochemicals, enzymes, vitamins, minerals, and other disease-fighting, health-promoting micronutrients. The sprouting process activates the life force of seeds and beans. A breakthrough sprouting technology naturally deactivates trypsin inhibitors and transforms soy into a fully enzyme-active 'live' food."

We will keep you updated on soy—check our virtual *Live It Or Diet Center* (LiveItOrDiet.com) for the latest information on this and many other issues.

More On Hormones

In their book entitled *The Superhormone Promise*, William Regelson, M.D. And Carol Colman discuss another alternative; estradiol. They write: "Some doctors prefer to prescribe pure estradiol—natural estrogen—because it is identical to the estrogen produced by a woman's ovaries; it may be better tolerated than Premarin (which, because it comes from horses, is not necessarily the best estrogen for humans) and cause fewer side effects. (In this case the use of the word 'natural' is misleading. In reality, both Premarin and estradiol are synthetic products in that they are both processed. The real difference between them is their chemical structure.)"

David Brownstein, M.D. writes in his book, *The Miracle Of Natural Hormones*, the following on estrogen: "There are three different types of estrogens manufactured by the body—estrone, estradiol, and estriol. Each of these different types of estrogen has very different properties in the body. Jonathan Wright, M.D., a pioneer in natural therapies, measured the serum levels and urinary excretion of the three estrogens and reported that of the three types of estrogen measured, 60-80% was estriol, 10-20% was estrone, and 10-20% was estradiol. If we are going to give estrogen hormone replacement to a woman, doesn't it make sense to give it in the same proportions as naturally made in the body? Premarin consists of 100% estrone. A natural estrogen preparation has been formulated by Dr. Wright and is known as

Triest. Triest is made from plant products and has the same chemical structure of the three types of estrogen produced in the human body—and mim-
ics the body's own production of estrogens by containing 80% estriol, 10%
estradiol, and 10% estrone."

Dr. Jonathan Wright's book, *Natural Hormone Replacement*, discusses many
aspects of natural hormone replacement therapy, and late-breaking research on
the dangers of synthetics such as Provera. At least three-fourths of post-
menopausal female deaths are associated with heart disease. Millions of women
have been taking Provera to minimize the risks of endometrial cancer when
taking estrogen replacement, <u>and recent studies show that they are putting
themselves at higher risk of suffering a heart attack by doing this!</u> Natural progesterone will provide cancer protection with <u>no such risk</u>. As far as Premarin
(estrogen replacement) is concerned, the proportions of estrogens are off the
normal human level (natural for horses—not humans!). In the chapter, "Why
You Should Consider Natural Hormone Replacement," Dr. Wright states the
following: "For the majority of women who have used Premarin, Provera, or
other patentable or synthetic hormones to ease the symptoms of early
menopause, the results have been mostly positive. But in the absence of any
"medically accepted" alternatives to these drugs for the last four decades,
women have been asked to gamble with their lives, accepting a small risk of
cancer in return for a large chance of preventing atherosclerosis, osteoporosis,
and possibly senility and memory loss. Natural hormone replacement (NHR)
greatly improves women's odds of 'winning' that gamble.

NHR is the next logical step in menopausal hormone replacement therapy. The concept of replacing hormones with identical hormones in the correct proportions at the correct time makes obvious sense. How could the
human species have survived if normal levels of every woman's reproductive
hormones predisposed her to a fatal disease during her fertile years? For
some, close observation of nature and creation is reason enough to switch
from HRT to NHR. For those who need 'proof,' scientific evidence continues
to build in favor of using a balanced combination of natural estrogens, plus
natural progesterone, and in many cases, DHEA and testosterone. The
advantages of NHR for menopausal and premenopausal women are now
quite clear. They include: Prevention of osteoporosis and restoration of bone
strength, reduced hot flashes and reduced vaginal dryness and thinning, better maintenance of muscle mass and strength, protection against heart disease and stroke, improved cholesterol levels, reduced risk of endometrial and
breast cancer, reduced risk of depression, improved sleep and better mood,
concentration and memory, prevention of senility and Alzheimer's disease,
improved sex drive."

Whether or not you opt for Hormone Replacement Therapy (as opposed to Natural Hormone Replacement) is up to you. I strongly suggest not only consulting with your physician, but reading everything you can get your hands on regarding the subject (see my list of resources, as well as pulling up information on in the Internet, etc.). Based on what I have read, my personal experience with Premarin and Provera, blood and saliva tests (and consultations with Dr. Gary), my own personal choice is still <u>natural estrogens and progesterone</u>. Dr. Lee explains the difference between natural and synthetic progesterone in his book: "If a drug company discovered a naturally occurring medicine, anyone else was free to capitalize on the discovery. These days, when a plant with medicinal value is discovered, the 'active ingredient' is isolated and transformed. This new molecule can be patented. The history of creating synthetic drugs consistently shows that separating the so-called active ingredient from the rest of the plant to create substances not found in nature almost always creates harmful side effects. Most of the progestins are synthesized from progesterone or from another hormone called nortestosterone and are not found in any living forms. Because progesterone is a natural hormone, the body is normally able to produce it, use it, and eliminate it as needed. The synthetic progestins, on the other hand, are not well processed by the body. Their activity is prolonged, creating reactions in the body that are not consistent with natural progesterone."

About his new book, *What Your Doctor May Not Tell You About Premenopause*, Dr. Lee says: "If you want to know what this book is about in a nutshell, I'll give it to you in one word—**balance**—a theme that recurs through every chapter. If your diet is imbalanced, your hormones will be imbalanced. If your emotions are out of balance, your hormones will be out of balance. If you are working too hard and not nurturing yourself, your hormones will be out of balance. **As you seek balance in your life, your health will improve.**"

I read Dr. Lee's new book. It is an incredible work that shoots straight from the hip. Dr. Lee, along with his co-authors, Jesse Hanley, M.D. and Virginia Hopkins, are angry. They are out-spoken advocates for women's health, and tell it like it is. They want you to learn about premenopause syndrome and understand your body and your emotions. They want you to stop behaving like cattle led to slaughter (those are <u>my</u> words). Dr. Lee writes: "As a doctor in family practice for thirty years, I learned early on that my patients' problems had as much to do with their emotional well-being as their physical well-being, and that is perhaps even more true as it applies to women suffering from premenopause syndrome. The prospect of aging is much more daunting for a woman than it is for a man, so those first signs of hormonal imbalance that a woman experiences can give rise to emotional issues that can make physical problems worse. To add insult to injury, if a woman goes to a doctor who practices conventional medicine, the solutions she is offered are likely to fall into two categories: Surgery or drugs. Both are likely to make her problems worse instead of better."

What is premenopause syndrome? The authors of *What Your Doctor May Not Tell You About Premenopause* explain it this way: "If you're a woman between the ages of thirty and fifty, you know a woman, maybe yourself, who has fibroids, tender or lumpy breasts, endometriosis, PMS, difficulty conceiving or carrying a pregnancy to term, sudden weight gain, fatigue, irritability and depression, foggy thinking, memory loss, migraine headaches, very heavy or light periods, bleeding between periods, or cold hands and feet. These symptoms are part of premenopause for a majority of today's women, and are the result of hormone imbalances, most of them caused by an excess of the hormone estrogen and a deficiency of the hormone progesterone.

However, premenopause symptoms are not just about biochemistry. They are also about women who are out of touch with cycles and rhythms of their bodies, their feelings, and their souls. These are women who struggle to balance families and work, women who forget to take care of themselves, and women who aren't getting the help they need from their health maintenance organization (HMO)."

In spite of what a conventional doctor will tell you, you can do something about the symptoms of premenopause besides antidepressant drugs, synthetic hormones, and surgery. Since *What Your Doctor May Not Tell You About Menopause* was written, the amount of new research and clinical information we have about premenopause syndrome has grown exponentially. The authors of this new book still maintain that: Taking one of the strange, not-found-in-nature synthetic hormones created by the drug companies is one of the best and quickest ways to confuse your body and throw it into a state of imbalance. They also warn us against Xenohormone. Against what? "Xenohormones, also called xenobiotics, are synthetic chemicals such as pesticides and plastics, which exert hormonal influences on all living creatures."

When I read *What Your Doctor May Not Tell You About Premenopause*, I was blown away by the section called *Xenohormone Hell*, that describes how these toxic substances we use in everyday life (including nail polish and nail polish remover, solvents, adhesives, car exhaust, and meat from livestock fed estrogenic drugs to fatten them up!) cause all kinds of harmful effects— including early puberty in girls!! Get this—doctors are preferring to view these premature pubertal changes that are becoming a trend as a *new 'norm,' rather that an abnormality*. I find that scary. Don't you? By all means, let's not look for the cause of this shift in nature. Let's just create yet another classification of normal that is <u>not natural</u>. Women——please!

Dr. Lee tells us that what is happening in this time of our lives is that "all involved systems, from the brain to the uterus, are down regulating. If you maintain balance in your life, it will be a gradual, barely noticeable process. If you are out of balance, all of the systems will not be getting the message that down-regulation is in process, and they will, in effect, be shouting at each other to try to provoke a response, causing night sweats and hot flashes. The biochemical over-reaction or under-reaction to this shouting causes high libido, low libido, acne, allergies, tender breasts, water retention, insomnia, and mood swings. When a premenopausal woman enters a doctor's office with these complaints, she is highly likely to leave with a prescription for estrogen or a birth control pill, which is probably the last thing in the world she needs."

Should I Just Use Wild Yam?

The authors of *What Your Doctor May Not Tell You About Premenopause* caution us about products identified as "wild yam extract." These products contain diosgenin, not progesterone. Dr. Lee tells us: "In the chemistry lab scientists can make progesterone from diosgenin. That does not mean that your body can make progesterone from diosgenin—or any other hormone for that matter. Those who sell diosgenin or diosgenin disguised as 'extract of wild yam' in creams or capsules and claim that it has the same effects as progesterone are not speaking the truth. Please make sure your source of progesterone cream is reliable." *What Your Doctor May Not Tell You About Premenopause* contains a list of progesterone creams.

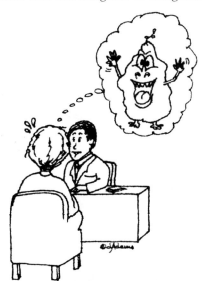

Have you tried Wild Yam Cream?

What About Herbs?

More and more doctors (alternative and medical) are using herbal medicines to help balance hormones. Dr. Jesse Hanley, M.D. (co-author with Dr. Lee and Virginia Hopkins of

What Your Doctor May Not Tell You About Premenopause), in a June 1998 inter-view with Dr. Lee, in his medical newsletter says: "During my medical train-ing I saw clearly that pharmaceutical drugs were a heavy-handed way of heal-ing and they often had so many undesirable side effects that they did more harm than good. During medical school I began my studies of Chinese med-icine—acupuncture and herbal medicine—which I've studied and integrat-ed into my practice ever since. Diet, nutritional supplements, herbs, natural hormones, and prescription drugs all have their place in a medical practice, depending on what the individual patient's needs are. Very often I find that in younger premenopausal women—say from age thirty to forty—achieving hormone balance is more a matter of <u>bringing the whole body into balance rather than supplementing a deficiency.</u> I start with diet, exercise, nutrition-al supplements and stress management, and if that doesn't solve the problem, I'll often try some herbs. Herbs, and particularly skillfully crafted herbal combinations, tend to have a gentle regulatory effect that can help move the body into balance in a few weeks, at a reasonable cost. Supplementing nat-ural hormones has a more powerful effect, and I use them when there's clear-ly a deficiency present." (Turn to *Appendix G* for more information on Dr. John Lee's Medical Letter.) In *What Your Doctor May Not Tell You About Premenopause*, the authors tell us that: "The use of herbs as medicines is gen-erally preferable to most prescription drugs because they tend to have a more gentle action and fewer side effects. The human body has spent millions of years evolving, and in that evolutionary process it has adapted elegantly to use the foods and medicines the earth provides in the form of plants. If you are going to use herbs to balance your hormones, it is recommended that you consult with a qualified and experienced herbalist."

The most effective test for hormone levels is the saliva test I mentioned (more sensitive and indicates cellular levels—consult *Appendix E*). Should you decide to take *natural progesterone*, there are many creams and oils on the mar-ket that contain natural progesterone. Some are processed properly, some are not. I use a cream called Pro Gest. So far, so good. The symptoms that first led me to investigate super-hormone replacement therapy, and then became more dramatic after starting on Premarin and Provera (spotting and hemorrhaging, night sweats, extremely painful cramps, radical bloating, intolerable PMS, etc.) are not present now. But, remember, this is <u>my</u> jigsaw puzzle. Please do not just do what I do, but investigate your own personal issues.

Dr. Christine Northrup, Assistant Professor of Obstetrics and Gynecology at the University of Vermont College of Medicine, and author of *Women's Bodies, Women's Wisdom*, lectured at the Chautauqua Institute in New York State in November of '96. She is a dynamic force in the arena of women's health, and an inspiring speaker. I want to share the following excerpt from that lecture with you:

"The body and its processes are seen as uncontrollable and unreliable, requiring control. Natural processes are seen very many times as diseases. Right now we are teaching OBGYN residents that the female body and female hormones are so unreliable that you want to get someone on the pill from about the age of thirteen to take away their cramps and any irregularity—I mean so that they'll never have a period on the weekend because you know that's important—and then you want them on the pill except for little blips now and then for your 1.8 children—and then about the age of 49-50 you just switch them over to a substance made from the urine of pregnant horses called Premarin—and then they can be on hormonal auto-pilot for the rest of their lives.

I had a woman come in who told me that after her first child was born her doctor suggested that she go on the pill to 'prevent ovarian cancer.' And, why would she get ovarian cancer? Because of 'chronic, incessant ovulation.' Once a month folks! Once a month! Notice culturally we don't have any concern for 'chronic incessant ejaculation,' do we. Nope—doesn't bother anybody. But we have this kind of 'cradle to grave' hormonal control thing for women.

My friend Bethany, who is an obstetrician, said that we should invent a new hormone because—really—if you look at the studies—there are a lot more studies to show that excessive testosterone is more dangerous than estrogen and progesterone. So, she said, 'I think we need to invent a new drug because what we have shown in mice (and you know if you want to know what's going on in humans you just want to show it in rats or mice first) that the less testosterone the mouse or the rat has, the more nesting behavior it displays.' So, we were thinking, if you could get young boys on this drug, you know, and call it 'Testaway' or 'Androstat' or something— you'd only take them off it to reproduce and the rest of the time they'd do the laundry.

Now, I only say that because, when you take this line of thinking—you know—that everyone should be on the pill because it protects us against these awful hormones—and apply it to men—it seems totally ridiculous, doesn't it? And, it's much harder to buy. But women buy into it all the time."

Testosterone—For Women?

Testosterone is also a female sex hormone.
—Susan Rako, M.D.
The Hormone Of Desire

When we are about twenty years old, women are producing peak levels of estrogen, progesterone, and testosterone. By the time we are fifty, we are producing much less. Then, most of us feel certain symptoms, go to the doctor, and receive a "standard treatment" which includes estrogen and progesterone. The authors of *The Superhormone Promise* say that at this point we still probably do not feel like "ourselves." They contend that "for many women who feel they are not quite themselves, the ingredient missing from the blueprint is testosterone."

We usually think of testosterone as a male hormone, but it is also a vital hormone for us women as well. Dr. Regelson and Ms. Colman explain it this way: "The ebb and flow of testosterone controls sex drive for both men and women. It is time to shatter the myth that testosterone is exclusively a male hormone. It is not. Testosterone is produced in both the ovaries and adrenal glands of women, just as a small amount of estrogen, the so-called female hormone, is produced in men."

Men make approximately ten times the amount of testosterone that women do, but it still is a key hormone in our sexual development. As we age, the production of testosterone declines. By the time we are forty, we have about half the amount that we had at age twenty. To quote Dr. Regelson and Ms. Coleman again: "One factor contributing to this decline is that at this age a woman's adrenal glands are pumping out less DHEA (see, *DHEA,* ahead in this chapter). DHEA is broken down into a small amount of testosterone when it is metabolized, and for women this is a main source of testosterone. By the time they reach menopause, many women are testosterone deficient."

Wait a minute. Won't testosterone make me more—masculine? Well, I guess we wouldn't have gotten some of it in the first place if it didn't balance out our "female" hormones. Lord knows we could use that balance.

Growth Hormone

What if you were promised "eternal youth;" that you could stop—even reverse the signs of aging by injecting yourself with a hormone that used to be present in your system to a much greater degree when you were younger? What if you were told that by raising your serum levels of Growth Hormone to those levels that were present when you were 25 years old, you would turn back the hands of time on your face and body? Pretty seductive, isn't it? Sound a little like Lestat's "dark gift" in *Interview With A Vampire*? Maybe a little too good to be true—or there could be some serious down sides (like never again being able to see the light of day).

Actually, there has been significant research and published studies regarding Growth Hormone and its supplementation. In The New England Journal of Medicine, published July 3, 1990, Dr. Daniel Rudman and his team presented their study: "The Effects Of Human Growth Hormone In Men Over 60 Years Old." Dr. Rudman's abstract stated the following: "The declining activity of the growth hormone-insulin like growth factor 1 (IGF-1) axis with advancing age may contribute to the decrease in lean body mass and the increase in mass of adipose tissue that occur with aging." To test this hypothesis, Dr. Rudman and his team studied 21 healthy men from 61 to 81 years old, twelve of whom were injected with synthetic growth hormone for six months. When comparing lean body mass, skin thickness, body fat, and bone density before and after in both groups, the following results were cited: Increased lean body mass, increased skin thickness, decreased body fat, and increased bone density in the twelve men that received injections of synthetic growth hormone.

Subsequently, The United States National Institute On Aging issued a mandate to conduct research "with the aim of improving the quality of life and maintaining the independence and vitality of people well into their later years." In late 1992, the institute launched a series of studies around the country to evaluate the safety and efficacy of "trophic agents" (human growth hormone and sex steroid hormones) for older people.

Also, in an International Workshop On Adult GH Deficiency conducted in May of 1991 in Stockholm, Sweden, the following features of adult GH deficiency were highlighted: Increased cardiovascular mortality, abnormal body fat, dehydration, low bone density, and impaired physical performance, and the following benefits of GH therapy were cited: muscle/fat ratio consistently improved, reduction of body fat observed, fluid balance restored, bone density increased, and exercise capacity improved.

On July 18, 1995, The New York Times published an article in the Science Times segment announcing: "Restoring Ebbing Hormones May Slow Down Aging." The article stated that "Growth hormone therapy may help people stay stronger and leaner."

In his book, *Turning Back The Aging Clock*, Lord Lee-Benner, M.D. discusses the possibility of stimulating the release of our own body's growth hormone through supplementation of certain amino acids such as L-ornithine,

L-phenylalanine, and L-tyrosine. (Flashback—remember *Life Extensions* by Dirk Pearson and Sandy Shaw?) Dr. Lee-Benner also has a program through his "World Health Foundation" where he monitors blood levels and prescribes a full spectrum Hormone Replacement Therapy (which includes synthetic growth hormone, and DHEA—see, *Appendix H*).

When I attended The American College Of Sports Medicine Conference in 1996, I heard some very interesting discussions (debates) on whether to connect "youth enhancement" observations to the increased presence of growth hormone, or to another hormone—DHEA.

DHEA

DHEA is short for dehydroepiandrosterone, a hormone made by the adrenal glands. The levels of this hormone (like growth hormone) also declines as we age.

DHEA is the precursor to androgens and estrogens. In his book, *DHEA— A Practical Guide*, Ray Sahelian, M.D. tells us that; "It is thought that at least half of the androgen and estrogen precursors in our body comes from the adrenal glands' DHEA. The rest are made in the testicles and ovaries. After menopause, when the ovaries are practically no longer functioning, 100% of the estrogen precursors come from the adrenal glands' DHEA." In his book, Dr. Sahalian presents a series of arguments and observations on the replacement of DHEA. Dr. Mortola, from the Department of Reproductive Endocrinology at Beth Israel Hospital and Harvard Medical School, is quoted as saying: "I'm only speculating, but if women are on estrogen replacement therapy and they want to add DHEA, they can probably decrease the estrogen dose by half."

Dr. Sahalian's book cites numerous studies on the impact of DHEA therapy. Among some of the findings are the following: Enhanced tissue insulin sensitivity, increased bone density, and body fat reduction. In addition, many of the doctors quoted in *DHEA—A Practical Guide* report satisfaction with their patients' results on DHEA therapy. Other doctors are not as enthusiastic, recommending caution and further investigation.

If you are interested in exploring the possible benefits of DHEA supplementation for yourself, I urge you to consult your doctor, and get your DHEA levels tested. Based on your evaluation, you can discuss the effective forms, the appropriate dosage, and the proper time to take DHEA (I've read that it should be taken both *with* food—and *without* food, and that it should be taken in the morning to follow the normal circadian rhythm). But—in any event—DHEA supplementation should not be taken *lightly*.

Pregnenolone

This hormone is a very important player in the "hormonal orchestra." According to William Regelson, M.D. and Carol Colman in *The Superhormone Promise*, "Pregnenolone is a superhormone that is key to keeping our brains functioning at peak capacity." Along with improving memory and mental function, it is said to enhance our performance abilities and increase our feelings of well being.

Like the other steroid hormones, DHEA, testosterone, and estrogen, pregnenolone is synthesized from cholesterol. *Cholesterol?* Right. While having too much cholesterol puts you at higher risk for heart disease, having too little may be dangerous. (Dr. Barnard in *Live Longer, Live Better* recommends that you keep your cholesterol level at 150.) Your body makes cholesterol. Simply put—you cannot live without cholesterol. Dr. Regelson and Ms. Colman write: "Cholesterol is a critical component in the production of steroid hormones. In a complex series of steps, cholesterol is broken down into different steroid hormones as the body needs them. It is first synthesized into pregnenolone and used by the body in that form. What is not utilized undergoes a chemical change that 'repackages' it into DHEA. DHEA, in turn, is used by the body as DHEA and is also broken down into estrogen and testosterone. This chain of hormones is known as the "steroid pathway." Because pregnenolone gives birth to the other hormones, it is sometimes referred to as the 'parent hormone,' which is probably the origin of its odd-sounding name.

Pregnenolone is produced both in the brain and in the adrenal cortex, the glands that sit above the kidneys. Like the other superhormones, pregnenolone production declines with age. By the time we are seventy-five, we are making 60 percent less pregnenolone than we did in our thirties. As our pregnenolone production drops, so does production of the other hormones in the steroid pathway. Pregnenolone provides the raw materials for these other hormones, and as levels of pregnenolone decline, so will the levels of the other hormones that are made from it."

Recently, pregnenolone (like DHEA) was made available over the counter in health food stores.

Melatonin

Not too long ago we all heard about this "linchpin" hormone and the studies that concluded the following: Melatonin "extends life, maintains youthful health and vigor, enhances sexual vitality, strengthens immune system, is a potent anti-oxidant, protects against stress, protects against cancer, prevents heart disease, restores normal sleep patterns, cures jet lag."

Quite a list. No wonder health food stores could barely keep jars of the stuff in stock. Everyone rushed out to buy another miracle in a pill.

This is not to say, however, that the research on melatonin and the other "superhormones" was not (and does not <u>continue</u> to be) very exciting. Obviously, I am personally following it very closely (and will continue to keep you updated on all that I learn about this and other compelling issues in my newsletters). There are many claims that make supplementing melatonin a very tempting option. In their book, *The Melatonin Miracle*, Walter Pierpaoli, M.D., Ph.D., William Regelson. M.D., and Carol Colman write that their experiments with Melatonin demonstrated that it is possible not only to "halt the downward spiral that far too many of us have come to accept as a normal part of aging, but also to actually extend the length and to improve the quality of our lives." They also say that one of their goals in writing *The Melatonin Miracle* was to "focus public attention on melatonin and the aging clock and to encourage other research organizations to undertake studies of this superhormone."

Okay. As you have read so far, each of our hormones functions in its own way to keep our bodies "resilient and strong." According to the distinguished doctors and scientists that I have cited, by restoring these hormones to their peak levels, we can "preserve the proper functioning of these rejuvenating agents." According to the authors of *The Melatonin Miracle*, however, there is only one hormone that can actually reverse aging by "resetting the body's aging clock"—Melatonin.

The hormone melatonin is released by the pineal gland, a "pea-sized structure" located deep within the brain. It is here where instructions are issued to the body telling it how and when to age. Just about all of our vital functions (including production of other hormones) are controlled by the pineal gland. The book *The Superhormone Promise* explains that "when the pineal begins to run down, so do all the systems under its control. Melatonin is a buffer hormone because, unlike other hormones that target and directly affect specific organs, it operates indirectly to affect all organ systems. Its job is to maintain homeostasis (or balance of the body) and thereby help the other hormones do their job more efficiently. About the age of forty-five, when our aging clock strikes middle age, melatonin levels begin their steepest decline, and the pineal gland itself begins to shrink and lose the cells that produce melatonin. Production of melatonin becomes erratic, and our nighttime melatonin peaks are not as high as they once were. By age sixty, we produce half the amount of melatonin that we produced in our twenties. And once we lose the ability to properly cycle melatonin, we begin 'aging' in the bad sense of the word. The drop in melatonin alerts the other glands and organ systems of the body that the time has come to wind down. In women, the ovaries stop functioning, levels of estrogen drop, and women enter menopause."

The chapter on Melatonin in *The Superhormone Promise* highlights how Melatonin can: *Enhance The Immune System, Restore Thymus Function, Strengthen Antibody Response, Fight Viruses, Block The Damage Caused By Stress, Be Used As A Cancer Treatment, Protect Against Heart Disease, and Be An Effective Sleep Aid.* This book offers advice on how to take Melatonin, but it also mentions that salivary testing has recently become available (check *Appendix J*) that will provide you with a more precise measurement of your melatonin levels. *I strongly urge testing before you take any supplements of this magnitude.*

CAUTION! DO NOT STOP READING NOW!

What, what, what ?

Before you pick up your keys and head to your car (armed with your little shopping list of new miracles), please read the following urgent message:

If you have paid attention so far, please do not tune out on me now. Listen. *Do not just run out and start taking all of this stuff!* Remember your Jigsaw Puzzle! Remember *my* journey! You have to learn what your needs are, what you are deficient in what your current hormone levels are before you start playing chemist and administering your own uneducated and potentially dangerous version of a "Superhormone Cocktail." Remember that I have undergone numerous tests. I knew what all of my hormone levels were before I began experimenting in this arena. And I continue to have them monitored to stay on track.

You must follow a similar course before you run to the store to buy some of the over-the counter products that are still available. I say *still* available because as I write this, the FDA is considering pulling (among other products) DHEA, and making it available by prescription only. They are doing this because people are just popping DHEA pills without discerning whether or not they need additional DHEA. Some of the noticeable side effects of this irresponsible self-diagnosing and prescribing are; facial hair and other masculinization in women, and developed breast tissue in men. Oops.

Careful, my friends. In *PUTTING IT ALL TOGETHER*, Dr. Gary and I begin your journey into the realm of "self-identification." None of this should be approached arbitrarily—not what you eat, how you need to exercise, and certainly not what hormones you should be supplementing. If you are a candidate for any type of hormone replacement, the tests that we recommend will let you know.

Thank you for your attention. Now, if you want to go shopping, I'm sure you could use some organic produce.

CHRONOLOGICAL AGE VERSUS BIOLOGICAL AGE

"Decreases and losses are odd things because much depends on how we perceive them. With age our skin may lose its smoothness and 'acquire' wrinkles. From the standpoint of the major function of skin, which is to enclose our organs and protect us from the environment, it matters little whether our skin is wrinkled or smooth. Wrinkled skin is not unhealthy skin, but we are taught to believe that smooth skin is preferable. A pessimist might say that with time the skin loses its smoothness; an optimist might say it gains wrinkles. The pessimist sees the change as negative, and calls it a loss; the optimist sees it as an affirmative and calls it a gain. Same change, different viewpoint. If we acquire wisdom with age, that is surely a gain."

—Leonard Hayflick, Ph.D.
How And Why We Age

What is aging? Is it the passing of "time?" Or, would a more accurate definition be "the clear indication of biological modifications that occur with the passage of time?" How good are you at guessing someone's age? Personally, I hate that game. I think it belongs in a carnival right along side the "guess your weight" booth. People love to introduce me to others with the inevitable "guess how old she is!" This makes everyone clearly uncomfortable. The new acquaintance peers at me just knowing there is something unusual here, but I can tell that they are thinking; "Either she is very, very young and extremely accomplished for this very, very young age (but she looks older) or, she is very, very old but she looks really, really good (for her age). I save them the agony of a 50-50 chance of being embarrassed, and blurt out my age. "Wow. You look really good!" "Thank you."

Dr. Hayflick, in his book, *How And Why We Age*, tells us that: "Subjective determination based on appearances are frequently wrong and, more importantly, age in years <u>does not directly correlate with biological age</u>. We all age biologically at different rates. Unlike the passage of time, biological aging, sometimes called functional aging, defies easy measurement."

It really all comes back to individuality. There are too many variables between people for us to make blanket statements about aging. Dr. Haflick compares the phenomenon of aging to a clock shop: "Each of our many tissues and organs behaves like an independent clock ticking at a rate different from that of the others. Because of this, a person of a given chronological age could be considerably younger or older biologically, depending on the average of how quickly or slowly all his or her clocks are ticking."

Did you know that technically you are a *younger* on a cellular level with each birthday? Therefore, when we celebrate a number on our birthdays, what does this number actually represent? Dr. Hayflick puts it this way: "Ordinarily we think not about the aging of our cells, but rather about how we relate to our family and friends or to what we perceive that society expects of someone our age. But if you say figuratively that you are not the same person you were five or ten years ago, you are quite literally right. All of us are composed of billions of individual cells and the products that cells make. Most of the cells present in our body today were not present five or ten years ago. In fact, some were not present yesterday. If many of your cells turn over in less than ten years, then how old are you, really? After all, the cells that turned over during the last ten years are gone and new ones may have replaced them several times, so your present cells may be younger than the cells that were present a decade ago." In fact, some people are actually biologically younger than their children!

As far as the subject of Hormone Replacement Therapy goes, Dr. Hayflick brings up an interesting point in his book. "We could seek to elevate our serum levels of certain hormones in an effort to retard the impact of aging, but what of the receptors on cells that receive these hormones?" Dr. Hayflick says: "The secretion of many hormones—including testosterone, insulin, androgens, aldosterone, and thyroid and growth hormones—has been found to decrease with normal aging. To complicate the picture, hormones act by first attaching to a receptor on their target cells; experimentation has shown that these receptors also frequently decline in numbers or efficiency with age. It is therefore possible that changes that have been attributed to decreases in hormone production are really due to decreases in the ability of target cells to respond to hormones."

"Siempre Viva?"

Let's face it. Chronologically, we are all getting older. But, do we have to age? And, if we do, how much of aging is a matter of applying *science*, or *attitude*?

As far as *science*, I am still intrigued and cautiously optimistic that we can evaluate and control certain aspects of the aging process. I don't want to put a damper on your excitement, but please hear me as I say (once again) that the importance of testing and professional evaluation in this arena *cannot be overstated.*

All that I have written here is admittedly seductive. How many of us would opt for "The Dark Gift," a "Siempre Viva" potion, a "Deal With The Devil" and "damn the torpedoes?" But, my friends, remember that this is not a game—this is your body, and it is your responsibility to treat it with respect. Yes, the prospects are thrilling, but take a deep breath, count to ten, consider all I have said, and arm yourself with knowledge before you proceed.

As far as *attitude*, I believe it has a lot to do with this. I have a very young attitude. In fact, it's been said that it is an *inappropriately* young attitude. Oh well. But, that's me. To be honest, there are signs of aging on me. Every morning, when I look into the magnifying mirror that I now need to use to put on my makeup, I see the reminders of the time I have logged on this planet. In my walk through life, however, I am perceived as a much younger person. It is the character of that walk—the youthful character—that has a lot to do with this perception. I move like a young person. I have boundless energy (because I exercise), I have a youthful physique (also because I exercise!), and I am usually optimistic and idealistic—very child-like qualities. I dress young, I don't wear "sensible" shoes, or a hairstyle that is "suitable" for a "woman my age." I don't say things like "In my day," or, "When I was your age." And, I know that I am growing, not declining—that I am better than I've ever been, but not as good as I will be—and, that I am a *force to be reckoned with.*

WHAT IS AGING GRACEFULLY?

Tough question. And, I think the answer is an individual one. We all want to look as good as we can, for as long as we can, but I think for each of us the degree of intervention will vary. Personally, I think it's a tough break to have come all this distance in life only to look in the mirror and go "yuck." Something is wrong with that.

So, what about plastic surgery? I wanted to briefly discuss this option here, not because I advocate it, but because it's out there big time, and there is a tremendous amount to learn about it. We, as a society, have adopted a very cavalier attitude towards plastic surgery. It is considered normal. Ah, but is it *natural*? Well, if you believe that technology is evolving *naturally*, then I suppose you could make a case for a "yes" to that question. No, I have not yet had a facelift, and people are always looking for the scars. (Exercise is a "fountain of youth," not just for your body, but your face as well—trust me.) But, my take on the plastic surgery issue is I believe that it's fine to extinguish the marks of time, as long as your face goes with your body. And, I also believe that it's fine to want your outside to reflect your inside.

Inside me resides a very young person.

In researching this subject, I read a very interesting book called, *The Youth Corridor*, written by Dr. Gerald Imber. Dr. Imber is a renowned plastic surgeon, but he presents a program in his book that includes diet, exercise, and supplementation to slow down the aging process. He says that if you start making lifestyle changes early enough, you can control "aging accelerators." His routines include some aggressive skin-care regimens, and the following general rules: "1. **Don't Smoke**—it reduces blood flow to the skin, resulting in a decrease in nutrients and oxygen, and an oxidation and denaturing of collagen. 2. **Don't Gain And Lose Weight**—this avoids stretching and laxity of skin, and at some point, we can no longer get away with this. 3. **Don't Get Too Thin**—there is nothing attractive about the look of anorexia, and besides, normal subcutaneous fat plumps out wrinkles and helps skin look and feel healthy. 4. **Don't Run**—the constant rising and pounding down lifts and pulls the facial skin away from underlying muscles and bone. 5. **Facial Exercises Are A Wrinkle Workout! Don't Do Them!** 6. **Avoid The Sun**—this is the primary accelerator of the breakdown of collagen and elastic fiber, causing loosening and wrinkling of the skin. 7. **Change Your Diet!**—anyone old enough to be interested in this book has been nurtured on overindulging in an unhealthy pattern devised for us by authority figures and condoned by government. 8. **Understand Antioxidants and Free Radicals**—various activities, as well as environment, have been shown to increase the presence of protein denaturing, destructive, oxygen free radicals. Along with the knowledge of the destructive capability of free radicals is the knowledge that they are products of normal metabolism, and are normally neutralized by antioxidant enzymes and diet-derived antioxidants."

Of course, Dr. Imber does discuss in detail the many procedures that are available, should you be considering this course of action. But, I found his thoughts on the "normal" versus "natural" aging process compelling. The following is an excerpt from his book:

"'When did all this happen? What do I do now?'

That question, and the frustration that accompanies it, provide much of the impetus for this book. For anyone who reads fashion magazines, or discusses the subject with friends, the bottom line is simple: Once the damage has been done, nothing short of surgery can restore what has been lost. And even then, the ravages of time cannot be fully undone. Worst of all, so many good years have been spent helplessly watching the changes add up, instead of fighting back. It's frustrating, it's annoying, and yet we simply write it off as the legacy of genetics and the effects of time. There seems nothing worth doing but to grind our teeth and wait for things to get worse. But is that really true?

It seemed to me that there had to be a better strategy than watching the horse leave the barn before closing the door. But what to do. I was fully aware of the problem; and the solutions, such as they were, were purely surgical, and aimed at correcting accumulated damage. A case of too much, too late. Or perhaps of appropriate therapy for the stage of aging confronted. Ideally, we would like to alter the speed at which these changes occur, if not prevent them completely. The concept of controlling the signs of aging, if not the process itself, became an issue to which I have devoted a great deal of my professional interest and energies. Some years ago, when I first began to question the conventional approach, I was particularly struck by the absence of treatment options for early changes in younger people, and by the attitude among colleagues that these early changes weren't worth dealing with. It made no sense. If we were going to influence the eventual outcome, the earlier we become involved, the better. Attention must be paid to caring for and preventing the earliest signs of aging, preventing wrinkles, not just curing them, and not solely to reversing the established signs of middle-age. Couldn't we rearrange the way we apply our knowledge to the problems of aging? Couldn't we use what we know of anatomy, surgery, medicine, and the chemistry of skin care to help maintain vigorous, good looks, instead of sitting around helplessly watching youthfulness slip away?

How wonderful if people could maintain their youthful appearance throughout adulthood and middle age. Quality of life counts, and when one has reached a stage of confidence and achievement, why not welcome it looking as good as you feel?"

Amen.

IT'S THE LITTLE THINGS

I have a very beautiful friend who is a doctor. Her name is Helene Friedberg, M.D. She is French. She is fascinating. She is full of "joie de vivre." I cannot believe her energy, her commitment to her work, to her son, and to our community. Where she finds the time to do all that she does is beyond me. She is confident and sexy. She is 42 years old, and when she walks into a room, all eyes are on her, all ears are tuned to her voice. She has a great attitude. She has a great accent.

Helene is a board-certified physician (internal medicine) and award-winning artist. She gave up a very successful internal medicine practice in 1992 to specialize in beauty enhancement and facial rejuvenation of women. The following is how we met:

I am a *fanatic* about makeup application. I am a perfectionist. And so, when I accent my mouth, I am extremely precise. One day I was asked, "Are those Dr. Friedberg's lips?" "No," I replied. "They are mine." Duh. Anyway, I learned that Helene did extraordinary permanent makeup and my work resembled hers. Well, the thought of not having to apply lip stuff 50 times a day to feel good about the way I looked really appealed to me. Long story short—I became a client of Helene's, and she of mine. Kiss me. My mouth does not smudge, or worse—disappear. As we age our lips become thinner (as our hips become fatter—if only that were reversed). Helene's procedure gives the illusion of a fuller mouth—permanently. She also does many other beauty enhancement procedures that are subtle, non-invasive ways of giving your self-esteem a little boost. There is nothing wrong with looking in the mirror and feeling better about your reflection. It's healthy. It builds a positive attitude. It may motivate you to pursue working on your body if you like your face. I asked Helene her opinion based on her experience with hundreds of women seeking to feel better about themselves. The following is our conversation:

. "Helene, why did you give up a successful practice to go into, well, beauty?"

"Because, first, I was unfulfilled with my life as an internist. It lacked creativity and I was a slave of my work. Second, I love beauty and always have. When I was a teenager I used to apply makeup on my mother, my sister, and my friends, and everyone thought I was great."

"What is your opinion on our society's preoccupation with youth and beauty?"

"I used to think it was very vain, and a very materialistic preoccupation. Unfortunately, we live in a very material world, where people judge us on our appearance first, like it or not. By making the most of our health and our appearance, not only do we feel better within ourselves, but within society as well. It has an enormous impact on our self-esteem."

"Do you believe it is healthy emotionally and mentally for a woman to augment her appearance with procedures such as yours, or even surgery?"

"I believe in balance in everything. If a woman truly has an easily correctable 'handicap,' and she has a complex about it, then there is nothing wrong with doing something about it."

"Do you feel that acceptance of the aging process is natural for a woman, or difficult?"

"Most women have a hard time with it, which is too bad. One should embrace fully each part of our life as a precious gift, and honor the One who gave us such precious gifts by making the most of ourselves, being the best we can be, and enjoy it!"

"In your experience, Helene, have the changes you have made for women's faces also facilitated a change in their attitudes?"

"Absolutely. A lot of my patients tell me, 'Dr. Friedberg, this is the best thing I have ever done for myself.' Not only do they look better, but their confidence is greatly enhanced. They move about differently in life. They feel 'attractive,' and so they are perceived as such. We all like that."

"What is the typical age group of your patients?"

"Anywhere between 25 to 85, with most of them 'baby boomers' in their 40's and 50's.

Donna, tell your people to enjoy life. Have a little 'lift' if it suits them. Just do not go overboard. Respect your gift. Moderation, balance, and love—above all, in everything you do. You must love yourself as you are, and proceed from there."

I love my lips.

Helene's practice is in Fort Lauderdale (see, *Appendix H*).

SLEEPING BEAUTY...THE SLEEP FACTOR
Don't Wake Me Before Eight (Hours Sleep, That Is)

"Rest is the unassailable beauty remedy. "
—Catherine Deneuve

Catherine Deneuve is one of the most beautiful women in the world. She is in her 50's. When questioned about her beauty secrets, she said, "I try to respect my basic needs—eight hours of sleep at a minimum."

Doctors all concur that sleep is a restorative process. I know I need eight hours of sleep to look and feel my best.

Sleep is acknowledged to be an effective healer for anything from the flu to depression. It boosts your immune system and it makes you feel better.

And we now have research that indicates it can make you look better as well.

Why have we been designed to spend nearly one-third of our lives in a practically unconscious state? It doesn't seem right, does it? Life is too short as it is. We are always looking to shorten the time we sleep, to have more *time*. But consider that there is a purpose to <u>this</u> aspect of living, just as there is a purpose to all of the others. The quality of your waking life will be seriously impaired if you do not get enough sleep. When we are sleeping, our bodies are nearly as busy as when we are awake. This part of the cycle must be effective for the <u>other</u> part to be effective. This is when we regroup, rebuild, restore, and release that wonderful Growth Hormone.

Dr. Paul Galbraith, a British chiropractor, writes in his book, *Reversing*

Aging: "Sleep is essential for the rejuvenation of every cell in the body. It is especially important for the rest and rejuvenation of the nervous system, including the brain. This is because the nervous system controls and coordinates all the other systems of the body, such as the digestive system, glandular system, immune system, and reproductive system. During sleep, nature restores and heals the body by eliminating toxins, tissue rebuilding, the replenishing of enzymes, and so on. The mind is given rest, and stress is released. In short, you recharge the batteries."

How much sleep do we need? Dr. Galbraith tells us that the average adult requires between seven and nine hours a day (children need more sleep, while people over 60 need less). He also tells us that the most natural and effective sleep occurs between the hours of 10pm and 6am, and that sleep must be deep and unbroken to attain *maximum rejuvenation.*

Dr. Galbraith continues: "Natural deep sleep depends upon the integrity of the sleep center in the brain." And the integrity of the sleep center depends on the health of your whole body. Good nutrition, eliminating sugar and other refined and processed foods, avoiding caffeine and alcohol at night, and exercise all support the sleep center. Also, try not to drink too much at night, as you will need to get up to go to the bathroom and disturb the sleep cycle.

Bottom line, my friend—you <u>will</u> look younger (and feel better) if you get enough sleep.

BEAUTY SCHOOL DROPOUT...HOW DO WE STAY MOTIVATED?

"The 'Power Zone' is not an every day thing—at least not for me. Despite its charms and mystery, it isn't what keeps me training. It's not even my greatest joy. I honestly find more pleasure in the ordinary magic of day-to-day practice. I like mundane reality, pushing through PMS, traffic jams, rainy days and my own mental and emotional short-comings, into the simple majesty of a humbling workout and doing my best for today."

—Karen Andes
A Woman's Book Of Strength

First, let's acknowledge that you are in a highly motivated state right now because you are reading this book. But how do you stay here?

Allow me to give you some extremely non-patronizing encouragement. I have trained (or supervised the training of) hundreds of women in my years as a fitness professional. Some of them worked out with me for years. "Oh sure," you say, "If I could afford a trainer I'd probably stick with exercise for years too."

Okay. I knew you'd say that. So, I investigated how many of my former clients have stayed with some type of exercise after they stopped training with me. Get this—better than 75%. Not only that, but several of them went back to school and became trainers themselves. Now, that really excites me. They were so inspired by their own results that they wanted to share what they found with others. That's exactly how it was for me!

What about my male clients? Well, for the most part they have been powerful, successful, and financially secure individuals. And, for the most part, they came to me out of fear. They created their empires, and it cost them their health. Many of them sought exercise only after a wake-up call (cardiovascular disease, cancer, pulmonary illness, you name it) frightened them into calling me. They desperately wanted to buy some time to enjoy the fruits of their success. This is an entirely different motivation from my female clients. The women in my life, including myself, have been motivated by a desire to be desired...physically. We want to look better than we do. And, we are never satisfied. So, we always want to look better than we do right now. And, there's always tomorrow, and another opportunity for improvement. So much of our self-esteem is woven into our physical selves. We need to address that.

Most successful men that I've met have perceived that their attraction lies in their *success*, and the accouterments of that success. I like "stuff" as much as the next person, but I cannot have a meaningful conversation with a Masaratti (although I wouldn't mind having one in one). My point is, women are moved by a fit male body, just as a male is moved by a fit female body. But, for *some* reason, men are in denial over that.

Okay, guys. Then explain "Chippendales."

Anyway, I really don't want to oversimplify our reasons to exercise. Yes, we are motivated to look better. But, we are also motivated to feel better. How many of us watched our mothers get drawn into the fitness craze by Richard Simmons and ecstatic promises of increased energy and vitality? (Gosh, he does seem to have a lot of energy.) But, what we frequently saw happen was a great commitment out of the box being replaced by complaints of increased fatigue and dubious results not being worth the price. For many of us, exercise competes with other interests and responsibilities. And, there is only so much time in a day. So, to fit it in, many of us wake up earlier, or go to sleep later. We are not weak-willed, undisciplined failures. We are tired. Compound that with the fact that the results of our valiant efforts usually lack drama, and there you have it—we're dropouts. If exercise is punishing rather than reinforcing, why do it? After all, it isn't something we have to do.

I am a classic case. I could never stick with anything. I have the attention span of a gnat. I require instant gratification. I get bored easily. I have lofty expectations and I'm usually disappointed. I set myself up for failure. When I tried sports or some form of exercise when I was younger, it always ended in disaster and humiliation. Talk about negative reinforcement—it became a self-fulfilling prophesy. I expected failure, so I failed. Even when I joined my first health club and tried a combination of stationary bike/sit-up board/leg-lift routines that I devised myself (fitness diva that I was... Duh...clueless), my payoff was nominal. Certainly not worth the time, or the membership. The turning point for me was <u>finally</u> getting the right training. I blasted off.

Only overt drama gets my attention, and only the continuation of that stimulus keeps it. Ask anyone who knows me. This applies to every aspect of my life. I'm almost impossible to please, but for 20 years I have been encouraged and motivated to do what I do every day...*one day at a time.* For 20 years, I have never dropped out. It is as much a part of my life as my grooming rituals. But, just as I make a choice on a daily basis to shave my legs or tweeze my eyebrows, I make a choice to exercise and eat right. It is a constant negotiation with myself. It is something I must choose to do every day. The trick is to celebrate each little daily victory over destructive options. "Just for today I got out of my own way enough to take a step in the direction of my dream. Today I topped what I did yesterday. One day...one moment at a time...to a new me."

Now, I am not saying that it won't be difficult at times. And you will experience setbacks—I won't mislead you. But there are signs you can look for—little red flags that will alert you that you are about to start sandbagging. And once you get into that mode—you know it's quicksand. Quagmired—sucked into the great abyss of lazy-land where the mantra is "Tomorrow is another day." You will find yourself making excuses. You will choose to do *anything* (including cleaning the house) over exercising. You will figure, once you have messed up your eating in the beginning of the day, there is absolutely no sense in working out—this day's a "write-off."

Nuts to all of that. The following is a paragraph that you can stick on your mirror to remind you anew each day of your commitment to yourself:

I am on a mission. I recognize the land mines along the way. I won't let them blast me off course...off purpose. I am connected to my world by a thread from above. I am grateful for the incredible gift of life, and breath in this body. I acknowledge my responsibility to my Creator and myself to keep my body in the best shape that I can. Today I will not procrastinate. I will find time, make time, steal time if I must——to exercise. I deserve to look and feel my best. Nothing less

*will do for me. Starting with the morning light, I choose to eat smart, move vig-
orously, and think positively. I am resolved to be victorious over my demons.
They are no match for this new me.*

—Go girl.

THE EMPOWERMENT...A WOMAN'S VOYAGE HOME

*"True Love begins with yourself. Each day I put forth the effort to take care of
myself, work out, eat healthy food, deal with my feelings and not bury them in a
giant bag of Dorito's, confront people when necessary, tell people the truth, and tell
myself the truth. This has changed my life—I have been freed from my own personal prison. I feel free. Free to live in the moment. When pain, betrayal, judgment,
or adversity come—I can live that too. I can face it straight up and know that it,
too, shall pass—every moment does."*

—Oprah Winfrey
Make The Connection

Do you know that "being in the moment" is something we are born with, and
with time we "unlearn" it? Psychologists say this process occurs around the
age of five. Up until this age, we are spontaneous and creative. We have
unbridled curiosity and enthusiasm, and challenging attention spans. Then,
routine takes over our lives. We go to school. Clocks abruptly intrude on our
worlds. We have to consider agendas, schedules, and *what people think*.
Suddenly, we worry how we are perceived. We do not want to wear that outfit because we were picked on the last time we wore it. Our thoughts are no
longer in the moment, but bounce from the past to the future.

We get a little older, and with adolescence, self-esteem drops dramatically. We are really a mess around the ages of twelve and thirteen. Hormones are
surging. We look strange. Most of us are no longer "cute." The difference
between a nine-year-old girl and a twelve-year-old girl is profound. We
become "young ladies" and we are told our behavior is not "lady-like." We
don't know how to act anymore.

I remember how painful my adolescence was. While the rest of the twelve-
year-old girls in my class were showing up at school sporting their new bras,
I was still in an undershirt. I *begged* my mother for a bra. "But, you don't *need*
one," she'd reply. Oh Lord, school was agony for me in those days. Not grad-
uating to a bra meant not being initiated into "The Bunny Rabbit Association"
(where the ritual was snapping your bra strap in class—signaling to all of the
boys that you have "come of age"). Staying in an undershirt meant staying a
"little girl," not becoming a "woman" like my classmates. So, of course, that
meant being ostracized. On top of <u>that</u> misery, I also was not allowed to

shave my legs. Hormones may have skipped over my breasts, but not the hair on my legs. I was met with daily chants of "Dirty Knees Donna" at school. None of the "cool" kids would talk to me. I was a geek, and banished to geeksville with the other school geeks.

This is when I began my "parking lot transformation." Using my allowance, I bought the required accessories of a "popular" girl of the day— pointed white Keds sneakers (polished even whiter), black nylons, a bra, and makeup. I would leave the house looking as I should—pleated skirt below my knees, undershirt and blouse, socks and *saddleshoes*. (Does it get any geekier?) Then, in the school parking lot, I would transform myself from child geek to grownup "Hitter Chick." I hiked up my skirt to way above my knees, replaced the undershirt with a bra, replaced the saddleshoes and socks with the black stockings and impossibly white sneakers, ratted my hair into the appropriately tortured style, and applied eyeliner and white lipstick (remember that look?). I even managed to shave my legs before I left the house, which (mercifully) escaped the notice of my busy, stressed-out Mom. The first day of my transformation resulted in being accepted by "all the right people." I, who had finally "gotten with it," became a part of the coveted "Hitter" crowd. I performed this little transformation behind cars in that parking lot until the end of junior high.

(Establishing a little pattern for life, do you think?)

Dr. Christine Northrup has said, "One of the ways you create health is to look at yourself and all the parts you don't like and say 'I accept myself unconditionally right now.' And it works. You don't actually have to like what you see, and you can love it."

The Model's Project

As I mentioned in *The Roller-Coaster Ride From Hell*, Twiggy was the standard of beauty when I was young. I would have to have a "near-death experience" to come even close. Well, unfortunately, nothing's changed for the young girls of today. Statistics show that girls as young as <u>eight</u> are beginning to obsess about their weight. We are all still looking at our impossible role models...models. But, in many cases, being a model and achieving that anorexic aesthetic requires just that...an eating disorder.

A few years ago I began a project that got some national attention. At the time I had my office on South Beach, and I decided that the modeling community there needed to get healthy. I knew they were trading in their health for a fleeting moment in magazines, and I wanted to educate them on how they could be slim while honoring their bodies' needs. I interviewed over

100 models, and every one of them had the same comment: "I'm starving!" Most of them lived on coffee and cigarettes and one sorry meal at the end of the day that was mostly junk. They were nutritionally bankrupt.

These are the women America worships. We are miserable trying to look like them—and the truth is <u>they</u> are miserable trying to look like them.

I chose six girls. I taught them nutrition—healthy alternatives to their current lifestyle that would keep them lean, give them energy, and secure their positions on the covers of magazines. I developed a circuit that was non-threatening (guaranteed not to "bulk them up"—models are terrified of "muscle"). I trained them, taught them boxing and other fun conditioning events, and actually made some changes. They lost body fat (yes, they had body fat to lose—models are usually "skinny fat people") and toned up, while increasing their energy.

After the news and magazine articles appeared, I received letters from distraught mothers of models from around the country asking for help. They described the nightmare of having a beautiful young daughter (some as young as 13) being ravaged by an eating disorder—just to keep working in the industry. What are we doing to our children, America???

Models are beautiful, though...I must admit. Most of them have superior genetics. I know what it takes (now), but I used to really envy them when I was younger. It wasn't until I entered my thirties that I finally began the agonizing process of *learning to love myself*. But, even still, I catch myself being manipulated by the current notions of "beauty." Just when I think I'm looking pretty good, I'll walk behind the inevitable row of tiny young butts doing the "Stairmaster Rhumba" at the gym, and I have to fight the impulse to be discouraged, and be thankful for the blessings that I have. I am the best I can be, and it's all been worth the work, the discipline, and the sweat—but, I am here to tell you that being fit is a <u>part</u> of *who I am* —it is not *all I am*. It's the part I know best, granted, but I am discovering that it is a very *tiny* part of <u>me.</u> As I pass 50, I realize that it's probably a good thing that I'm finding a new perspective. I may not be "middle-aged," but I am a grown-up. And, I can do anything I want.

Let's face it, my friend. We are here. Another stage of life—that is both normal and natural. How we view it will affect how it treats us. In *What Your Doctor May Not Tell you About Premenopause*, we read: "It's easy to believe that you're immortal up to your mid-thirties or mid-forties, when the evidence is piling on that aging is in process. But, if you take care of yourself now, your aging process will happen later in life and will be more gradual and less debilitating. If you do your best to maintain your physical, mental, and emotional balance through the midcycle of your life, aging will be more graceful and less painful." Dr. Hanley puts it this way: "I like to call the process of a woman moving from her premenopausal years into her menopausal years 'wisening.' When you're wisened, you're in a position to say, 'My dears, now that I know I have options, and I can see there are twenty-five different ways to do this, to hell with that one.' What we're able to do in those wisening years a twenty-one-year-old could not do, regardless of how savvy she is. A younger woman does not have the distance, the perspective, the bangs, the bruises, the experience, the emotions, and the objectivity that a forty-year-old has to evaluate, discriminate, and make decisions."

"When I hear myself saying, 'if only this, if only that, I might have been,' I stop listening to that voice and direct myself to take an action toward my desire."

—Maureen Brady
Mid-life—Meditations For Women

CHAPTER VII

EATING FOR HEALTH, HEALING, AND HARMONY

MACROBIOTICS IN PERSPECTIVE

MACROBIOTICS IS NOT A CURE-ALL.

Nothing is.

Any healer who tells you that his methods will absolutely cure your symptoms is a fool. If you believe him, you're a greater fool.

Symptoms come and go.

But real healing happens when we dare to breathe in the universe, stretching both body and soul to reach for balance and truth.

Everybody has minor symptoms. Aches and pains, tension, upset stomachs, headaches, skin eruptions, mood swings, occasional colds and flu.

A self-healing lifestyle starts with recognizing that minor symptoms don't just happen to us. We have an active hand in creating them, by the choices we make in our daily lives.

How we exercise, how we cope with stress, what we eat. All of these contribute to our bodies' natural ability to maintain equilibrium and health. Especially how we eat.

But the truth is, most of us don't want to make changes in our diets, just for the sake of healing minor symptoms...unless they start to happen too frequently. Or, until they escalate into bigger symptoms.

—Kristina Turner

Where are <u>you</u> in this scenario? Are you ready to make changes in your diet? Are you ready to make changes that require thought and planning? Are you ready to make changes that are 180 degrees from the way you are eating now?

If the answer is "yes," then you will be ready to begin your Live It Or Diet Lifestyle System at a higher level.

I love this section of my book. But, if it just doesn't "resonate in your current frequency," leave it and return when it does. Here I am presenting the work of three women I greatly admire: Kristina Turner, Annemarie Colbin, and Judith Lynne. I believe their work takes what I am discussing in this book to another level...one you just may want to investigate. It is powerful, effective, and uplifting.

First of all, there is natural weight loss when you switch to whole, unprocessed foods, even though the calories seem higher. Most Americans are overweight, and they eat a diet that is almost completely void of whole grains. However, 40% of the American diet is comprised of fat, and 20% is comprised of sugar! Unlike high-calorie (disguised as low calorie—read labels—who eats one tiny ounce of anything!) foods loaded with fat and sugar, whole grains are packed with nutrition. They are rich in vitamins and minerals, and they contain protein and fiber. We have already discussed the importance of fiber in the diet for efficient elimination of wastes and disease prevention. It is recommended that we have between 20 and 50 grams of fiber a day. Believe it or not, this is easy to do when you follow a diet of natural, organic, unprocessed foods. However, the typical American manages to go through an entire day without as much as one gram of fiber!

Think about it.

Breakfast: A cup of coffee on the run, maybe some refined carbohydrate like toast or Danish or bagel. Fiber—0.

Lunch: Fast food from a drive-through. Fiber—0.

Dinner: Refined pasta with meat, maybe some vegetables from a can. Fiber—0.

Got problems with your digestive system?

Got problems losing weight?

Try filling your day with whole foods. Your body will balance out and function more efficiently, and you will lose weight naturally.

KRISTINA TURNER

EATING IN HARMONY WITH NATURE

In the past 200 years, since the advent of modern agricultural and food processing techniques, our diet has progressively gotten farther and farther away from natur-

al foods which sustained traditional peoples all over the earth for centuries...primarily whole grains, beans, locally grown vegetables and fruits—and fish, sea vegetables, wild and range-fed animals, and natural condiments.

Instead, we eat mostly from colorful boxes and cans. We spray our vegetables and fruits with deadly chemicals, then we ship them halfway around the world before we eat them. We keep chickens awake with electric lights, and feed them hormones to get them to lay eggs constantly.

It's been a grand experiment in the wonders of technology...
but what a price we are paying in our health!

—Kristina Turner
The Self-Healing Cookbook

The Self Healing Cookbook Recommendations

SELF-HEALING PRINCIPLES:

Principle # 1: Eat in harmony with nature—traditional, whole, unrefined foods with locally(and organically) grown produce.

Principle # 2: Balance natural forces in cooking—warm and cool, heavy and light, wet and dry, hard and soft, salty and sweet, quick and slow, ordinary and inspired.

Principle # 3: Use foods to create desired effects—in your body, in your moods, in yourlife.

WHOLE FOOD SOURCES OF NUTRIENTS:

Complex Carbohydrates: Whole grains, beans, vegetables, fruits

Protein: Beans, meat, poultry, fish, seeds, nuts, whole grains, seaweeds

Fat: Seeds, nuts, oils, beans, fish, tofu, tempeh, oats

Calcium: Dark greens (kale, collards, etc.), soybeans, seaweeds, seeds

Iron: Dark greens, seaweeds, millet, lentil, garbanzo beans, seeds

Vit A: Dark leafy greens, carrots, squashes, seaweeds

B Vitamins: Whole grains, sea vegetables, lentils, fish, fermented foods

Vit B-12: Fish, grain-fed poultry, meat, eggs

Vit C: **Dark greens:** (kale, parsley, broccoli, etc.), local fruits

Vit E: Whole grains, unrefined oils, seeds, leafy greens

Trace Minerals: Sea salt, seaweeds, organic produce

BALANCE

Your body has a natural urge for balance.

All life on earth is busy balancing two complementary/opposite natural forces: **Expansion** and **Contraction** (known in the Orient as Yin and Yang).

To stay in good health, our bodies need to keep both forces in balance.

•Expansive foods fuel: Mental, spiritual, psychological activity, and relaxation. Some expansive foods are: Roots, winter squash, tofu, leafy greens, seeds, local fruits, nuts, potato, tomato, and tropical fruits, spices, and honey.

•Contractive foods fuel: Physical activity, purposefulness, focused work, and tension.

Some contractive foods are: Fish, poultry, cheese, red meat, miso, tamari, eggs, and salt.

Have you noticed that when you eat foods on one extreme (expansive), it often creates cravings for foods on the opposite extreme (contractive) for balance. *The Self-Healing Cookbook* tells us that a steady diet of extreme foods can lead to mood swings, and even serious physical symptoms.

Beans, vegetables, and whole grains fall in the middle, and The Self-Healing Cookbook tells us that a steady diet of these foods renews energy, relieves stress, and prevents illness.

THE FOOD-MOOD CONNECTION

Eating in the extreme throws both your body and moods off balance. One of the easiest ways to evaluate if your diet is too expansive or contractive is to listen to your moods.

•Too Expanded: Too much sugar, chocolate, alcohol, fruit, etc. Can make you feel briefly elated and energized, then—spaced out, confused, forgetful, worried, sad, overly sensitive, no will power.

•Too Contracted: Too much salt, meat, cheese, or eggs can make you feel aggressive and competitive, then—impatient, frustrated, stubborn, resentful, insensitive, compulsive, driven, controlling, angry.

Use food to create desired effects. Most people are unaware of the fact that the kind of food they eat has a direct impact on their ability to accomplish their goals.

If you feel boxed in, tense, and overworked, and you want to feel more creative, intuitive, sensitive, mellow and relaxed—eat less: Salt, meat, eggs, cheese, and hard, baked goods, and eat more "Gently Expansive Foods."

If you feel confused, fatigued, spacy, moody, crave sweets, and susceptible to everything, and you want to feel more focused, assertive, physically active, and down-to-earth—eat less: Sugar and honey, raw food and juice, potato and tomato, and alcohol, and eat more "Mildly Contractive Foods."

TO CLEANSE AND REBUILD

Feeling low energy, overwhelmed, or irritable? Trying to cope by eating unhealthy snacks? Time to pause and take positive steps to renew yourself, before you get sick.

Start by listening closely to recurring signals from your body and moods. These are nature's way of telling you when stressed internal organs need cleansing and rebuilding.

Spleen, Pancreas, and Stomach

Feel scattered, anxious with mood swings—have erratic energy levels, bingeing on sweets, gas, upset stomach, low resistance to infections?

- Foods that stress these organs: Sugar and honey, high fat foods, tropical fruits, juices, food additives.
- Foods that support these organs: Millet and sweet vegetables (turnips, carrots, onions, pumpkin), arame, kombu, miso, occasional local sweet fruit.

Lungs, Large Intestine

Feel sad or depressed, nostalgic, stuck, weary—fatigued, stuffy sinuses, phlegm, gas, constipation, diarrhea, pale complexion?

- Foods that stress these organs: White flour, yeasted breads, high-fat foods, sugar and honey, antibiotics, food color and additives.
- Foods that support these organs: Brown rice and dark leafy greens, roots, winter squash, onion, leek, ginger, garlic, hijiki, wakame, miso soup, apples, pears.

Kidneys, Bladder

Feel overwhelmed, confused, afraid, and insecure—with frequent pale urine or scant dark urine, lower backache, low sexual energy, bags under your eyes, and often feel cold?

- Foods that stress these organs: Ice cold food and drink, milk and dairy foods, too much raw food, sugar and honey, over-salting.
- Foods that support these organs: Brown rice, buckwheat, aduki beans, sturdy greens, roots, winter squash, kombu, hijiki, arame, miso soup, watermelon or berries (in season).

Liver, Gall Bladder

Feel impatient, frustrated, angry, and blocked creatively—with headaches, often overeating, eyes irritated or bloodshot, oily or dry skin, and restless from 11PM to 2AM?

- Foods that stress these organs: Overeating (especially eggs, meat, cheese, and ice cream), alcohol and drugs, chemicalized foods, coffee and chocolate, sugar and honey.
- Foods that support these organs: Barley, quinoa, wheat, rye, daikon, spring

greens, broccoli, cabbage, cauliflower, parsley, wakame, sea palm.

Heart, Small Intestine

Feel over-excitable, can't relax, chronic tension, workaholic—with aching or tense chest, backache between shoulders, high blood pressure, and red complexion?

•**Foods that stress these organs:** All of the above.

•**Foods that support these organs:** Corn, quinoa, pot-boiled brown rice, bitter greens and summer veggies, sea palm, nori, and occasional strawberries and other local fruit.

SLIMMING DOWN GUIDELINES from The Self-Healing Cookbook

1. Emphasize digestible grains: Brown rice, millet, barley, quinoa, or buckwheat. (Minimize oats, they're highest in fat.)

2. Try the following "fat dissolving vegetables": Radish, turnip, onion, leek, shiitake mushroom, or daikon. Eat dark leafy greens 2 to 3 times per day—they are high in minerals and are great for improving metabolism (try kale, bok-choy, collards, turnip greens, watercress, mustard greens, etc.). Eat local fruits in season, but to minimize weight-producing sugars, eat less fruit, more vegetables.

3. Eat low-fat, light-proteins such as beans, fish, and tofu, and minimize meats.

4. Use the following "special cleansing foods": Sea Vegetables (cleanses blood, tones intestines, provides vitamins and minerals to improve metabolism), Burdock Root (cleanses the blood and helps build will-power), and Hato Mugi Barley (a tasty, cleansing grain used in Chinese medicine—use when you feel frustrated, bloated, or sluggish).

THE 5 PHASE THEORY
A 5000-Year-Old System Of Balance

The flow of life. What is that? It is <u>many</u> things. *The 5 Phase Theory* offers an understanding of them as they apply to creating balanced meals. Chinese culture has long incorporated these principals into many arenas of existence.

According to this theory, there are five tastes in the mouth that need to be stimulated for us to have a satisfying meal. Each "taste" targets a different set of organs in the body, and nourishes it. When we incorporate each taste in our meals, we are satiated and nourished. For example: Sweet vegetables like squash and sweet corn nourish the stomach, spleen, and pancreas organs. *The 5 Phase Theory* also describes common foods that weaken corresponding organs and internal balance. For example: <u>White sugar and refined chemical sweeteners weaken the stomach and pancreas.</u>

In *The 5 Phase Theory* we read: "The body will always strive to stay in balance. If it isn't getting enough of the taste that it needs in the form of healthy foods, it will crave the unhealthy foods. For example: Leafy greens are a nourishing food. If one isn't eating enough greens, the body might crave chocolate, coffee, tobacco, or alcohol. By simply choosing healthy foods including bitter leafy greens, sweet vegetables, sharp seasonings, salty condiments, and sour pickles or dressings—we insure that our bodies are satisfied and nourished."

Balance is so important in all aspects of life. Most of us charge through a day without paying attention to what we are putting in our bodies. We don't have the time or the energy to deal with it, and so a day turns into a week turns into a year turns into decades of unhealthy habits. The aging process is accelerated, stimulants are needed for energy, depressants are needed to calm down, *anti*-depressants are needed to cheer up! What in the heck are we thinking about? Certainly not our bodies.

If you didn't already know about this ancient paradigm, I wanted to introduce you to it. If you already know about it, take another look. It is worth the consideration. Annmarie Colbin discusses The 5 Phase Theory in her book, *The Natural Gourmet.*

Annemarie Colbin

Early Chinese philosophers described the world in terms of the movement of energy. Upon emerging from Infinity, energy first split into two opposing forces, Yin and Yang. The energy flow of these two opposite but complementary principles was then further subdivided by points where it changed direction. The Chinese called these points Wood, Fire, Earth, Metal, and Water, and assigned to them various characteristics.

Basically, the idea of the 5 Phase Theory is that balance is attained when energy flows smoothly from one phase to the next, neither blocked nor hastened. Theoretically, we should eat more or less equal amounts from all the phases—about 20% from each, so as to equally nourish the different organ systems and thereby achieve balance.

The ideal is to eat from all phases, so as to allow the energy to move around. A well balanced meal in terms of this system has each phase represented as a major (the principal foodstuff of a dish) or a minor (as a secondary foodstuff or condi-

ment). To plan a balanced meal, choose your main dish (say a whole grain entree) from one of the phases, and then pick beans, vegetables, soup, and dessert from the other phases.

Have fun. It may take you a little while to get used to this system. In fact, you may even ignore it when you first encounter it! I did. However, my students and I have found that it beats every other system when it comes to menu planning and giving zest to your meal.

—Annemarie Colbin
The Natural Gourmet

THE 5 PHASES

WOOD
ORGANS: Liver, Gallbladder
TASTE: Sour
FOODS:

Grains	Vegetables	Fruits	Misc.	Meats/Fish
Barley	Bell Peppers	Avocado	Rice Vinegar	Chicken
Oats	Artichokes	Currants	Umboshi	Chicken Liver
Rye	Lettuce	Grapefruit	Sauerkraut	
Triticale	Parsley	Lemon	Yeast	
Wheat	Rhubarb	Lime		
Quinoa	Swiss Chard	Orange		
Beans	Sorrel	Sour Cherry		
Mung Beans	Sprouts	Kiwi		
Split Peas	Broccoli			
Peanuts	Carrot			
Green Lentils	Green Beans			
Black-eyed Peas				

FIRE
ORGANS: Heart, Small Intestine
TASTE: Bitter
FOODS:

Grains	Vegetables	Nuts & Seeds	Fruits	Meats/Fish
Corn	Red Pepper	Sunflower Seeds	Apricot	Shrimp
Amaranth	Brussels Sprouts	Sesame seeds	Raspberry	Squab
Popcorn	Chicory	Pistachios	Strawberry	Lamb
Beans	Chive		Persimmons	
Red Lentils	Dandelion Root			
	Dandelion Greens			
	Endive			
	Escarole			
	Tomatoes			

FOODS:

VEGETABLES(CONT.)
Collards
Kale
Bok Choy
Snow Peas

EARTH
ORGANS: Stomach, Spleen, Pancreas
TASTE: Sweet
FOODS:

GRAINS	NUTS & SEEDS	SWEETENERS	FRUITS	MEATS/FISH
Millet	Pumpkin Seeds	Rice Syrup	Raisins	Anchovies
Vegetables	Caraway Seeds	Barley Malt	Prunes	Carp
Jerusalem Art.	Almonds	Maple Syrup	Tangerine	Salmon
Eggplant	Filberts	Carob	Cherry	Swordfish
Pumpkin	Pecans	Honey	Grapes	Tuna
Squash:	Pine Nuts	Apple		Pheasant
Acorn	Banana			
Butternut	Dates			
Crookneck				
Hubbard		**MISC.**	**BEANS**	
Spaghetti		Arame	Chickpeas	
Sweet Potato		Kombu		
		Kuzu		

METAL
ORGANS: Lungs, Large Intestine
TASTE: Sharp
FOODS:

GRAINS	VEGETABLES	BEANS	MEATS/FISH	FRUIT
Rice	Cauliflower	Navy Beans	Cod	Pear
Sweet Rice	Cabbage	Soy Beans	Flounder	Peach
	Celeriac	Lima Beans	Haddock	
SPICES	Chinese Cabbage	Northern Beans	Halibut	
Bay Leaf	Cucumber	Tofu	Scrod	
Cordamon	Daikon	Tempeh	Turkey	
Cayenne	Garlic	Beef		
Clove	Ginger			
Coriander	Lotus Root			
Dill	Mustard Greens			
Fennel	Radish			
Horseradish	Potato			
Nutmeg				
Thyme				

WATER
ORGANS: Kidney, Bladder
TASTE: Salty
FOODS:

GRAINS	VEGETABLES	FRUITS	MISC.	MEATS/FISH
Buckwheat	Agar Agar	Blackberry	Salt	Crab
	Beets: Greens	Blueberry	Miso	Clam
BEANS	Burdock	Boysenberry	Shoyu	Lobster
Black Soybeans	Hijiki	Cranberry	Tamari	Duck
Kidney Beans	Shitake Mushrooms		Salty Pickles	
Pinto Beans	Wakame		Tekka	
Aduki Beans	WaterChestnut	**NUTS & SEEDS**	Salty Pickles	
		Black Sesame Seeds	Gomasio	
		Chestnuts		

INCORPORATING MACROBIOTICS AND THE 5 PHASE THEORY

Remember, if this isn't for you (right now), that's okay. It will be here waiting for you when you are ready.

As you already know, there are many other considerations in constructing the blueprint for your Phase I Plan, so you mustn't forget them in working within *Macrobiotic Principles* and *The 5 Phase Theory*. (For example, if you have Candida, you must stay away from yeast and all fermented foods such as vinegar until you are rid of the condition.) Apart from such minor adjustments, constructing meals in this manner will be relatively simple. And, proportionately, the payback is huge. Your cravings will virtually disappear. If you find you have a "need" for alcohol, that too will vanish. The instant you put this food into your mouth, your body will react with a silent but resounding "YES!" You will find your energy increasing, along with your mental acuity. You will sense a strengthening and a power surge through you that you wouldn't think was possible from "just food." This was my experience when Judith Lynne prepared meals for me using these principals. Remember, we have already acknowledged that food is one of the most powerful "drugs" you will ever put into your body. Eat inappropriate foods for you, and your energy will be drained, you will have uncontrollable cravings, and your mind will be in a dense fog. Eat the foods that your body wants and needs, and they will act like "medicine," supporting you and lifting you to a whole new level of wellness. Wow.

JUDITH LYNNE

Judith Lynne is the natural food educator and owner of *Cooking Comes Naturally with Judith Lynne*, in Louisville, Colorado. She teaches introduction to natural food classes and gives store tours for people who want to change from the Standard American Diet (SAD) to whole natural foods. Judith also offers group and private cooking classes to those who want to experience her unique style of teaching, which brings humor and fun into the kitchen. Her practical knowledge comes from 21 years of experience using natural foods to deal with her own special dietary needs and those of her family. Judith has helped many people during their transitions to whole natural foods.

I found Judith through Doc Gary. She counseled his patients on natural cooking, and really impacted his practice. What an addition to our team! Judith has been a great help to me in launching *Live It or Diet Lifestyle Systems* in Fort Lauderdale. She takes our clients shopping, and educates them on natural, healthy alternatives to the foods that are sabotaging them. At our monthly support group meetings, Judith prepares something wonderful for us to sample, and shares quick, easy and delicious recipes that make the passage into another way of thinking about food smoother and a lot more scrumptious! I have asked her to contribute some of her wonderful recipes to this section of the book. I wanted you to experience what it was like to eat this way. Sample these easy recipes—listen to your body—and you will never want to go back to eating sliced turkey rolled up in a piece of lettuce over a sink again!

Introducing...Judith Lynne

COOKING COMES NATURALLY
with Judith Lynne

Welcome to the world of whole natural foods! Shopping in a health food store, or natural food store, might be new for some people. Having worked in natural food stores I understand the concern that a beginner could feel. What are all these new words? What is all this STUFF?

How do I cook it?

What does it taste like?

And...how is it going to make me feel?

These are all valid concerns. Having been through several dietary transitions myself, I have lived all of the questions. And, working in a natural food store, I have heard many people recite the same thing.

It all starts with your attitude. It's actually a lot of fun. If you make it a big deal, it will be. If you make it an exciting adventure, it will be.

It is actually quite simple. Annemarie Colbin states in her book *Food and Healing,* "Whole foods are simply fresh, natural, edible things, as close to their natural state as possible: Fruits, fresh vegetables, unrefined cereal grains, beans, nuts, seeds, sea vegetables. Animals can be eaten whole by one person at one sitting if they're small enough (smelts, oysters, sardines, soft-shell crabs, small fowl), or by a whole group or tribe over a few days' time, as is done by hunting communities. Whole foods provide not only certain amounts of basic nutrients in the natural proportion to each other; the nutrients in them are also bound together by that subtle energy that animates all living systems.

Whole foods, then, give us not only nutrition, but energy—'wholesomeness,' that is."

We have all heard the phrase "garbage in-garbage out." Change it to "wholeness in-wholeness out." We become more of a whole person when we begin to ingest whole, natural foods. Our emotions begin to calm down, and we could possibly even become more patient with our fellow man. When we are properly nourished it touches us emotionally, mentally, physically and spiritually. It is all connected and it all starts with what you do or don't put in your mouth.

So, are you ready to start your adventure? Before we begin with my simple, quick recipes, it's best that we deal with at least one of those questions: "What is all this stuff?" Let's start with a glossary of ingredients.

Knowledge is power!

Aduki beans: A small red bean with a slightly sweet flavor that is said to be beneficial for kidneys in the Oriental traditions.

Agar agar: A sea vegetable that is a natural gelling agent. The vegetarian alternative to gelatins.

Bragg Liquid Aminos: A brand name for a non-fermented soy sauce.

Brown rice syrup: A hypoallergenic moderate sweetener that won't overpower the foods with which it is used. It is a slow digesting complex carbohydrate sweetener that doesn't affect the blood sugar like refined sugar does.

Burdock: A long, thin, firm root vegetable that supplies many minerals, purifies the blood, tones and strengthens intestines, and it's alkalinizing to your system.

Ginger: A fibrous root that can be grated, chopped or made into a tea. It's best used to settle stomachs and stimulate blood circulation. Ginger is also a good source of minerals, such as calcium. Ginger juice is made by grating the root and squeezing the pulp.

Great northern beans: A white bean that is relatively high in protein and fiber.

Kale: A hearty green leafy vegetable that contains large amounts of vitamins and minerals. It provides the bitter taste that some people feel those that crave sweets are lacking. (In other words, if you are constantly craving sweets, try giving your mouth some bitter greens!)

Kamut: A whole grain that is an ancient Egyptian wheat. Many wheat sensitive people can eat it without a reaction. (I find it sweeter than spelt, another whole grain that is similar to wheat.)

Kombu: A sea vegetable that is high in minerals and is used to tenderize beans, rendering them more digestible.

Kuzu or Kudzu: A white root starch that is used as a thickener. It needs to dissolve to room temperature or cool water, and thickens in hot. It renews vitality and is very alkalinizing and soothing to your stomach.

Miso: A fermented soy bean paste that has enzymes that aid in digestion. It is mainly used for soups or stews.

Mochi: A cake of pounded sweet brown rice that puffs up when it's baked and melts like cheese when grated.

Mung beans: Small green beans that do not hold their shape when cooked. The beans can be sprouted and are very nutritious.

Parsnip: A root vegetable that has a sweet flavor. It is a good source of minerals and vitamin A.

Quinoa: (Pronounced keen-wa) is the fruit of the plant related to lamb's quarters, but it is used as a whole grain. It is naturally high in lysine and protein. Be sure a rinse well before using, as quinoa has a bitter protective coating that is easily washed off.

Tahini: Peanut butter is made from ground peanuts...tahini is made from ground hulled sesame seeds. Tahini is naturally high in calcium as well as phosphorus, niacin and iron.

Tamari: Is a fermented soy sauce that has glutamic acid, which is the natural form of monosodium glutamate. Unlike shoyu, tamari is wheat- free. It is traditionally the result of miso production.

Tempeh: Is made from whole soybeans that have been cultured and formed into cakes. It is very high in protein and packed full of wonderful enzymes that help with your digestion.

Toasted sesame oil: The result of roasting sesame seeds prior to pressing for oil. It imparts a wonderful toasted flavor to stir-fries. Sesame oil is one of the oldest oils.

Umeboshi plums/pickled plum paste/ume plum vinegar: Umebosi plums are made from a green fruit that resembles an unripe apricot. They are repeatedly pickled in salt and exposed to the energies of the sun's rays. They get their red color from the beefsteak plant that is added to the pickling brine. Umeboshi plums are very alkalinizing and help to relieve intestinal upsets. It is available in whole plums or in a pickled plum paste. The ume plum vinegar is not really a true vinegar, but rather a brine. It is the result of the pickling process of the umeboshi plums.

Wakame: A green sea vegetable that gently sweetens soups, stews, and baked casseroles. High in minerals, especially calcium.

Now that we have the "What is all this stuff?" question under control by reading the glossary, you might have noticed that all of these foods have properties that enhance your health. Food literally becomes your medicine. It's an exciting realization that food can be used to build our health and that we have the free will to choose what we allow to pass between our lips. It's up to us!! Freedom! It's a sweet thing.

THE HEARTY SOUL

The recipes that follow were inspired by: 1- my need to create good-for-me "fast food," 2- my recent stay at the Kushi Institute (KI), and 3- my road trip across America cooking on a one burner portable gas stove.

I love to cook, but who has the time to spend in the kitchen? I need quick and easy recipes that use as few tools and machines as possible. You will notice that a few recipes are just basic ideas for you to expand upon. I created these recipes while I was on the road, so I didn't measure and figure. They are the ones in this book without the values. These recipes just sorta happened to me, so let me introduce the art of "eye balling it." Don't worry...it will be easy!

My drive across America involved a one-month stay at the Kushi Institute. The KI is the premier learning center for macrobiotics. Studying macrobiotics is not about contemplating the different ways of cooking brown rice. It is a lifestyle that involves the principles of balance and change. The material that was presented to me inspired me by the simplicity of their food preparation. Measuring is not always necessary. Tailoring your recipes to your individual needs comes first.

One of the most important points that I left with was the importance of proper chewing. Your food needs to be thoroughly mixed with your saliva for optimum digestion. From this vantage point, I can't help but appreciate my teeth. Regular dental visits protect my investment in my health by taking care of my teeth and gums...and may your floss be with you!

I had the best time cooking on my portable stove during my stops while driving across the wonderful US of A. It was proven to me that one can cook anywhere and under almost any condition. I was creating incredibly quick, easy and delicious meals using the simplest ingredients and journalizing my adventures. During this process I wrote a mission statement vowing to cook for myself even when I didn't want to. It is my commitment to myself on paper...it felt powerful. I encourage you to write your own dietary mission statement.

UPON THIS ROCK I BUILD MY CHURCH

While camping on the South Dakota prairie, it came to mind to say this simple prayer before I eat as a way of focusing my mind on the process of chewing (which can also be called "eating"). After trying it several times I noticed that there was now a feeling of deep purpose behind my chewing. It was building my church upon the rock of health that is created from ingesting whole natural foods. WOW...it felt awesome. I found repeating this phrase 3 times brought me into a clear mindset...transporting me from food preparation to eating, helping me to be in the moment. My body would do the rest. Team work!

Now, with all that said and done, let's begin!

Let's start with a simple sauce that is wonderful on bitter green leafy vegetables (which help with our sweet cravings), on cooked quinoa rolled in a boiled collard green (another bitter green leafy vegetable), or even all by itself on your finger!

GINGER UMEBOSHI SAUCE

4 tablespoons tahini

1 tablespoon fresh lemon juice

1 teaspoon umeboshi paste

1/2 teaspoon Bragg liquid aminos (non-fermented soy sauce)

1/4 teaspoon onion powder

1/2 teaspoon fresh ginger juice.(grate fresh ginger and then squeeze the pulp over the measuring spoon)

sea salt to taste

1/4 cup water

Put all the ingredients in a small blender.(Braun hand held blender comes with an attachment that is perfect) and blend until creamy.

Serving size: 1 teaspoon   Makes 16 servings

Values per serving
37 cal   1 g protein   1 g carb   3.3 g fat

By reading the glossary you can understand that this sauce is a good source of calcium (sesame seeds), has alkalinizing ingredients (umeboshi paste and ginger), and the ginger and umeboshi paste could help to settle your stomach as well. Can't beat that...and it tastes great, too!!

Let's keep going with the bitter leafy green vegetable ideas. Let's face it..we all crave sweets. Let's try throwing it a curve ball by introducing more bitter tastes into our diet.

KALE WITH GINGER

1 bunch kale, washed and chopped

small amount of water

pinch of salt

Boil 1/2" water and salt, adding kale, cover and cook for 3-4 minutes. Remove from pot and drain any remaining water.

2 teaspoons toasted sesame oil

1/4 teaspoon ginger juice (grate fresh ginger and then squeeze the pulp)

1/4 teaspoon tamari

Heat oil over medium high heat. Sauté cooked kale quickly to coat with oil. Add ginger juice and tamari, adjust to your taste. You can use BraggLiquid Aminos in place of the tamari if you need an unfermented soy sauce.

Serving size: 1 cup Makes 3 servings

Values per serving

71 cal   2.5 g protein   6 g carb   3.5 g fat   2.5 g fiber

We can expect some peaceful energy after eating this dish since it is high in minerals...and minerals are known to calm us down. The kale can help keep us from the ice cream store too! See, if we start to appreciate what the food is doing for us, we will want to work with this process of self-healing.

vvv

Wheat is a grain that has been used and abused in the SAD (Standard American Diet), especially refined wheat. Tabouli is traditionally made from bulgar, which is made from whole wheat. Wheat, either whole or refined, is still a reactive food for many people. The following tabouli recipe is made with quinoa, for a light and nutritionally power salad.

QUINOA TABOULI

1 cup quinoa (rinse well as the outer kernels have a bitter coating that needs to be washed away)
2 cups water
pinch of sea salt

Bring the water to a boil and add quinoa, cover and simmer until done, approx. 20 minutes. Place in a large bowl to cool.

2 medium tomatoes, chopped
1/2 cup chopped parsley
1/2 teaspoon crushed garlic
1 1/2 tablespoons extra virgin olive oil
3 tablespoons fresh squeezed lemon juice
sea salt to taste

Add tomatoes, parsley, and garlic to cooled quinoa. In a small bowl, mix together oil and lemon juice and pour over quinoa mixture, stirring well to coat well. Salt to taste. Serve cold.

One large peeled cucumber can be substituted for the tomatoes. Try some scallions with it as well, or even some diced raw purple onion.

SERVING SIZE: 1 cup Makes 4 servings

Values per serving

117 cal   4 g protein   19 g carb   7 g fat   3 g fiber

Everyone loves pasta. Unfortunately, it is usually made from refined wheat. Those of us who must now say "no thank you" to refined wheat pasta can say "YES" to a company named SOYBAYA that makes a variety of delicious whole grain pastas from kamut.

Along with wheat, cow's milk is another food that can be a reactive food. Cheese is a tough one for people to let go of. Goat milk cheese is a lovely alternative. There are some really good ones out there that don't taste "goaty"....no kid-ding!

BROCCOLI PASTA SUPREME

2 large stalks of broccoli, chopped and steamed

1 package SOBAYA kamut and brown rice pasta

1 4 oz. Package SALADENA goat cheese crumbles...Provencal flavor

2 tablespoons ume plum vinegar

1/2 teaspoon salt

1 teaspoon grated onion

Cook pasta according to package directions. After draining, cut with a knife into bite-size pieces. Combine all ingredients in a large bowl and adjust salt to taste. Serve warm.

SERVING SIZE: 1 cup Makes 4 servings

VALUES PER SERVING

313 cal   16 g protein   8 g fat   46 g carb   9 g fiber

This recipe was the result of cooking on the run. My daughter, Heidi, was visiting from Portland, OR, and we had places to go and things to do! There seems to be a real attitude problem when it comes to cooking..."It takes SO much time!" Not so my friend. If we could give it a new word to describe the process of cooking that negates the image of aprons, a sink full of dirty dishes and the rest of your life on hold until you escape from your dungeon called your kitchen, it would be...ummm...

Processing? No, that conjures up images of equipment.

Creating? Well, it is truly an art. You are taking separate ingredients and tastes and combing them to create a new form. (And gosh, I hope it tastes good.)

Well, I guess it all comes down to COOKING...so get a grip and deal with it.

Okay, I tried.

During my trip I had grown tense from all the driving. I wanted to soothe my nerves the natural way, with sea vegetables. Wakame is naturally high in minerals that my body needs to help me to relax. Soup is soothing to my soul as well as my tummy. Try this delightfully easy to prepare soup:

CORN "OFF THE COB" SOUP

2 cups water

6" piece of wakame, broken into pieces

1/2 carrot, diced

1/2 onion, diced

1 ear corn, kernels removed

2 teaspoons dark miso

Bring water and wakame to a boil. Add carrot and onion and cook for approx. 5 minutes. Add corn kernels and cook until corn is done to your liking. Remove from heat. Using a small mesh strainer, add miso so that it dissolves into the soup as you stir it through the strainer. This will prevent lumps of miso from being in your soup.

This simple recipe was the result of seeking a replacement for couscous, which of course, comes from wheat. Necessity really is the mother of invention!

I have served this to a wide variety of folks, and the result is always the same...This is:

GREAT KAMUT "KAKE"

3 cups organic apple juice

1 cup BOB'S RED MILL Pharaoh's Pharina (kamut cereal)

1/4 teaspoon sea salt

1/4 cup brown rice syrup

1 cup fresh raspberries

Bring apple juice, brown rice syrup and salt to a boil. Slowly stir in kamut cereal, turn heat down. Cover and cook 15 minutes stirring occasionally. Remove from heat—fold in raspberries and put in 1.5 liter glass dish, or dish that resembles a loaf pan. Cool before putting in refrigerator. Serve cold.

Serving size 1 piece Makes 5 servings

Values per serving

188 cal   4 g protein   44 g carb   .064 fat   3.2 g fiber

This kamut kake is fantastic because it is so simple to make. The flavor will knock your socks off, too. But the best part of it is that the Pharaoh's Pharina will help you to a-Nile-ate your refined sugar needs.

Since we have started to create sweet treats, let me present a fast and easy recipe that is simply delightful. It blends up to be a smooth, creamy refreshing snack.

AGAR FRUIT DELIGHT

4 cups organic apple juice

4 tablespoons agar agar flakes

1 tablespoon brown rice syrup

Put juice, agar agar and brown rice syrup in a pot, boil, reduce heat and simmer 5 minutes, stirring occasionally until agar dissolves. Pour into glass Pyrex dish and allow to cool before placing in refrigerator.

When nice and cold, put 1 cup into blender with either 1/2 banana or 4 large strawberries. Blend until smooth, adding a few drops of water or juice to get the blender moving...if needed. Be sure and blend thoroughly as the agar can sometimes leave little lumps.

Try using assorted fruit juices such as apple-banana, or apple-strawberry juice.

Serving size: 1 cup   Makes 4 servings

Values Per Serving
272 cal   1.2 g protein   41 g carb   .5 g fat   2.7 g fiber

Wind! The South Dakota prairie was so windy. How will I cook? Boy, those french toast and pancake smells coming from the KOA (national camp grounds) outpost smell so good. It had been raining the night before so the next morning took more time to pack up then usual. And I was really hungry. No time to wait for food to cook. I wanted it now! But the wind...how could I possibly cook in this?

I was faced with a choice. Life is full of them, ya know. Suddenly my mission statement was way up front in my mind. NO...I will NOT eat that food. I believe that when we make a conscious effort to "build my church on this rock," options open up that weren't noticed before.

By backing my car up next to the picnic table I was able to create a wind shield by opening the door and using a few other items. I did it. I cooked in what seemed to be a hopeless situation. The following recipe is what was divinely inspired and I gratefully consumed it. I was enormously proud of myself.

WINDY'S APPLE MOCHI MELT
enough dried apple slices for a serving

water to cover apple slices

the juice of 1/2 of a small lemon

enough water and kuzu to make a medium thick sauce

pinch of salt

grated plain mochi

Cook dried apple slices in water until apples are soft. Squeeze lemon juice on top. Make kuzu sauce. Turn heat to low and top with enough mochi to cover apples thoroughly. Put lid on the pot and when the mochi has melted, remove from heat. Enjoy!

It could have been so easy during my drive to wimp out. You know, cheat.

Refined sugar and wheat products were calling my name at every gas station and rest stop. I wanted sweet! I had been in my car for what seemed an eternity, my back and shoulders ached and my hind end was loosing its hind sight. I would scope out the counters and freezers hoping that maybe there would be an "allowable food"...a treat...please? I had to keep repeating, "I will NOT do that to my body." It worked. I stopped at a rest area and took another inspired look at my food supply. Here's where the unnoticed becomes noticed. I had all the ingredients right there before me to pull this together...

TOFU LEMON PUDDING

1 package Mori Nu silken tofu, firm

juice of one lemon

enough finely grated lemon peel (zest) for your taste

enough brown rice syrup for your taste

1/2 teaspoon barley miso

Blend all ingredients, adding any water necessary for processing.

Food used as healing can be a new concept for some people. Even the herbs and spices that one chooses to enhance their food have an important place in the "whole" picture.

The following two recipes use sage and bay leaves—not only for their flavor, but for what they can do for one internally. Sage has been said to be good for canker sores, bleeding gums, sore throat, lungs, wounds and digestion...just to name a few. Bay leaves have been used for infections.

The following recipes are made from soaked beans and one from canned beans. While it is always better for you to use the fresh beans, canned beans do have their place. Try and purchase organically grown beans which ever way you choose.

I created the following recipe as the result of needing to "rotate my food." I was eating too many of the same beans. Who had ever heard of mung beans?? I had never cooked them before. The result of my experiment is the following soup. A few years later Donna was introduced to my cooking with this recipe, so it is extra special to me. She took a few bites and didn't want to stop eating it...it made her feel that good.

Back to the concept of food rotation. By rotating my food I am assured of getting a wide variety of nutrients and not setting the stage for food sensitivities. Rotating your food is very simple. If you eat mung beans today, don't use them again for a few days. With the grains, if it can be as simple as rye bread on Monday, spelt on Tuesday and rice on Wednesday.

So are you ready for a new taste? You won't be disappointed.

MUNG BEAN SOUP

Soak overnight:

1 cup mung beans

Use enough water to cover the beans, and to allow them to double in size

Soak beans overnight in the water

The Next Morning:
Prepare:

1 medium acorn squash

Cut the squash in half and remove seeds. Bake at 350 (until soft. You can bake it whole, too. Just poke with a knife and remove seeds when done.

Add:

5 cups water

1 large bay leaf

1 medium onion, chopped

Pour off the water that the beans have soaked in. Place mung beans and the 5 cups of water in a pot. Bring to a boil. Skim off any foam that may occur during boiling. Add bay leaf and onion. Cover and cook on medium heat for approx. 45 minutes, or until soft. Stir and check periodically to watch water level.

The squash component:

1 cup baked acorn squash

1/2 teaspoon sage

salt and tamari to taste (approx. 1/2 teaspoon salt and 1/2 teaspoon tamari)

Add squash, sage, salt and tamari to the mung beans. If you have a BRAUN hand-held blender, put blender in pot. Blend up large chunks of squash and some of the beans to make the creamy texture, keeping about 1/2 of the beans whole. (Just use a regular blender if you do not have a Braun.)

Serving size: approx. 1 1/2 cups

Values per serving
195 cal   8 g protein   40 g carb   0 fat   12 g fiber

Mung beans do not need to be soaked. I always do it for better digestibility. You need to decide what is best for you. Which ever way you choose, the end result will be worth the effort.

Now, this next recipe is a 15 minute no-brainer-open-a-can-o'-beans type dish...and it's really good! I call it:

TOTALLY GREAT NORTHERN BEAN SOUP
1 (that's one) 15 oz. Can organic great northern beans
1/2 can of water
1 small bay leaf
1 medium onion, chopped
1/2 medium carrot, chopped
6" piece of wakame
1/4 teaspoon sage
Bragg Liquid Aminos

Place all ingredients in a pot and simmer for 15 minutes. Remove bay leaf and discard. Remove wakame and chop into small pieces. Put back into pot and, using hand blender, blend some of the soup. (Just use a regular blender if you do not have a hand-held) Stir and add Bragg to taste. Enjoy!

Serving size: 1 cup Makes 2 servings

Values per serving
135 cal   9 g protein   24 g carb   0 g fat   6 g fiber

Food can help to create moods. If you feel you need to become more grounded instead of feeling spacy, try getting to the "root" of your problem with the following recipe...

BURDOCK AND PARSNIP STRENGTHENER

1 teaspoon toasted sesame oil

1 cup burdock, shaved

1 cup parsnips, shaved

water

1 teaspoon tamari

Scrub burdock and parsnips. To shave, hold burdock and parsnip in your hand straight away from your body. Shave by cutting away from you as if whittling a tree branch. Heat oil in skillet over medium high heat and sauté burdock for 2 minutes. Add parsnips. SautÈ a few minutes and add just enough water to cover veggies half way. Season with tamari and cover to simmer until any liquid that remains has been absorbed. Adjust tastes if necessary. A 1/4 cup serving of this should be enough to get your feet back on the ground!

Serving size: 1/4 cup   Makes 4 servings

Values per serving
70 cal   1.1 g protein   14 g carb   2.2 g fat   2 g fiber

I was in the Upper Peninsula of Michigan where the air was fresh, the sky was blue, but the air was chilly...man did I need some stew! And so it was...

ADUKI BEAN SQUASH STEW

1 cup aduki beans

small piece of kombu

3 cups water

1 small squash (butternut, buttercup, etc.)

salt to taste

Bring beans, kombu and water to a boil. Skim off any foam that may occur in boiling. Add squash, cover and reduce heat to low. Check the water level, adding more, if necessary. Add salt when beans are done, approx.. 1 hour. A dash of nutmeg is optional, and yummy.

The mayonnaise that is used in the following "chicken" salad recipe is made with grape seed oil. Grape seed oil is the by-product of wine production. It helps to raise the good cholesterol and is an excellent natural source of Vitamin E and essential fatty acids that are necessary for normal metabolism and maintenance. The brand name is FOLLOW YOUR HEART and is available to you in the refrigerator case at most natural food stores. Be sure and look for the purple label, as this is the one made from the grape seed oil. But, try not to serve it in a wine glass!

TEMPEH "CHICKEN" SALAD

1 8 oz. Package organic tempeh (sesame quinoa works well)

1/3 cup FOLLOW YOUR HEART grapeseed oil vegenaise

1/2 cup chopped celery

2 tablespoons chopped scallions, green part only

2 tablespoons vinegar free, honey sweet pickle relish

1/4 teaspoon sea salt

Cut the tempeh into little cubes. Boil in 3/4 cups water for 20 minutes. Drain. Put into a bowl and add the rest of the ingredients. Mix well and adjust taste, if necessary. Serve cold.

Serving size: 1/2 cup   Makes 4 servings

Values per serving

118 cal   7 g protein   12 g carb   10 g fat   4 g fiber

I served this to some friends of mine who had never even heard of tempeh, let alone know what it tastes like. Imagine my excitement when I spoke to them some time later and they told me that they had made the chicken salad several times.

I love to teach people about natural foods. There are so many wonderful "new" foods available to us. Please try at least one new food a week, month, or whatever is comfortable for you. Using whole natural foods will broaden you horizons, not your hips!

There are some really great whole food cookbooks available either in the bookstores or at the library. You can literally check them out before you buy them to see if they are worthy of being in your personal library. Let's face it, books can be expensive. It's a good idea to invest in a few until you are creating your own recipes. It's going to happen, you know. You will begin to tap your creative juices while cooking with natural foods.

The following two recipes were inspired by reading cookbooks. The first one is *The Natural Gourmet* by Annemarie Colbin. In her recipe, Aduki Bean Dip, she uses aduki beans that she has cooked from scratch. For all of us workin' folks, openin' a can of beans could be all we have time for. But, that's the beauty of reading cookbooks...IDEAS! While reading her recipe I figured out that this could be made even simpler by using a can opener instead of a pot with a lid.

The second cookbook is *The Self Healing Cookbook* by Kristina Turner. In her Sweet Squash Pie recipe she gives suggestions for different types of squash and spices to use. I enjoy acorn squash, but don't enjoy cinnamon, plus I don't digest pie crusts very well. I just inserted my needs into her recipe and created the following Acorn squash pudding.

This is how you begin to create your own recipes. Know thyself, know what you need to feel good. Read cookbooks and experiment. But please do what my friends are always yelling at me to do..."WRITE IT DOWN"! I am always asked, Judith did you write it down? And once again my head falls in humility and I have to say..."Nope."

Before I begin with my version of Aduki Bean Dip...just a word about eating beans. If there were such a thing as picnic police, citations would be given for eating baked beans followed by watermelon! Your digestive system deserves respect, as well as the guests attending the picnic! Avoid what could be embarrassing moments by understanding proper food combining. If ever there was a food that was not combined correctly that could speak to you after you ingest it, beans would be the one. Beans mix well with whole grains and veggies. Save the watermelon for another time. It's been said: "Melons...eat them alone or leave them alone." If you don't want to be sitting alone, properly combine your beans!

So, here is the quickest, simplest and mostest delicious dip that's good for your kidneys, too...and of course, beans made from "scratch" are always tastier and better than canned beans, so once you get cooking, try making the aduki beans this way. I made this recipe for the Live It or Diet Support group and we did our own "scratch" test. I presented one batch of beans made from scratch, and the other from canned beans, and had them guess which one was which. No one in the room had ever tasted aduki beans so the room was divided, but in the end both bowls were empty!

ADUKI BEAN DIP

1 15 oz. Can of EDEN aduki beans, drained, save liquid in case you need it for blender

1 tablespoon ume plum paste

1 tablespoon KAUAI ORGANIC FARMS organic ginger puree

Blend all together in a food processor or blender, using any liquid to help the blender move, if necessary.

Serving size: 1/2 cup   Makes 2 servings

Values per serving

220 cal   14 g protein   38 g carb   0 g fat   10 g fiber

This is a great dip to serve your dinner guests. For a colorful and nutritious arrangement, use this red dip for the center, summer squash for the yellow, carrots for orange, and leaf lettuce for green. I find I have the most fun in presenting my food. Make it pretty and they will come!

And now, last but not least in my contribution to Donna's wonderful, inspiring book, I present:

ACORN SQUASH PUDDING

2 cups cooked acorn squash

4 tablespoons brown rice syrup

1/4 teaspoon allspice

1/4 teaspoon sea salt

1/2 cup water

2 tablespoons kuzu

Process squash, brown rice syrup, allspice and salt in a food processor. Dissolve kuzu in room temperature water, stirring to dissolve lumps of kuzu. Pour water and kuzu into a pot and bring to a boil, stirring with a wire whisk. Stir until it thickens and add to squash mixture in the food processor.

Process, adjusting tastes if necessary. Bake at 350(for 25 minutes. Serve cold. It's just that simple. And it is simply delicious!

Serving size: 1/2 cup   Makes 4 servings

Values per serving
37 cal   1 g protein   1 g carb   3 g fat

One last pointer. Food and emotions are affected during dietary changes. Try and create look-alike meals that are visually appealing to you. If you love bacon, try a product called "Fakin Bacon" made from tempeh. Replace ice cream with blended frozen bananas. They become a wonderful creamy desert that satisfies my own ice cream relationship.

It has been an absolute pleasure introducing you to what may be alternative ingredients. I trust that once you get cooking, it will come naturally to you as well.

Try these recipes out for yourself before you serve them to guests. Get to know your ingredients. Experiment with different tastes. When you take a bite, think about ways in which you could improve upon it, or what you could serve it with to enhance the overall meal. By the time you have made each recipe 3 times, you will probably not be measuring, and will be adding something that you enjoy that is not even in the recipe! Fear no more! Happy cooking—and before you know it—Cooking Comes Naturally!

Oh, one last quickie:

NATURAL BREATH FRESHENER

For a natural breath freshener, try putting a small piece of a cardamom seed in your mouth. It's not loaded with the refined sugars that most breath fresheners are, and can actually help to boost your energy.

IT ALL STARTS IN THE KITCHEN
Let's Go Shopping!

Well, here we are—where it all begins. After everything we have explored in this book, it comes back to taking responsibility for what we eat. So, my friend, remember the old scout motto and "be prepared." No more random food-shoving. Arm yourself, and your kitchen. Shop!

Now, shopping the way I am recommending can be an adventure, so it might be an adjustment for you. Most of us are used to grabbing familiar boxes and bags off of supermarket shelves, looking only for bold print that promises "fat free" or "reduced fat." I hope you now realize that these items are not the ticket to a healthy and fit body (and in fact, could produce the opposite results). So, where to start?

First, make room in your kitchen. Prepare a box for a homeless shelter or local food drive, and fill it with the refined and processed foods in your cupboard. Ouch. I know. But, believe me, the best way to begin is to begin, and that can't happen if you feel you must first consume what you currently have stocked in your kitchen. You have enough information after reading the preceding chapters to recognize the culprits on your shelves. Be brutal. Get rid of the stuff.

Thank you. I'm proud of you. Now, to the store for some "power shopping."

You can get some of your "basic" items in a traditional supermarket, but you might need a "health food market" to find most of the foods that we are introducing to you. We may be getting into uncharted territory here for some of you. It was at first for me, too, but I now do 90% of my shopping in health food markets like *Wild Oats Community Market*, *Bread Of Life*, and *Mother Nature Natural Foods* in Fort Lauderdale. Charlie (a great lady) and Matt are the managers of *Mother Nature* in Fort Lauderdale, and have both been there for six years. They have a combined 45 years in the natural food and supplement industry. They both have degrees (Matt was even pre-med) and are incredibly knowledgeable and helpful. If they don't have the answers (or the products) you are looking for, they will get them for you. Nick, the manager of Fort Lauderdale's *Wild Oats*, makes sure his store is well-stocked and well-run. He really cares. I ask him for something, and it appears. Charlie, Matt, and Nick are the types of passionate professionals you will find in many stores like theirs (see *Appendix G* for health food markets). I encourage you to find a market that specializes in natural, whole, and organic foods. Get to know it and the people who work there. It will be your stomping grounds.

WELCOME TO A "WHOLE" NEW WORLD!

Get In Touch With The World, And Your Food

"To eat is human, to digest divine."

—Mark Twain

The following information comes from the wonderful educational literature distributed by Wild Oats Community Market:

NATURAL—WHOLE—ORGANIC

Meat and Poultry

When it comes to protein, what does "natural" really mean? Meat and fish can be nutritious and pleasurable parts of your diet—if you know where they come from. Don't be fooled by the "natural" meats in conventional supermarkets. The USDA definition of natural applies only to processing and only guarantees that the product contains no artificial preservatives, flavors or colorings. The natural meats I buy at Wild Oats are guaranteed to be processed in a healthy way from animals raised humanely. The following words will tell you what "natural" means to us:

"Free-range." This means the animals roam and graze freely with the sun on their backs. These stress-free living conditions produce better-tasting, more tender meat than conventionally produced meat; free-range meat also has an average of 20% less fat.

"Humanely raised." Animals have room to move in a spacious barn or paddock, as opposed to the factory farm norm: Complete confinement in cramped cages, dark crates, and crowded feedlots that are often fogged with pesticides in order to control flies.

"Drug-free." Conventional meat producers use a wide array of FDA approved drugs—and an unknown number of other substances that are available without a vet's prescription.

"Antibiotic-free." Animals should receive antibiotics only when they are very sick. Most conventional livestock receive antibiotics to counteract the stressful and unclean living conditions on factory farms. As a result, many strains of bacteria—including E. Coli and salmonella—are becoming increasingly resistant to all known antibiotics. Antibiotics ingested through meats have been linked to lowered human resistance to bacterial infections (including many new super germs), and yeast infections.

"Artificial growth-hormone free." The use of growth hormones can produce larger and leaner animals more rapidly than nature ever intended, but these hormones may produce even more dramatic effects in people—including breast growth in five-year old children and breast cancer in women.

"Vegetarian-fed." Most of the meat that we eat comes from animals that are innately vegetarian. The "Mad-Cow" disease that swept Great Britain was linked to cows that had been fed tainted feed made from sheep and other cows.

"Stress-free." Fear rules the modern-day factory farm. An animal's adrenaline turns into sugars that darken and toughen meat.

"Organic." According to the EPA, 90% to 95% of all pesticide residues are found in meat, fish and dairy products. Organic standards for meat still vary from state to state. Until national organic standards go into effect, meat may not be labeled "organic." You may buy "natural" meat that comes from animals fed organic grains from birth, however. Natural meats are rich in protein, zinc, iron, and B vitamins, and can be an important part of a balanced diet if you choose the leanest cuts.

The main problem with beef is the high amount of fat. That is why most of us are turning to white-meat poultry. An even more important reason to go natural and lean is because toxic pesticides and drug residues concentrate in the fat of animals. (These chemicals are also passed on through dairy products.)

What about game meats? Game meats are exotic and healthier red meat choices, with fewer calories and less fat and cholesterol than conventional beef—and no residues of antibiotics or growth hormones. One of my favorite discoveries is Buffalo! It is sweeter than beef—leaner, and very tender.

Choosing organic can help reverse the trend toward large corporate, chemical-based farming. Organic farmers are working to keep our land fertile. They follow environmentally responsible business practices. Organic farmers treat their animals with dignity, honoring the special role of these animals in a full agricultural cycle. Cows feast on alfalfa, hay, and other feed grown without pesticides for at least one year before a dairy farm receives organic certification.

I recently spent two weeks in rural (extremely) Minnesota, and believe me, it was a revelation for this city girl. I saw hundreds and hundreds of miles of the most beautiful farm country imaginable. I saw animals grazing and hay bales (round *and* square). I even had the incredible experience of running in the fields around these hay bales! (I know—"Escape from New York.")

*A note on digestion—if you feel bloated after eating meat, avoid the antacid route. What you might really need is <u>more</u> acid. As we age our bodies produce less hydrochloric acid (HCl) the stomach acid that helps us fully digest meat and fish so we can reap their nutritional benefits. Consider trying a HCl/bethaine supplement, or digestive food enzymes with pepsin and protease.

Eggs

The word is out: Egg yolks may not be the artery-antagonizing heartbreakers we thought they were. You'll find far more nutrients inside an egg yolk than in an egg white, including iron and vitamins A, D, and B12. (Protein and B2 are found in approximately equal amounts in both.) Eggs are high in dietary cholesterol (213 mg. per egg), but scientists now believe that saturated fat, not dietary cholesterol, is the main culprit in high blood cholesterol. Eating your yolks gives you a perfect balance of healthy, unsaturated fats and the lecithin, which helps break them down. The American Heart Association still recommends eating no more than four whole eggs a week.

Which egg is best? The following are some terms to consider:

"Free-range eggs" come from hens that are allowed to be real chickens. They happily dig, scratch, forage, and run, and often consort with roosters to produce fertile eggs. For the richest flavor, the best baked goods, and the happiest hens, choose fertile or organic eggs that come from free-range chickens.

"Fertile eggs" may be no more nutritious than non-fertile eggs, but the difference for the hens is like night and day!

"Organic eggs" come from hens not given antibiotics or drugs, and fed healthy diets of certified organic grains. Organic eggs must meet national standards as of 1997.

"Non-fertile eggs" have not been fertilized by a rooster. Generally, they come from hens that live very stressful, restricted lives. These hens are crammed into small wire cages and spend their short lives cranking out eggs under bright lights. Commercial producers often de-beak birds in order to control the fighting and chaos that their frustrated natural instincts cause.

New strains of salmonella bacteria don't need a cracked egg to flourish. They can spread from an infected hen right into her eggs. Make all of your egg-eating experiences safe by following a few simple guidelines:

1. Keep raw and cooked eggs refrigerated under 40 degrees F.

2. Avoid eating raw or undercooked eggs in foods like eggnog and Caesar salad.

3. Keep eggs stored in their carton, where they won't absorb other odors and flavors.

4. Use leftover cooked eggs within four days.

5. Serve freshly cooked eggs immediately, or refrigerate right away.

6. Never eat an egg that's been out of the refrigerator for more than two hours.

Fish

The main rule of choosing fresh fish is to trust your nose and your eyes. The fish should smell *briny*, not fishy, like it just came from the ocean. With filets and steaks, look for fish with pink to cherry-red color. Pass over fish in shades of tan or brown. If you do not live near the ocean, frozen fish may actually be fresher than some of the "fresh" catches.

As far as omega-3 fatty acids (the fat you want), the following are the fish that contain the highest amounts: Mackerel, anchovies, herring, salmon, sardines, lake trout, Atlantic sturgeon, and tuna. Moderate amounts of omega-3 are contained in: Turbot, bluefish, striped bass, shark, rainbow smelt, swordfish, and rainbow trout.

*Eat a variety of fish to lessen your risk of overdosing on one contaminated source. Eat fish two or three times a week. Don't eat the skin on your fish, the main storage place for toxins. If you are pregnant—don't eat more than seven ounces of canned tuna a week, and don't eat swordfish, shark, fresh tuna, or fish from inland waters more than once a month.

Beans

Beans are loaded with Phytochemicals and protease inhibitors that are being studied as anti-cancer agents. Although a bean's protein is considered incomplete because it is low in the amino acid methionine, your body will transform it into high quality, complete protein if you eat grains. A good ratio of beans to grain in a meal is 1 to 4 (more grain). Beans are one of the best sources of soluble fiber. There are many different kinds of beans. Sample the following:

Adzuki, Anasazi, Black-eyed Peas, Black, Canellini, Fava, Garbanzo, Great Northern, Kidney, Lentils, Lima, Mung, Navy, Peas (whole and split), Pinto, Red, Soybeans. (If you have a "problem" with beans, try *Beano*. It works!)

Grains

Whole grains are the seeds and fruits of cereal grasses, filled with energy ready to germinate into a plant. Whole grains are high in fiber, complex carbohydrates, vitamins and minerals. The parts of whole grains are: Bran, germ, endo, and exosperms. Refined grains are stripped of the bran and sometimes the germ, which removes most nutrients (22 nutrients to be exact) and then enriched.

There are many wonderful grains to choose from, and many of these might be unknown to you. Try some of the following—you will be rewarded:
Amaranth, Barley, Buckwheat, Bulgur Wheat, Couscous, Kamut, Millet, Oat Groats, Quinoa, Rye Berries, Spelt Berries, Teff Berries, Triticale Berries, Wheat Berries, Yellow Corn.

Sea Vegetables

Sea vegetables grow in the world's rich oceans where they absorb 56 different minerals and trace elements that are as good as gold for your body. Did you know that your blood contains a proportion of minerals and trace elements remarkably similar to ocean water? With seven to ten times the mineral content of vegetables like broccoli, sea vegetables are an important part of the sea. Sea vegetables aid digestion, heal mucous membranes and joints, and are the traditional Japanese food for healthy skin and hair. Cook with them. I add them to just about everything! They are hard when you buy them, so just put them in with your meat, fish, or grains near the beginning of the cooking process. They will normalize the pH of these foods (as they are highly alkaline and grains and meats are acidic—see, *Acid -Alkaline And Toxic Wastes In Your Body*). They are also extremely high in fiber (see, *Sugar-Sensitivity*).

The following is a list of these remarkable foods:
Dulse, Nori, Hiziki, Arame, Wakame, Agar-agar, Kelp, Kombu.

HOT TIPS ON COOL MEALS AND SNACKS
Preplanned Portion Control

One tip for snacking (which is actually one of your little meals—your stomach doesn't know the difference between a meal and a snack—it's all nutrient feedings to your body) is to count or measure out a serving size of whatever it is and put it in a baggie...when the baggie is empty, *you're done*. Remember that *processing food* (eating) raises your metabolism, (not eating processed food, when part of the digestive process has been eliminated through refinement—thereby raising only your blood sugar!). So, if you can, preplan a couple of small "feedings" for the day.

The following are some of my ideas for quick and easy meals:

WHAT'S FOR LUNCH? TRY SALADS!

Quick salad meals can save you! Sometimes you just do not have the time to prepare balanced meals that bring in all the elements that support your dietary type. Try building a meal with field greens as the foundation. You can put anything you like on a salad—tofu, grilled chicken, turkey, fish (try canned tuna or salmon packed in spring water—rinse well). Add other vegetables, like snap peas, broccoli, zucchini, etc. A nice addition is to sprinkle on some goat's cheese and sun-dried tomato bits, or soy nuts, or spicy pumpkin seeds. You can find some great fat-free or low-fat dressings in health food markets (and sometimes even in supermarkets). Walden Farms, Spectrum Naturals, San-J (among others) make some good products to choose from. Or, you can make your own dressing. Try mixing the following: Balsamic vinegar (or rice vinegar, or Bragg Liquid Aminos), a tiny bit of olive oil, mustard, parmesan cheese, lemon, and a little apple juice.

Try adding grains and beans to your salad. Make your grains (be adventurous—try some grains like: Quinoa, kamut, millet, wild rice mixed with brown rice, etc.) with a sea vegetable (see, *Get In Touch With The World—And Your Food*). If soy is for you, then add some TVP (texturized vegetable protein—it comes as granules that soften when moistened. Great source of protein!) Add some *Bragg Liquid Aminos* while cooking. If you are in a hurry and cannot make beans from scratch, add some canned beans (adzuki, kidney—any of the ones on your supportive list—<u>make sure to rinse the beans before you use them</u>) at the end. Keep this mixture in the refrigerator (no longer than three days) and top your greens with it.

Try Beano if you have a problem with beans—it works!

OATMEAL AS A COMPLETE MEAL

Once again, the best rule to follow when buying any carbohydrate product is to <u>look for one with the highest fiber content</u>. Steel Cut Oats are higher in fiber than rolled oats because there is less processing. A product called *John McCann's Irish Oatmeal* has 6 grams of fiber. It comes in a tin (you might have to go to a health food market to find it). Another Steel Cut Oat product is from *Arrowhead Mills*. Remember, the oats in these products have not been "rolled," so they take longer to cook.

But wait—I'm going to tell you how to make this breakfast in a "minute." <u>The night before do the following</u>: Put 1 serving of the Oats into a Tupperware container. Add enough (good) water to cover them. Dice an apple and add that along with some cinnamon. Mix well. Put in the fridge.

In the morning, add 1/2 serving of Oat Bran (Arrowhead Mills), more water (lots), stir, and pop into the microwave for *two minutes*. Add a few raisons. Viola! (Now, if you are like us and do not like microwaves, you can eat this oatmeal cold, as it has softened through the night—or heat it on the stove for a minute. Also, the enzymes from the apple aid in the digestion of this food, along with neutralizing its pH).

For a more complete meal—add a protein powder to your cooked oatmeal. Before you add the protein, make sure to add more water to your cooked mixture and stir well. I prefer soy protein powders, but there are protein powders from other sources (such as rice, egg and whey) as well. Look for a protein powder with at least 20 grams of protein per serving (and no carbohydrates, sugar and other garbage). I have examined many products, and so far my favorites are *Genisoy 100% Soy Protein*, *Super Green Pro-96*, *Nature's Life Soy Protein*, *Wild Oats Soy Protein*, *Designer Protein*, and *Whey To Go Whey Protein* by Solgar. Spoon it into your oatmeal and stir well.

If you do not remember to prepare the night before, it still takes only 15 minutes to prepare in the morning. Microwave the Steel Cut Oats for 5 minutes without the Oat Bran. Then add the Oat Bran and microwave for another 10 minutes. Then add your raisins and protein powder.

Eat half of this if it is too large a portion for your meal plan, and save the other half for the following morning.

For 1 Full Serving
440 calories   35 grms protein   67 grms carbs   6.5 grms fat   12 grms fiber

For 1/2 Serving
220 calories   17.5 grms protein   33.5 grms carbs   3.25 grms fat   6 grms   fiber

Yet another way to have your oatmeal is to add cooked oatmeal to a protein shake. Or, simply a serving of uncooked Oat Bran (7 grams of fiber!). Try this: Make a protein shake with a recommended protein powder (see, the "Shake Off Fatigue" recipe), a little water and ice, and frozen strawberries (or any frozen fruit—I like using frozen fruits because they make the shake more like a "smoothie"). Add your oatmeal, oatbran, or Cream Of Rye and blend.

SHAKE OFF FATIGUE

This recipe is for one serving. This shake is designed for high protein intake, energy, and immune system boost. It can be used daily.

1 Serving of: Soy Protein Powder—Whey Protein Isolate—100% Egg White Protein Powder or Rice Protein Powder
110 calories   20-22 grms protein   0 carbs   1 grm fat

1/2 Serving (1 Tablespoon) Flax Seed Meal
35 calories   3 grms protein   3 grms carbs   1.5 grms fat   3 grms fiber

1/2 Serving of "Lite" Powdered Soy or Rice Milk (Optional, try 4 oz of fruit juice if you prefer)
40 calories   1 grm protein   8 grms carbs   1 grm fat

1 Serving of Fruit
60 calories   15 grms carbs   2 grms fiber

1 Tablespoon of Apple or Pear Butter
40 calories   10 grms carbs

Fill a blender half way with (good) water. Add ice cubes, Soy Protein, Flax, Powdered Soy Milk (or 4 oz fruit juice), Fruit, and Fruit Butter. Blend on high.

Total Values Per Serving:
285 calories   24 grms protein   35.5 grms carbs   3.5 grms fat   4 grms fiber

You can add 1/6 cup (1/2 serving) of Oat Bran (or 1/2 serving of Cream Of Rye) to your shake. This will add 75 calories, 4 grams of protein, 11 grams of carbs, 1 gram of fat, and 3.5 grams of fiber.

With Oat Bran (or Cream Of Rye)
360 calories   31.5 grms protein   46.5 grms carbs   4.5 grms fat   7.5 grms fiber

This shake is a complete breakfast. It can be used as another meal during the day. It can be used before a workout that consists of both strength training, followed by cardiovascular.

ΔΔ**Tip:** GO BANANAS! Try peeling a bunch of ripe bananas, then cut them in half, seal them in a freezer bag, and freeze them. One half of a medium banana supplies approximately 50 calories.

You can also try 1 serving of apple sauce as the fruit in your shake, or buy bags of frozen fruits (sugar-free, of course) to keep in your freezer.

GRAINS MIXTURE
A Complete Meal...A Complete Protein

This recipe is for 4 servings

8 Ounces of Dry Quinoa (or Millet)
800 calories 32 grms protein 152 grms carbs 16 grms fat 17.2 grms fiber

2 Cups of TVP
236 calories 44 grms protein 28 grms carbs .8 grms fat

Handful (1 ounce) of Arame Sea Vegetables
40 calories 2 grms of protein 8 grms carbs 7 grms fiber

1 Can of Health Valley Chicken Broth or Hain Vegetable Broth—No Salt Added
90 calories 14 grms protein 0 carbs 3 grms fat

Bragg Liquid Aminos

Seasoning To Taste

Bring 6 cups of water to a boil. Add Quinoa (or Millet), Arame, and a few squirts of Bragg

Simmer for 5 minutes—add chicken broth and seasonings

Simmer for 10 minutes—add TVP. If you need to add more fluid, add water and a little more Bragg. Stir well and cover. Turn off the heat and let stand for 5 minutes.

Per Serving:
290 calories 24 grms protein 48 grms carbs 5 grms fat 6 grms fiber

Per 1/2 Serving:
145 calories 12 grms protein 24 grms carbs 2.5 grms fat 3 grms fiber

Use this mixture as a side dish, on a salad, or as a complete meal. Divide a serving in half to use as a "snack." Add more protein such as chicken or turkey to make it a larger protein meal. Use spices such as paprika, garlic, onion, ginger, cumin, turmeric, etc.

SALMON SPREAD
1 Can of Chicken Of The Sea Pink Salmon in Water
150 calories 25 grms protein 5 grms fat

2 Slices of Soy or Rice Pepper-Jack Cheese
80 calories   8grms protein   2 grms carbs   4 grms fat

1/2 Cup Chopped Spinach
30 calories   2 grms protein   5 grms carbs   2 grms fiber

Dash of Rice Vinegar, Paprika, & Cayenne Pepper To Taste

Thoroughly rinse salmon and mix in a bowl with rinsed spinach, shredded cheese, rice vinegar, paprika and cayenne pepper (to taste). Cook in microwave until hot and cheese melts (about 2 minutes).

Yields:

One Full Serving
260 calories   35 grms protein   7 grms carbs   9 grms fat   2 grms fiber

1/2 Serving
130 calories 17.5 grms protein 3.5 grms carbs 4.5 grms fat 1 grm fiber

Use this mixture as a dip with brown rice crackers, as a spread on wheat-free, gluten-free whole-ground brown rice, spelt, kamut, or millet bread, or on a salad for a complete meal.

1/2 Serving on 2 Slices of Brown Rice Bread
330 calories   23 grms protein   43 grms carbs   5 grms fat   6 grms fiber

Note: Water-packed white tuna can be substituted for the salmon. The calories remain the same, however, the protein content will be 10 grams higher and the fat content will be 5 grams less for a full serving.

EXTRA QUICK TOFU STIR-FRY

8 Ounces of Extra Firm Low-Fat Tofu
200 calories 21 grams protein 2 gram carbs 4 grams fat

One Package Frozen StirFry Vegetables
75 calories 6 grams protein 18 grams carbs 6 grams fiber

Dehydrated Chopped Onion, Braggs Liquid Aminos, Paprika, Cayenne Pepper, Olive Oil

Dice tofu into small cubes. Defrost vegetables in the microwave for 3 minutes. Mist some olive oil in a pan. Sauté diced tofu in oil until lightly browned, adding onion, Bragg, and paprika. Add vegetables and Cayenne pepper (to taste). Cook until hot.

Serve with Grains Mixture or Brown Rice, Kamut, Spelt, or Quinoa Pasta. Recipe makes two servings.

One Serving
137 calories   14 grms protein   10 grms carbs   2 grms fat   3 grms fiber

With 1/2 Serving of Grains Mixture
282 calories   26 grms protein   34 grms carbs   4.5 grms fat   6 grms fiber

MORE TOFU!

Using a package of extra-firm, low-fat tofu, do the following:

Marinate tofu overnight in low-fat Italian dressing (if allowable).

Heat a sautè pan until hot. Blacken tofu with Cajun spices.

Put into oven at 450 degrees for 10 minutes.

Slice and serve...on salads, on grains, etc.

250 calories   21 grms protein   2 grms carbs   5 grms fat

GREAT EGGS!

3 egg whites
51 calories 10.5 grms protein 0 carbs 0 fat

1 whole egg
75 calories   6.3 grms protein   0 carbs   5 grms fat

1/2 cup TVP
59 calories   11 grms protein   7 grms carbs   0 fat

2 Tablespoons Rice Parmesan Cheese
15 calories   2 grms protein   1 grm carbs   .5 grms fat

1 slice Soy or Rice Pepperjack Cheese
40 calories   4 grms protein   1 grm carbs   2 grms fat

1/2 cup chopped spinach (or any allowable vegetable)
30 calories   2 grms protein   5 grms carbs   2 grms fiber

1 tablespoon of Rice Butter

Bragg Liquid Aminos

Seasonings: Herbs, Paprika

Scramble eggs in a heated pan with rice butter. When almost done, add TVP, spinach, Bragg, seasonings, rice parmesan and Pepperjack cheese. Cook until done.

Values

270 calories   35.8 grms protein   14 grms carbs   7.5 grms fat   2 grms fiber

Have a craving for sausage and eggs?

Try LightLife Lean Italian Links

1 Soy Sausage: *60 calories   5 grms protein   5 grms carbs   2 grms fat*

ENDLESS PASTABILITIES

4 Ounces Pasta (Spelt, Quinoa, Rice or Kamut)
380 calories   10-20 grms protein   60-80 grms carbs   3 grms fat   5-10 grms fiber

1/2 Can Adzuki, Black, Kidney, Black Soy. Or Great Northern Beans (Hain, Eden)
220 calories   14 grms protein   38 grms carbs   10 grms fiber

1/2 Cup TVP
60 calories   11 grms protein   7 grms carbs   0 fat

1 LightLife Lean Italian Links (Soy Sausage)
60 calories   5 grms protein   5 grms carbs   2 grms fat

1 Cup Chopped Broccoli (Or Favorite Vegetable)
40 calories   4 grms protein   8 grms carbs   4 grms fiber

Handful (1 ounce) of Arame Sea Vegetables
40 calories   2 grms of protein   8 grms carbs   7 grms fiber

1 Can of Health Valley Chicken Broth or Vegetable Broth—No Salt Added
90 calories   14 grms protein   0 carbs   3 grms fat

Bragg Liquid Aminos

Rice Parmesan Cheese, Paprika, Allowable Seasonings To Taste

Broil soy sausage for a few minutes until brown. Slice in small pieces. Boil Pasta (al-dente) with Arame. Drain and return to saucepan. Add beans (and liquid if you are using Eden brand) to pasta and Arame. Add TVP, soy sausage, vegetable, chicken or vegetable broth, Bragg Liquid Aminos, Paprika, and seasonings to taste. Heat, and serve topped with Rice Parmesan Cheese. Supplies 2 Servings—Complete High Protein Meal

Per Serving:

465 calories   23 grms protein   50 grms carbs   3 grms fat   17 grms fiber

(Try Beano to aid digestion of beans.)

PACK A LUNCH!
Turkey Sandwich on Wheat-Free, Yeast-Free, High-Fiber Bread

4 oz Sliced Turkey Breast
120 calories   20 grms protein   1 grm fat

2 Slices Wheat-Free, Yeast-Free, High Fiber Bread
195 calories   6 grms protein   30 grms carbs   6 grms fat   6 grms fiber

Values For One Sandwich
315 calories   26 grms   protein   30 grms carbs   7 grms fat   6 grms fiber

RECIPES FROM THE NOLTE COMPOUND

The following are recipes that I created for Nick Nolte. After Doc Gary tested Nick, we knew what was supportive for him. At his home in California, Nick has a magnificent garden filled with organic vegetables, fruits, and herbs (the herb garden belongs to his son, Brawley). It was a great joy to just go out back and pick what we would eat! We needed to be mindful of balancing pH values for Nick, so each recipe indicates if it is on the acid side or the alkaline side.

BRAWLEY BUFFALO BURGER (acid)
1 pound of ground buffalo (4 servings)
1/2 jar flavored tomato sauce (peppers, onions, etc.) or salsa
Parmesan cheese (or soy or rice alternative)
Spike or favorite seasoning
Bragg Liquid Aminos (few squirts)
one tablespoon olive oil
one egg
Mix buffalo, cheese, sauce, Bragg, egg, and seasoning in bowl and make patties. Sautè in olive oil and one tablespoon of sauce. *Serve with vegetables to balance pH

NOLTE GARDEN VEGETABLES (alkaline)

cabbage

zucchini

yellow squash

cherry tomatoes

green beans (or asparagus, or any other green vegetable)

sage

paprika

Miso dressing

one teaspoon olive oil

Sautè cut up vegetables in Miso, sage, one teaspoon olive oil, and sprinkled paprika. Only slightly cook until hot.

BRAWLEY'S ROSEMARY POTATOES (alkaline)

baby potatoes, yellow potatoes, red potatoes (favorite potatoes)

rosemary

sage

paprika

olive oil

Wash and pierce potatoes and bake until slightly cooked. Thinly slice and sautè in one tablespoon of olive oil and fresh rosemary and dash of sage— sprinkle with paprika—cook until browned.

BRAWLEY'S ROSEMARY CHICKEN (acid)

One pound free-range chicken (four servings)

fresh rosemary

sage

one tablespoon olive oil

paprika

Wash chicken and slice—sauté in olive oil, rosemary, sage (dash), and paprika until fully cooked. *Serve with potatoes and sautèed vegetables or salad to balance pH

TAMARI CHICKEN (balanced pH)

One pound free-range chicken (four servings)

handful of Arame sea vegetable

San-J Fat-Free Tamari-Mustard Dressing

Bragg Liquid Aminos (few squirts)

one tablespoon olive oil

fresh ground pepper

sprinkle of Cayenne pepper

Sautè chicken and arame in 1/2 cup dressing and olive oil. Sprinkle with peppers (use Cayenne sparingly).

GARDEN SQUASH (ACORN, SUMMER, OR ANY OTHER FROM GARDEN) (alkaline)

squash (1 whole acorn or spaghetti squash—cut in half—makes 2-3 servings)

low fat rice or soy butter alternative (or Miso dressing)

paprika

Layer glass pan with 1/4" of water. Wash squash, clean out seeds, quarter and pierce. Spread rice butter on each piece and sprinkle with paprika. Cover with clear wrap—microwave until soft.

GRAIN DISH (complete protein—balanced pH)

Quinoa (two servings)

TVP (Texturized Soy or Vegetable Protein—Optional

Lentils (two servings)

Arame Sea Vegetable

Miso dressing

Bragg Liquid Aminos (few squirts)

Boil Quinoa, Lentils, and Arame in water and Bragg for 20 minutes. Add Miso and handful of TVP. Simmer until TVP is soft (approx. 5 minutes).

*Serve with salad.

EGG WHITE OMELET (slightly acidic)

One dozen egg whites—three yolks

Fat Free Jalapeno Pepper Soy Cheese (approx. 2 oz-cut up in small bits)

Goat Cheese (approx. 1 oz)

Bragg Liquid Aminos (few squirts)

cut up vegetables of your choice (or a sea vegetable to change pH)

rice or soy butter alternative (approx. 1 tablespoon)

paprika

Beat eggs and Bragg and pour onto vegetables in pan frying in rice butter. Add both cheeses and continue to stir until cooked. Sprinkle with paprika.

*This is for three meals.

TURKEY LOAF (acid)

1 pound ground turkey breast (4 servings)

salsa—one jar (mild)

Fat Free Jalapeno Pepper Soy Cheese (approx. 4 oz-cut up in small bits)

Health Valley Lentil Chili (in a can)

Bragg Liquid Aminos (several squirts)

one egg

paprika

Rub a glass baking pan with olive oil. Mix all ingredients in bowl and flatten in baking pan. Bake at 350 (for 1/2 hour. Drain all water from pan, sprinkle with paprika, and continue to bake until done (approx. 15 minutes—keep checking).

NO TURNING BACK

When you finally know that there is a God, you are extremely humbled. Nothing is ever the same again. (Hallelujah!) Second only to the profound impact that that awareness has had on my life is the humbling education I have received on my "health" expedition. Nothing can ever be the same again. (Hallelujah!)

For many years as a fitness professional I developed exercise protocols, designed specific workout programs, and counseled on nutrition. (The latter I clearly had no business doing.) To the best of my ability and limited knowledge, I would guide clients on how, what, and when to eat. I knew this component must be addressed in order to get any gratifying results—and, although it was always a big improvement on their usual eating habits, it was not (I eventually discovered) optimum.

Researching this book stopped me dead in my tracks. Wait a minute! How can you tell people what to eat if you have no information? Who *are* they? What are their unique issues? Yes—eating soy products is a wonderful idea, especially if you're a woman in your 40's—but what if you have low thyroid function or you are on a drug like Synthroid? Yes, having at least two fruits a day and balsamic vinaigrette on your salad is a great plan, but what if you have Candida? I could not in good conscience function as I used to in the fitness arena. I realized I must cease the old ways, and fully explore this new path before I could continue working. There is no turning back. I'm committed. I'm a believer.

As I have said over and over again in this book hoping it will be the one huge concept you embrace—*there is no such thing as one program for all people.*

EITHER YOU LIVE IT—OR YOU DIET

You've gotten a lot of information so far, but understand that all I'm really doing is pointing out the iceberg in the ocean to you, and all we're really seeing here is just the tip of it. Once you've finished this book, it will be up to you to dive for a closer look at the rest of your iceberg.

This is a way of life. But, there is a process. It starts with a healthy internal belief system. From there, you make adjustments as you create your ability to do so in your mind. You have the power to "think" yourself restored and beautiful. No more diets. No more short-cuts. No more roads to failure and depression. Believe in you. Start the process.

"Thoughts are things; they have tremendous power. Thought crystallizes into habit and habit solidifies into circumstances."

—Brian Adams

CHAPTER VIII

THE CRASH OF '92

"Consciousness creates the body. Our bodies are made up of dynamic energy systems that are affected by our diets, relationships, heredity, and culture and the interplay of all these factors and activities. We're not even close to understanding how our bodily systems interact with each other, let alone how they interact with other people's. Yet over two decades of my practice, it has become clear to me that healing cannot occur for women until we have critically examined and changed some of the beliefs and assumptions that we all unconsciously inherit and internalize from our culture. We cannot hope to reclaim our bodily wisdom and inherent ability to create health without first understanding the influence of our society on how we think about and care for our bodies."

—Christiane Northrup, M. D.
Women's Bodies, Women's Wisdom

"Top o' the world, Ma!" I was 42 years old. I had an extremely successful fitness business, and a health and fitness segment on the local Channel 5 News Show. I was planning my own fitness facility. I was financially secure.

I had attained notoriety in my field. I was living my dream.

It was about to become a nightmare. I was working 24-7. I was drained, sleep deprived, and nutritionally unbalanced. And, as I worked more, slept less, and grabbed meals on the go, I felt worse and worse. My moods were dark and my temper was short. I had <u>no</u> coping mechanism. Once I began sliding, it became an avalanche. I drank tons of caffeine to keep going, and drank almost a bottle of wine a night to settle down. I was no longer enjoying my work, my family, my life. I was depressed, but I was driven. I began hating the way I looked. I was obsessing about getting older. I turned my exercise routine up a notch. Then another. I was making myself nuts. I had insomnia. I couldn't turn off the work in my head. I got sick all the time, but I worked anyway (until I had to watch the Gulf War flat on my back with a raging fever). Before I was well, though, I was back at it. I just wouldn't take a break. Until *I* broke!

It began with inappropriate behavior. I became unrecognizable to myself (not to mention others!). I couldn't seem to control myself. I did off-the-wall things. My family was alarmed. My conduct was bizarre, even for me. They considered Baker-Acting me. I lived without accountability. I listened to no one. Then, I began to feel very alone. I was thinking of suicide. I was losing my memory. I was confused. I started to feel that I had to find a way out.

I cashed in my entire life—marriage, family, and business—and ran away. I trashed everything that mattered to me—my loved ones, my work, my home. "Why am I doing this?" It was as if someone else possessed my body. My depression deepened. I could not function. All I did was cry, and try to find my way home. Finally I did, and for six months I could not work, or even look anyone in the eye. I was ashamed and humiliated. The whole experience was surreal and terrifying. With my family's help, I slowly began to rebuild my health, and my world.

A nervous break-down someone said. *Clinical depression* said another. *Hormone imbalance* said still another. *Manic-depression* was yet another diagnosis.

For the longest time I had no clue what happened to me, until I began researching this book. In the work of some of the brilliant minds that I have referenced here, I found *me*! I cannot tell you the relief I felt! How validating and liberating it was to learn that there were reasons for my actions! Was I eating supportively for my blood type and my genetics, or was I suppressing my immune function? Did I have the appropriate foods in the right ratios to balance my oxidative rate, or was I creating biochemical havoc that altered my personality? Was I aware of my hypoglycemia, insulin resistance, and sugar-sensitivity, or was I sabotaging my entire system by adhering to the prevailing diet "wisdom" of the day? Was I addressing my low thyroid function, or was I compounding it with severe adrenal fatigue? Did I know my body was in an extremely acidic condition which caused a toxic environment in my body? Did I know that my wine was making an opportunistic Candida condition a victorious enemy within me? Wow.

I am not a wacko! I am not alone.

One of the most significant works in this realm is *Nutrition And Your Mind* by Dr. George Watson. Although published in 1972, it still stands as a thought-provoking, ground-breaking book. Dr. Watson studied the biochemical response of nutrients and related it to personalities. (His work on oxidative rates is one of the foundations of *Live It Or Diet Lifestyle Systems*.) Dr. W. D. Currier wrote in his forward of *Nutrition And Your Mind*: "It is dangerous to classify mentally disturbed persons solely in psychological terms. The old saying 'You are what you eat' is not precisely true, although every function of the body, and especially mental activity, is dependent upon the quality and kind of food we eat, as Dr. Watson explains. Our genetic endowment plays a fundamental part in mental health, and some persons may be mentally disoriented when they eat or lack certain foods."

Dr. Watson chronicles several case histories in his book. His work with "normal" people who behaved abnormally is intriguing stuff. Dr. Watson writes: "When one knows nothing of nutrition, and eats merely from ignorance, habit, or learned prejudices, there is a steady decrease in physical—and often mental—performance as the years of youth go by. Your personality, what you think, feel, and do, depends to a great extent on the biochemical reactions which occur in the cells of the nervous system. Indeed, your present pattern of life may not really reflect the 'optimum you' at all, and this can result solely from nutritional needs that you know nothing about."

The next section is called *Putting It All Together*. I've given you a lot to study and think about. Now you must begin to look at how to apply this information to <u>you</u>.

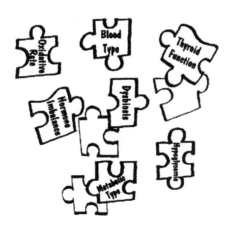

CHAPTER VIV

PUTTING IT ALL TOGETHER

YOUR PERSONAL GAME PLAN

"While true science is based on observation, experimentation, and continuous read-justment of thought processes and beliefs, depending upon its empirical findings, the same is true for trusting inner guidance. Ultimately, I've found it enormously empowering to realize that no scientific study can explain exactly how and why my own particular body acts the way it does. Only our connection with our own inner guidance (innate wisdom) and our emotions is reliable in the end. That is because we each comprise a multitude of processes that have never existed before, and will never again. My father used to say, 'Feelings are facts. Pay attention to them.'"

—Christiane Northrup, M.D.
Women's Bodies, Women's Wisdom

YOU ARE THE AUTHOR

In this section, I am going to leave it to you to sort out your own basic regimen. For more specific guidance (and to take this to the next phase), you can have <u>your</u> *Live It Or Diet Lifestyle System* constructed for you. There are many different types of tests and questionnaires that will take individualization to another level for you, but this book will start you at Phase I.

Phase I is about balance.
Some things are worth repeating, so I will reiterate Dr. Lee's words from the section, *Hormone Replacement Therapy and The Great Dilemma:*

"If you want to know what this book is about in a nutshell, I'll give it to you in one word—**balance**—a theme that recurs through every chapter. <u>If your diet is imbalanced, your hormones will be imbalanced. If your emotions are out of balance, your hormones will be out of balance.</u> If you are working too hard and not nurturing yourself, your hormones will be out of balance. **As you seek balance in your life, your health will improve.**"

In Phase I you begin to construct your blueprint for a healthier and more fit lifestyle. You begin the process. Don't look for your daily food lists. Don't look for the carbohydrate, protein, and fat gram amounts to count. Don't look for precise calorie and serving sizes. You won't find them in <u>Phase I</u>. Right now, I want you to *listen to your body.* You know if you are eating too much. When you are full...<u>stop eating</u> (see, *K.I.S.S.*). I have given you a great deal of information. Apply it. Trust that you have the knowledge to carry out <u>Phase I</u> (remember *"We Interrupt This Broadcast..."* ?).

"THE UNIFIED DIET"

An article published in The Palm Beach Post on July 5th, 1999, heralds the coming of the new "Unified Dietary Guidelines." The organizations endorsing the guidelines are: The American Heart Association, American Cancer Society, American Dietetic Association, American Academy of Pediatrics and the National Institutes of Health. The headline read "Experts Unite On Universal Diet That Works." The reporter, Shari Roan, writes: "Five of the nation's leading health organizations united to endorse a diet plan that, they say, represents the best and latest scientific advice for helping to prevent most major diseases. 'The good news is that we don't need one diet to prevent heart disease, another to decrease cancer risk and yet another to prevent obesity and diabetes,' said Dr. Richard J. Deckelbaum, a professor of pediatrics and nutrition at Columbia University in New York City who helped prepare the guidelines. 'A single healthy diet cuts across disease categories to lower the risk of many chronic conditions. Our idea was to first just meet to see if there were major differences. But (the groups' dietary recommendations) were all essentially in consensus with one another.'

Dr. Shelly Shapiro, a cardiologist with the University of Southern California Health Science Center and an American Heart Association spokeswoman said: 'The revolutionary part of this is that different groups choose to come together and try to reach a consensus.'

'We feel if we give the public similar messages they may have more incentive,' said Dr. Edward A. Fisher, director of lipoprotein research at New York's Mount Sinai School of Medicine's Cardiovascular Institute. When we come out with a recommendation, it's only because we have the evidence to support it. The problem with diet books is that the scientific evidence is lacking to support most of the programs.'

The unified guidelines are hardly sexy. Summarized in four major points, they are:

•Consume a variety of foods.

•Decrease fat intake.

•Increase consumption of fruit, vegetables. And whole grains.

•Consume only enough calories to maintain a proper weight.

The authors of the statement also point out that proper weight is best achieved with regular exercise. And they note that stopping smoking and consuming little or no alcohol are the cornerstones—along with the dietary guidelines—of good health behavior."

This is extremely basic stuff, okay? Remember "Lowering the water instead of raising the bridge" in the *Cardiovascular* section? The powers that be will come up with something—anything—you will do that is healthier than what you are currently doing now! You have demonstrated that you are resistant to any radical adjustments, so this is the dietetic version of "Exercise Lite." But, remember the thread that runs throughout this book—*understanding and addressing your individuality is the key to achieving any dramatic results!*

So, you want to know why I put this article in here?

Because my Mom called me all excited about it exclaiming, "Here's something I can do!" And, trust me, I have been working on my Mom for a looong time trying to get her to modify her eating and exercise behavior. (I'd like to keep my precious parents forever, ya know.)

So, does "The Unified Diet" sound simple to <u>you</u>? Well, if it's so simple, why are we as a country such a staggering distance from this (duh) painfully sound behavior? The truth is that one third of our adult population <u>still</u> smokes or drinks too much, and a third is *obese*.

I have been and done all of the above, my friend, and if a neurotic wing-nut like me can turn her life around, anyone can!

JUST THE BASICS

There is so much to know, and so much controversy. I wanted you to be aware of *all* that is out there. That's why it took me so long to complete this book. I felt this need to share with you all that I was learning—and I was learning something <u>every day</u>!

But, I do not want to overwhelm you, I want to jump-start you. Therefore, in the interest of *keeping it simple*, I'd like this book to accomplish one thing: To get you thinking and investigating in the right direction for <u>you</u>.

The following are some basic guidelines to help you begin your journey:

K.I.S.S... 12 LITTLE GOLDEN RULES TO FOLLOW FOREVER
(Basic Guidelines)

1. **Eat balanced meals,** with your appropriate ratios of Protein, Carbohydrate, and Fat (start with 1 gram of protein per pound of half your weight, figure in 15% fat, and fill in the rest with carbohydrates—see, *Back To Calories In-Calories Out* coming up in this chapter).

2. **Eat little or no refined and processed foods** (see, *Let's Go Shopping*, for information on whole and organic foods).

3. **Drink little or no alcohol,** especially distilled alcohol.

4. **Do not eat out of bags and boxes.** Count or measure out the serving size of any food so that you know how much you are consuming to help you stay out of that river in Egypt.

5. **Serve yourself like a person and sit down when you eat.** We are going to open up a chain of restaurants (for single people) that will have no tables and chairs, but rows of sinks instead. (These restaurants will have very low over-head as well because everyone will just wash their own dishes in their sinks when they are through.) Let's stop eating over the sink, okay? Don't we deserve a relaxed dining experience? Besides, we digest our food better when we are not rushed or stressed.

6. **Eat the bulk of your starchy carbs before six p.m.** (like brown rice or potatoes, etc.). Your last meal should contain mostly lean protein and vegetables. (There is never a good time to eat processed white bread!)

7. **Eat your last meal three hours before you go to sleep.** Your metabolism naturally slows down at night, and you will be more likely to store night-time calories as body fat.

8. **When you are full, stop eating.** Get up and do something else, and while you are doing that, ask yourself why you want to continue to eat.

9. **Drink the appropriate amount of water for <u>you</u>.** Divide your weight in half, and <u>that</u> number is how many ounces of water you should drink daily.

10. **Eat two servings of fruit and three servings of vegetables daily.** This is

important to supply your body with adequate vitamins, minerals, enzymes, and fiber.

11. **Consume between 20 and 40 grams of fiber daily.** The only way to effectively accomplish this is to stay away from processed foods.

12. **Follow the above eleven rules 80% of the time.** This 12th rule is that if you get off track 20% of the time, it won't harm you (particularly if you are in balance). But, if you are like most people, you will find that when you eat what you think you want 20% of the time, you feel so crummy compared to the other 80% of the time that you will gradually lower your "cheating" percentage. You will have discovered what it feels like to feel good, and it just won't be worth the price anymore to eat poorly.

PHASE I
Starting The Process—The First 28 Days

If you came here first hoping to "cut to the chase" and get the *Cliff Notes* version of this book—foiled again! This section will actually act as an index—taking you to key places in the text. I want you to know *why* I am asking you to do something. Sneaky, huh? Maybe. But, if you have avoided the contents of this book, you will be grateful for how this section is constructed once you are forced to go back and read what I have written. Trust me. You want to know this stuff.

Why 28 days? Because I do not want you overwhelmed by looking at a

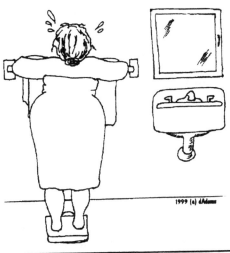

1999 (a) dAdams

TOWEL RACKS ARE A GREAT TOOL FOR WEIGHT LOSS!

loooong commitment in horror as if you've just been sentenced to 10 to 20 in solitary with no time off for good behavior. Falling off the wagon is easy when the road is long and bumpy. So, Doc Gary and I have constructed *The Live It Or Diet System* in phases. Also, <u>you can do a lot in 28 days!</u> You can make some real changes that will significantly impact how you look and feel.

During Phase I your body will begin to get into balance... approaching homeostasis...in harmony with itself so that it can begin functioning like the efficient machine it was designed to be. You cannot build anything that will stand without pouring a foundation first. Your first 28 days will be dedicated to that—building a strong and powerful platform on which to erect the new you. Focus only on attaining ground zero—that is eliminating all the culprits that you know are sabotaging you—and become determined to adopt a healthier lifestyle.

This is where you should begin using our Phase I support products. They will help to balance you, and address the gut issues that plague 99% of us. (See, *Live It Or Diet Phase I Protocol: Let's Get Started.*)

Cleaning House

When you begin a restoration project on anything, what is the first thing you do?

Clean! Out with the old—make room for the new.

Piles of accumulated junk and useless garbage you have been storing for years—outta here! Doesn't it feel great when you do that? You bet!

Now, apply the same principle to your body. You probably have years of accumulated junk festering in your body's basement.

During autopsies colons have been found weighing as much as forty pounds! Think about that! Yipes! You may easily be carrying around 10 to 15 pounds of encrusted debris (mucous, old fecal matter) on your colon wall, clogging up the works. This not only inhibits colon function, but it contributes to abdominal bloating and discomfort (as you can imagine). This garbage also affects peristalsis, (the contraction of the colon wall to move waste through) decreases nutrient absorption, and provides a toxic environment for disease to breed.

The intestinal tract is part of the digestive system. It is divided into two main parts; the small intestine and the large intestine (colon). The colon's primary function is to convert what remains after digestion into disposable waste. We must have proper elimination and maintain healthy flora to have a healthy colon. And the health of the colon is essential to the health of the body. **Every** health and fitness program needs to begin with addressing colon health. It doesn't much matter what else you do—exercise your brains out, eat more protein, cut out fat, chant or rant—if you are loaded with toxic wastes.

And so, I might be talking about unpleasant things in this section, but it is absolutely necessary to call your attention to this issue. It will mean the difference between a successful program and another disappointment. Believe me, I know. And you know I know if you have read this book.

Let me ask you a question. Do you eliminate twice a day? How about once a day, every day? IT IS NORMAL AND HEALTHY TO HAVE TWO ELIMINATIONS A DAY. IT IS NOT HEALTHY TO NOT HAVE ONE. Don't be in denial over this. You are being affected in ways you cannot even imagine if you do not eliminate wastes every day.

That's right. I'm gonna talk poop here.

You know the condition of your colon by your stool. What does yours look like? Do you ever look at it? Well, I want you to. No kidding. Here's what David Webster says it should look like in *Acidophilus & Colon Health*: "Your stool should be medium to light brown in color, free from foul odors, firm yet not hard, and most of it should float in the water." Does this describe yours? Also, you should not have to force your bowel movements. Waste should move from your body without much effort on your part. If you have to strain and force when you are on the bathroom, you have a problem.

Then there's "transit time," the time it takes for food to be completely digested. From the time you eat the food to the bowel movement normally takes between 12 and 20 hours. Transit time varies with dietary habits. It is not healthy when your transit system breaks down, leaving stuff stuck in a dark tunnel indefinitely (someone call maintenance!).

The latest statistics are that over 34 million people in this country alone suffer from digestive disorders! And the incidence is higher in women—23 percent of the female population as opposed to 15 percent of the male. Also, over 75 percent of women 65 years and older are frequently constipated!

Girls, we got trouble in River City with a capital P!

And this all leads to disease. According to the American Cancer Society, "Colon cancer is the number one cancer for men and women combined in America." David Webster in *Acidophilus & Colon Health* tells us that there is a combination of factors contributing to this condition: "Because the colon has no sensory nerves it is one of the body's most abused organs. This deficiency in sensory nerves means that colon problems usually only catch our attention when they are already advanced or chronic and begin to have an adverse effect on other bodily functions."

Detoxification And Cleansing

So what should we do?

In *Acidophilus & Colon Health* we read: "The first step in establishing colon health is to embark on a cleansing process. It is necessary to eliminate waste that has accumulated in the colon." Dr. Matsen in *Eating Alive* tells us that "the result of detoxifying the intestine will be increased absorption of nutrients, often very noticeable to a person as an improved sense of well-being." But know that once you start getting rid of that junk on your colon wall, you will become more sensitive. So, when you were once so insulated from "dietary indiscretions," now you <u>will</u> feel that cup of coffee at night, one glass of wine might go to your head, and you will <u>know</u> that that jelly-filled donut has just poisoned you!

Take It Slow!!!

Once again, more is not better! Especially in this case. (Remember, I know we're the same, you and I..."Oh yuck....I have what where??? Call Rotor-Rooter! Get it gone now!!!") Dr. Matsen says "If old toxins are stirred up faster than the elimination organs can handle them, a person will feel worse for a while." So, follow our directions, and take it slow.

Actually, some discomfort at first is inevitable. You are mobilizing some nasty stuff, and releasing toxins may temporarily cause some side affects, including: Headaches, sore muscles, and fatigue. <u>If</u> you experience any side affects, and <u>how severely,</u> depends on <u>how quickly</u> toxic wastes are eliminated (drink plenty of pure water!). David Webster in *Acidophilus & Colon Health* says that with colon cleansing "there are usually periods of great exhilaration. Listen for the body's messages. Be patient. If you desire to rest, do so. Don't over exert." You have been accumulating this toxic debris for years, so it will be challenging for your body to deal with it. Think about the way your body eliminates toxins—in your sweat, breath, urine, and stool. So all of these channels will be expelling toxins from your body as you cleanse. You might break out, or have an unfamiliar odor to yourself. This is <u>temporary</u>. And it's worth it, believe me.

Cleansing your colon produces a wide variety of elimination responses. You may experience gas or bloating, or even some diarrhea at first. This is your body adjusting to new stuff. It will pass (all puns are intended). You may have stronger-smelling eliminations because of the toxins in them. And you might notice that your toilet bowl is more full than usual. This is because the fiber that you have introduced in your diet is grabbing old junk and escorting it out. Also, fiber itself increases bulk. Now, because this junk has been residing in your colon for some time, you might notice that it has many different appearances: Dark, light, stripped, lumpy, and maybe even what looks like critters (see the section on *Parasites* in *Your Food Must Become You*).

The Rewards

You will begin to feel better, lighter, and more energetic than you have in a long time. You will think more clearly, move easier, and have an improved attitude. Your gut will begin to flatten and you will see your shoes. Your body's systems will begin to function better with less toxins to deal with, including the system that mobilizes fat!

Fiber

I have talked elsewhere in this book about fiber. There are many sections you can turn to that support the importance of fiber, among them: *Eat To Live, Glycemic Index Vs. "Effective Carbohydrate Content," Sugar Sensitivity*, and *EATING FOR HEALTH, HEALING, AND HARMONY*. There are two types of fiber—soluble and insoluble. Fruits and vegetables have cellulose (insoluble fiber) that is not broken down by the digestive process. You might have heard this referred to as "roughage." It helps to remove wastes from the colon. The fiber in brown rice, oat bran, and nuts, for example, are forms of soluble fiber. Research shows us that soluble fiber reduces blood cholesterol and supports fat metabolism. Safe, effective colon-cleansers are insoluble fiber-based products. And with increased fiber intake, you need to increase water intake. If you become constipated when you begin taking a colon-cleanser with insoluble fiber, it is probably because you are not drinking enough water. Think of insoluble fiber as a "sponge" in your colon that swells as it comes in contact with liquid. Proper hydration will keep this "sponge" moving through your colon, gathering junk along with it. Without enough water, the sponge could get stuck. Also, you may experience some "cramping" until you have passed the sponge. Increase your water intake to soften the sponge even more. Don't cut back on your water if you get diarrhea, as it is not a symptom of "too much water." Excess water is flushed through your kidneys, so if anything, you will just urinate more.

The Importance of Hydration

Drinking pure water is absolutely essential for the removal of waste products from your body. What is pure water? Well, I can tell you what it is <u>not</u>. It's not the water that comes out of your tap. Let's start there. The following is a quote from *An Analytical System Of Clinical Nutrition* by Guy R. Schenker, D.C.:

"Public water supplies contain large quantities of chlorine. Chlorination is essential to the distribution of sanitary water for household use. For household uses other than drinking, that is. (Although recent evidence suggests that bathing in chlorinated water may play some role in the recent dramatic increased incidence of Melanoma skin cancer.) Chlorinated water may be the most significant contributor to the atherosclerotic diseases. Chlorine sets off a free radical chain reaction that leads to plaque formation clinically resulting in degeneration, coronary, and stroke. Chlorine also results in the formation of chlorinated hydrocarbons in water (which are carcinogenic). A study by the California health department showed that chlorinated drinking water can increase the risk of miscarriage by 65%.

And what about fluoridation? Every country outside the U.S. which has tried fluoridating water to promote dental health has ultimately outlawed the practice due to it being ineffective and dangerous. Fluoridated water does not improve dental health; in fact it actually makes teeth more brittle. The quantities of fluoride found in may public water systems is toxic and inhibits cellular DNA repair. It is thus carcinogenic. It is also a causative factor in Down's Syndrome.

The case against public water is completed by noting the residues of aluminum salts, and the clinically significant quantities of pharmaceuticals found in water that has been through water treatment plants. Billions of pounds of drugs are eliminated annually in people's urine and feces. Waste treatment plants do not even touch much of this drug load, which is then 'recycled' to you in 'drinking' water. Giving one example—the concentration of antibiotics is 1000 times higher in U.S. water than German water. The Center For Adaptive Genetics And Drug Resistance at Tufts University speculates that this may contribute to the antibiotic resistance developed by so many bacteria. Antibiotics are only one of hundreds of drugs found in public water."

Wow. Think about that the next time you turn on your tap, or order a glass of water in a restaurant!

So, it is not just the quantity of water we need to drink (see, K.I.S.S. for guidelines) but the quality. Dr. Schenker says that "natural water" may be the most important nutritional consideration for everyone. Finding a good source of natural water is essential in preventing strokes, heart attacks, and kidney degeneration, and it is the best source of certain very valuable mineral nutrients. Considering this, we recommend that drinking water be from a natural source such as a spring or a well. And the water pH should ideally be 7 or above (see, Alkaline-Acid Balance). And what about filters or water purifiers? These are beneficial only in the rare instance that your public water has a pH above 7 and the desirable hardness. Then and only then will a <u>good</u> filter produce good drinking water. Otherwise you are wasting your time and money. Also, water softeners can be deadly, and under no circumstances should softened water be used as drinking water."

It seems you are better off finding a reputable source of spring water!

But is it getting to your cells?

Doc Gary tells us that you can drink two gallons of water a day and still be dehydrated on a cellular level. (Water is like any other nutrient—if it doesn't make it into the cell, it does little good.) He finds this is the case in 70% of his patients when they first arrive at the clinic. And most people are not aware of the effect that dehydration has on the metabolism of the body. Water regulates <u>all</u> functions of the body. Therefore, dehydration can affect any part of the body. We need water for spine, joint, and disc health. Also, it has been discovered that Attention Deficit Disorder, (ADD) Attention Deficit Hyperactivity Disorder, (ADHD) and all children that have difficulty in learning have one thing in common—dehydration! They are not getting water to the cells. In *The Homeopathic Review*, we read the following: "The difference at a cellular level is that a hydrated cell is like a grape that is full of water and is electrically charged and able to interact energetically. The dehydrated cell is like a raisin that is lacking water and is not electrically charged and unable to interact energetically. When dehydrated, the right side of the brain works independently of the left side. The charge that makes the electrical connection is missing. As a result, the right hand does not know what the left hand is doing." We have assumed that because we *drink* water we automatically *absorb* water. Recently, scientists have been introducing the theory that water needs to be "carried" to be assimilated. "The key to achieving hydration is to provide a transporter that will facilitate the uptake of water into the body," according to *The Homeopathic Review*. Adding small quantities of "transporters" can increase water uptake. Examples of transporters are: Apple, pear, and watermelon juice, caffeine, and dandelion. Years of research has lead to the development of a product called Hydrate that is part of our Phase I Protocol, *Let's Get Started*. Hydrate contains the right dilute amount of caffeine, dandelion, Germanium (acts as an anti-oxidant) and silica. Hydrate also enhances the flow of electrical current in your body. (See, *Live It Or Diet Phase I Protocol*.)

Most people think they are drinking water when they drink coffee, soda, tea, or fruit juice, but most of these drinks actually speed up water *loss*.

So, once again, drink pure, natural water.

For more information on water, refer back to section on *Water* in the chapter *NOW WHAT DO I EAT?*

LIVE IT OR DIET PHASE I PROTOCOL:
Let's Get Started

We have an optional starter kit for you that will make Phase I and your 28 days a more dramatic and successful event. The protocol is called *Let's Get Started* and it includes the following:

Lifestyle Colon-Cleanser
> Contains soluble and insoluble fiber to assist in removing intestinal debris, and probiotics to balance intestinal flora.

Lifestyle De-tox Tea
> A natural blend of herbs to gently encourage regular elimination.

Lifestyle Hydration Formula
> To assist cellular hydration.

Lifestyle Liver Formula
> Herbs to support and cleanse the liver.

Seasilver Foundational Health Formula
> A nutrient formula designed to balance body chemistry, cleanse vital organs, purify blood and lymphatics, nourish body on cellular level, oxygenate body's cells, protect tissues and cells against toxins, and strengthen the immune system.

(See, *Appendix F* for how to order the *Live It Or Diet* Phase I Protocol, *Let's Get Started* .)

WEEK ONE: First Things First
Your Gut

I want you aware of a possible underlying condition that could sabotage your efforts. Its nasty, relentless presence was doing me in (see, *15 Rounds—My Championship Bout,* page 143) so I recommend that you investigate if it is lurking within you.

Answer the following questionnaire before you continue:

DYSBIOSIS/CANDIDA QUESTIONNAIRE

1. Have you ever taken antibiotics?   yes/no

2. Have you ever had persistent prostatitis or vaginitis?   yes/no

3. Have you ever been pregnant?   yes/no

4. Have you ever taken birth control pills?   yes/no

5. Have you ever taken prednisone or   yes/no
   other cortisone-type drugs?

7. Are you sensitive to perfumes, pesticides, cleaning products, tobacco smoke and other chemicals? — yes/no

8. Are you more uncomfortable when it's humid or where it is moldy? — yes/no

9. Have you ever had athlete's foot, fungus under your nails or other similar external conditions? — yes/no

10. Do you crave processed carbs such as sugar and bread? — yes/no

11. Are you frequently tired, drained and lethargic? — yes/no

12. Do you find you have memory loss? — yes/no

13. Are you easily confused? — yes/no

14. Do you "zone out" and lose focus or concentration? — yes/no

15. Do your extremities become numb, burn or tingle? — yes/no

16. Do you have trouble sleeping? — yes/no

17. Do your joints swell or have pain? — yes/no

18. Do you have cramping or aching in your muscles? — yes/no

19. Do your muscles occasionally go weak or lose control? — yes/no

20. Do you have pain in your stomach? — yes/no

21. Do you ever suffer from constipation? — yes/no

22. Do you ever suffer from diarrhea? — yes/no

23. Do you frequently have gas, indigestion or heartburn? — yes/no

24. Do you ever feel bloated and swollen in your abdominal area? — yes/no

25. Do you have vaginal discharge, itching or burning? — yes/no

26. Do you have prostatitis? — yes/no

27. Do you suffer from impotence or loss of sexual desire? — yes/no

28. Do you suffer from endometriosis? — yes/no

29. Do you have severe menstrual cramps and PMS? — yes/no

30. Do you cry easily or have anxiety attacks? — yes/no

31. Are your extremities frequently cold? — yes/no

32. Do you get irritable or lose your temper easily? — yes/no

33. Do you have mood swings? — yes/no

34. Do you get headaches or feel pressure in your head? — yes/no

35. Do you ever get dizzy, lose your balance or have spots in front of your eyes? — yes/no

36. Do your eyes burn or tear easily? — yes/no

37. Do you get rashes or have itching? — yes/no

38. Do you have food sensitivies?   yes/no

39. Is there mucus in your stools?   yes/no

40. Do you have rectal itching?   yes/no

41. Does it burn when you urinate?   yes/no

42. Do you ever have a feeling of incontinence   yes/no
(urinary urgency or frequency)?

43. Do you have build up of wax or fluid in your ears?   yes/no

44. Do you have frequent ear infections, ear pain or   yes/no
reduction in hearing?

45. Do your eyes burn or itch?   yes/no

46. Do you have chronic sinus congestion or post nasal drip?   yes/no

47. Do you frequently get a sore throat, cough or have laryngitis?   yes/no

48. Do colds frequently turn into bronchitis?   yes/no

49. Do you have a coating on your tongue?   yes/no

50. Is your mouth frequently dry?   yes/no

51. Do you have bad breath?   yes/no

52. Do you have foot or body odor?   yes/no

53. Do you get "canker sores" or blisters in your mouth?   yes/no

54. Do you ever have shortness of breath?   yes/no

55. Do you ever have pain (tightness) in your chest?   yes/no

56. Do you bruise easily?   yes/no

57. Does your diet consist of mostly   yes/no
refined and processed foods?

58. Are you under stress?   yes/no

If you have answered half of these questions "yes," there is a strong probability that you have a condition of the gut that requires a special protocol.
Adhering to the following recommendations will be of additional benefit and
will provide dramatic changes in your weight and how you feel. In *Live It Or
Diet Systems* this condition is a "red flag" that overrides many other recommendations for about a month.

Dysbiosis/Candidia Protocol

Follow this protocol for one month if you answered "yes" to more than half of
the questions in the previous section. Try and stay strict if you can. The greatest benefits come from totally eliminating offending foods for one month.

Candida—A Review

Candida Albicans is not a disease. It is a stress-related condition of imbalance. It is exacerbated by anti-biotics (as opposed to pro-biotics which you can take to help combat this condition). Antibiotics kill the friendly as well as the harmful bacteria, allowing this condition to flourish. Candida also flares up in people who have taken birth control pills, have had chemotherapy, or have taken cortico-steroids.

Candida is not a germ or a bug. It is a parasitic strain of yeast-like fungus that rapidly multiply in the gastro-intestinal and genito-urinary areas of the body when resistance is low, and the immune system is overworked. These yeast reproduce by feeding on sugars and carbohydrates in these tracts. As it does, it further weakens the immune system, causing the infection called Candida Albicans or Candidiasis.

Many toxins are released in the bloodstream when this fungus travels throughout the body, and this causes extensive disturbances. These disturbances manifest themselves in numerous ways, creating a wide-range of symptoms that appear in the questionnaire. Even hypothyroidism, adrenal fatigue, and blood sugar regulation conditions such as hypoglycemia and diabetes have been traced back to Candida. Frequently, allergies to foods are present in people with candida infections. The symptoms of a food allergy or an environmental sensitivity are often the same as the symptoms of Candida. Because Candida symptoms mimic other conditions and diseases, it is often misdiagnosed.

People who have a nutritionally poor diet, (high in refined and processed carbohydrates, sugar, and alcohol) who do not get enough rest, and are stressed out are at risk for Candida.
(Turn to the section on *Candida Albicans*, page 174 for more information.)

It is important that you completely eliminate the following foods for 4 weeks:

• Sugars or sweeteners of any kind (Stevia okay)
• All products containing sugar (read labels)
• All products baked with yeast
• All gluten grains (wheat, oats, rye, and barley)
• Dairy products (except kefir or yogurt with live cultures)
• Smoked, dried, or pickled foods
• Mushrooms
• Nuts or nut butters (except almond and almond butter)

•Fruits, fruit juices, canned and dried fruits

•Coffee, black tea, and caffeine

•Carbonated beverages (the phosphoric acid binds up calcium and magnesium)

•Alcohol

•All things containing vinegar

•All fermented products, such as wine and soy sauce

•Ham and other processed luncheon meats

•All aged cheeses

The following are recommended foods:

•Lots of fresh and steamed vegetables. Include the following:

1.Onions	4.Cabbage	7.Kale
2.Garlic	5.Broccoli	8.Boc-Choy
3.Ginger root	6.Greens	9.Fennel

•Gluten-free grains such as brown rice, millet, amaranth, and buckwheat

•Pastas made from the above grains

•Poultry

•Seafood

•Sea vegetables

•Beans (especially soy)

•Tofu and tempeh

•Plain yogurt with live cultures

•Rice cakes/crackers

•Herb teas

•Some citrus fruits (such as grapefruit and lemon) after the first 4 weeks

This is an incredibly restrictive list, we know. But, the first 4 weeks are critical because these energy-draining yeasts must be starved of the foods they live on so they "die off." It is an option you need to consider if you want to feel better.

Determining Health Consideration Adjustments

There are certain considerations to be aware of that must modify your eating plan. When we construct a *Live It Or Diet Lifestyle System* for you, these and others will be factored in to an optimum regimen for you to follow. For now, however, without us to advise you one-on-one, please review the following issues and their compensations. This will help make Phase I more specific to you. Refer to the corresponding sections in this book.

Leaky Gut/Dysbiosis

If you have these or related conditions (and <u>most</u> people do) try the food combining in the related chapters to aid digestion, while adding the supportive formulations recommended for Phase I. (See, *Digestion*, page 148 and *Leaky Gut and Dysbiosis*, page 190).

Blood Type

Knowing your blood type will lead to basic awareness of foods that are supportive, benign, and detrimental, based on D'Adamo's (and earlier) research. If you do not know your blood type, you can go to your doctor, give blood, or order our blood-typing kit off our website (or call our hot line). (Review *Blood Type Recommendation*, page 340).

Food Sensitivies

If a food is supportive for you based on the above considerations—but you have a sensitivity to it—it must be rotated out of your food planning. (Go to *Food Allergies*, page 153).

Hypoglycemia

Your meal patterning must consist of meals spaced no more than three hours apart. Foods with a high glycemic index must be avoided. (See *Hypoglycemia*, page 164 and *Glycemic Index* in *Appendix*, page 373).

CHD

If you have a history of cardiovascular disease, high blood pressure, high cholesterol, (anything above 180) or you are at high risk because of your family history, you would follow a low fat diet with very limited animal protein. This would cancel out any blood type recommendations for red meat and override any fat recommendation over 15%. (Go to *Eat To Live*, page 196).

Diabetes

This condition would indicate protein recommendations no higher than 20% of your daily calories. Also, research shows that diabetics (and people at risk for diabetes) should reduce fats and oils, and limit dairy. (See, *Can I Give Myself Diabetes?*, page 168).

Hypertension

This condition would indicate protein recommendations no higher than 20% of your daily calories. (Again, return to the section addressing *Cardiovascular Disease*, page 196).

Drug Interactions And Drug Depletion

Certain drugs and foods have a negative interaction (ex: Synthroid and soy foods) while other drugs seriously deplete certain nutrients from the body. Check with your pharmacist—and refer to *Drug Depletion*, page 92.

Sugar Sensitivity

If you feel you are sugar-sensitive, you could try the food combining recommended in that chapter to raise serotonin levels. Foods with a high glycemic index must be avoided. (See, *Sugar Sensitivity*, page 170 and *Glycemic Index* in *Appendix*, page 373).

Food Rotation

Do not eat the same foods day in and day out to reduce the risk of developing sensitivities, and to maximize nutrient absorption. (Return to the section on *Food Allergies*, page 153.)

Low Thyroid Function

If your basal temperature falls below normal range, your calories must be adjusted down to compensate (throws off the "calories in-calories out" balance equation). Basal temperature testing is done based on Barnes' protocol. Low thyroid function also effects protein requirements—hypothyroidism would indicate a lower protein ratio in your daily calories. Supportive nutrition is also required. (Return to *Thyroid Hormone*, page 177)

Checking Your Thyroid Function

Remember, thyroid function is a first-string player in your "hormonal orchestra" (see, *Thyroid Hormone*). Because of this, we recommend the following simple test. If your thyroid function is low, it could be a significant link in the chain of issues that are putting you out of balance. If your thyroid function is *very* low, it could throw off your caloric requirements because your metabolism is severely affected.

Broda O. Barnes, M.D., in his book *Hypothyroidism: The Unsuspected Illness*, writes the following: "Thyroid secretion is essential for the operation of the cell and, in effect, determines how hot the fire gets in the cell and the speed of activity in the cell. The term 'metabolism' refers to the fires within the body cells."

Dr. Barnes continues that when the thyroid gland is removed from an otherwise normal animal, all metabolic activity is reduced, and metabolism can reach levels as low as 35 to 40 percent of normal. So, as you can see, when looking at these "requirement" and "expenditure" charts, you'll want to know if your thyroid is functioning normally.

Dr. Barnes maintains that axillary, or underarm temperature (basal temperature) is one of the more accurate methods of testing thyroid function. (Basal means that the body is <u>totally</u> at rest.) Dr. Barnes offers the following guidelines (you will need a basal thermometer—one that is used under your armpit):

"Take your basal thermometer to bed with you. Shake it down well and place it on the night stand. Immediately upon awakening in the morning, (do not get out of bed—*do not sit up—move as little as possible*) place the thermometer snugly in the armpit for ten minutes by the clock. A reading below the normal range of 97.8 to 98.2 strongly suggests low thyroid function.

The basal temperature can be taken by a man on any given day. Not so for a woman. During the menstrual years, temperature fluctuates during the cycle. Basal temperature is best measured on the second and third days of the period after flow starts." (Dr. Gary recommends that you take your temperature days 2 through 5 of your cycle.) "After menopause, the basal temperature may be taken on any day." If you test hypothyroid (low thyroid) there are nutrients that will support the thyroid. *Live It Or Diet Lifestyle Systems* incorporates formulations developed by Dr. Gary and Dr. Jack Hinze that specifically address different issues, such as low thyroid function. These formulations will stimulate different glands and processes to function more efficiently.

Moving On

Once again, this is just <u>Phase I</u>...the first step in your journey. I do not know you or your specific issues, so the most I can do in this format is present some basic guidelines. First, it is important that you understand that there is more to all of this than just jumping in with reckless abandon. As I told you in the *Cardiovascular Conditioning* chapter, I urge you to turn to *Appendix A* for **The American College Of Sports Medicine Risk Factor Checklist.** Certain factors put you at higher risk for certain conditions and diseases. I recommend that you consult your physician before you engage in any new programs.

During this 28 day period you can track your progress (and remember, I recommend that you do) in a journal. Writing down your experience daily will help you to gain perspective and keep focused. (See, *Appendix F* for the *Live It Or Diet Daily Journal*). I am not saying that this is a "28 day program"—it is a program for life. However, I want you to track your progress for four weeks to make certain that you are sure-footed and well-armed on your new path. Celebrate your victories (and defeats—we all have them) in your journal. Write down what you eat, and how it makes you feel. This is very important! Remember what it says in this book—food is the most powerful drug you will put in your body. It always makes you feel something: Energized, lethargic, happy, depressed, re-vitalized, bloated—you name it—when you put something into your body, it responds. Record how that food made your body react so you remember it.

Also, weigh yourself only once a week, not obsessively every day. Baby-boomer women have the ability to bloat by 2 to 5 pounds in a matter of hours as a result of about a billion things! Track only your fat loss—not your sputtering hormones—or you will lose your mind!

And...remember to have fun.

Embrace the process—enjoy the journey—stay in the moment!

THE NEXT THREE WEEKS - Burn Fat For Fuel!

You may be disappointed if you fail, but you are doomed if you don't try.
—Beverly Sills

Do not be discouraged if you did not drop any significant "weight" during your first week. You are probably dealing with metabolic issues and gut problems that need correction. This next three weeks will turn up the heat in your program.

During these next three weeks of Phase I you will be concerned about caloric guidelines, and energy expenditure (while integrating the considerations you put in place in week one). I just want you to begin thinking in simple, basic terms. Although I say in this book that I do not subscribe to the concept of "Calories In-Calories Out,"(See, *Calories In-Calories Out And Other Fairy Tales*, page 98) I do want you to be aware of energy requirements.

Before you begin the next three weeks, you will assess: The approximate daily caloric intake required to stay as you are, the energy cost of certain exercises, and what you need to do to attain your "ideal" weight.

Although we all do possess that "metabolic mystery" that throws off these numbers, it is just an approximation to get you on track. These calculations do not take into account your body-fat to lean tissue ratios and most of your specific issues. But, I believe it is important that you are <u>aware</u> of just how much you require to run your body at its current weight, and what adjustments are needed to <u>lower</u> your current weight. Again, I hate talking in terms of "weight" and such, but until we build your *Live It Or Diet System*, this is a good place to start.

In *Calories In-Calories Out... And Other Fairy Tales* it says that, "being sedentary is a very good way to gain fat... you need to expend calories above your daily basal metabolic requirements to efficiently lose body fat." But remember, it also says that if you are *strength training*, you will be gaining muscle... and that is a good thing! Although it weighs more than fat, muscle takes up less space than fat, and is *metabolically active*. That means your metabolism will increase with each pound of muscle you gain! (Go to *The Truth You've Been "Mything" About Muscle*, page 13). So, it is <u>not about the scale</u> my friend. Do not "diet" and look for pounds lost on the scale. Without exercise, those pounds could be your precious muscle!

Meanwhile, stick to your *Blood Type Recommendations*.

Stay focused on any *Health Consideration Adjustments* that applied to you from Week 1.

And keep that body moving! If you follow the plan, you will begin to BURN FAT FOR FUEL!

Record what you eat, how you feel, and your exercise regimen for the next three weeks in your journal.

BACK TO CALORIES IN-CALORIES OUT

Alright, maybe it is a fairy tale, but let's say we believe in them for a moment—just to keep it simple. You must be aware of how much you <u>consume</u>, how little you actually <u>burn</u>, and what you <u>need</u> regarding calories (remember *The Unified Guidelines*). Although this approach homogenizes much of the information in this book, and it is flawed (what <u>is</u> "ideal" body weight?)—it will probably be extremely enlightening anyway.

We usually do not pay enough attention to this stuff, so bear with me. If this is complicated for you, do not panic. I understand. Some people look at this stuff and glaze right over. That's why people like me have a job! However, if you are good with numbers and a calculator and you like figuring things out, you will love what is coming up. It may even seem like a game to you. If you are frustrated, don't worry. All of this and much more will be determined in Phase II when you have a *Live It Or Diet Lifestyle System* built for you. Just by-pass this section and go straight to *Appendix C* to start at Phase II with a *Live It Or Diet* councilor.

All I want to accomplish here is to get you out of Egypt (denial) again. I need for you to know that if you weigh 150 pounds, that one hour walk that you take will only burn 180 calories—not enough to offset that 500 calorie dessert!

Since I do not have you here with me to properly evaluate you, I have included charts (which I modified from *Nutrition For Fitness and Sport* by Professor Melvin Williams). Again—height and weight charts will not tell you about your body's composition. And...do you have a small frame, a medium frame, or a large one? Well...look at your wrists. Are they "tiny?" Be honest now.

Or, try this: Measure your elbow bones. Extend your arm—bend your elbow at a 90 degree angle with your wrist facing your body—place your thumb and index finger on the two prominent bones on either side of your elbow—measure the space between your two fingers with a ruler. If a woman measures more than 2 1/4 inches to 2 5/8 inches, she probably has a medium to large frame, and if she measures less, she probably has a medium to small frame. If a man measures more than 2 3/4 inches to 3 1/8 inches, he probably has a large to medium frame, less—probably medium to small.

Ready? Take a deep breath—here we go...

TABLE 1:

DETERMINATION OF "IDEAL" BODY WEIGHT:

Females age 25 and over. (If you are between 18 and 25, subtract one pound for each year under 25.)

Height	Lbs (Small Frame)	Lbs (Medium Frame)	Lbs (Large Frame)
5'10"	134-144	140-155	149-169
5'9"	130-140	136-151	145-164
5'8"	126-136	132-147	141-159
5'7"	122-131	128-143	137-154
5'6"	118-127	124-139	133-150
5'5"	114-123	120-135	129-146
5'4"	110-119	116-131	125-142
5'3"	107-115	112-126	121-138
5'2"	104-112	109-122	117-134
5'1"	101-109	106-118	114-130
5'0"	98-106	103-1151	11-127
4'11"	95-103	100-112	108-124
4'10"	92-100	97-109	105-121
4'9"	90-97	94-106	102-118

TABLE 2:

APPROXIMATE CALORIC EXPENDITURE PER MINUTE FOR BICYCLING AND WALKING:

Calories Burned Per Minute Per Pound Of Body Weight
Weight In Pounds:
100 105 110 115 120 125 130 135 140 145 150 155 160 165 170 175 180 185 190 195 200

EXERCISE:
Calories Burned Per Minute In Bicycling

5 mph
1.9 2.0 2.1 2.2 2.3 2.4 2.5 2.6 2.7 2.8 2.9 3.0 3.1 3.2 3.3 3.4 3.5 3.6 3.7 3.8 3.9
10 mph
4.2 4.4 4.6 4.8 5.1 5.3 5.5 5.7 5.9 6.1 6.4 6.6 6.8 7.0 7.2 7.4 7.6 7.9 8.1 8.3 8.5
15 mph
7.3 7.6 8.0 8.4 8.7 9.1 9.5 9.8 10 10.5 10.9 11.3 11.6 12 12.4 12.7 13.1 13.4 13.8 14.2 4.5

Calories Burned Per Minute In Walking to Light Jogging

2 mph
2.1 2.2 2.3 2.4 2.5 2.6 2.8 2.9 3.0 3.1 3.2 3.3 3.4 3.5 3.6 3.7 3.9 4.0 4.1 4.2 4.3
3 mph
2.7 2.9 3.0 3.1 3.3 3.4 3.5 3.7 3.8 3.9 4.1 4.2 4.4 4.5 4.6 4.8 4.9 5.0 5.2 5.3 5.4
4 mph
4.2 4.4 4.6 4.8 5.1 5.3 5.5 5.7 5.9 6.1 6.4 6.6 6.8 7.0 7.2 7.4 7.6 7.9 8.1 8.3 8.5
5 mph
5.4 5.7 6.0 6.3 6.5 6.8 7.1 7.4 7.7 7.9 8.2 8.4 8.7 9.0 9.2 9.5 9.8 10.1 10.4 10.6 10.9

OKAY...REALITY CHECK. GO TO..."YOUR BASIC CALORIC REQUIREMENTS"
(Take your calculator, and a clear head, okay? If you have brain fog, save this for another day.)

YOUR BASIC CALORIC REQUIREMENTS

1a. The approximate daily base-line calories needed for your current weight: _____

To maintain your current weight, multiply the weight you are now by:
- 12 calories per pound if you are sedentary
- 13 calories per pound if you are moderately active (most people)
- 14 calories per pound if you regularly participate in some form of recreation

2a. The adjustment for your metabolism: _____% or -_____calories

Based on your thyroid function. Using Barnes' protocol of basal temperature testing, deduct a percentage of calories from your daily requirements (1a) depending on where your basal temperature falls. If it is between 98.2 and 97.8 it is normal (no compensation)—between 97.8 and 97, deduct 10% from your base-line calories (1a)—between 97 and 96, deduct 15% from 1a—below 96, deduct 20% from 1a.

3a. Specific dynamic action of foods: +_____calories

Calories needed to digest different macronutrients (5% for fats, 10% for carbs, 20% for proteins—but you will average it out to 10% of total calories after thyroid compensation -2a).

4a. Your approximate daily caloric requirements for maintenance:

_____

Factoring in all of the above. (1a-2a+3a=4a)

1b. The approximate daily base-line calories needed for your "ideal" weight: _____

Using table 1, figure your ideal weight, then multiply it by the following:
- 12 calories per pound if you intend to remain sedentary
- 13 calories per pound if you will be moderately active

2b. The adjustment for your metabolism: _____% or_____calories

Based on your thyroid function. Using Barnes' protocol of basal temperature testing, deduct a percentage of calories from your daily requirements for ideal weight (1b) depending on where your basal temperature falls. If it is between 98.2 and 97.8 it is normal (no compensation)—between 97.8 and 97, deduct 10% from your base-line calories (1b)—between 97 and 96, deduct 15% from 1b—below 96, deduct 20% from 1b.

3b. Specific dynamic action of foods: +_____calories
Calories needed to digest different macronutrients (5% for fats, 10% for carbs, 20% for proteins—but you will average it out to 10% of total calories after thyroid compensation).

4b. Your approximate daily caloric requirements for "ideal" weight:

_____

Factoring in all of the above. (1b-2b+3b=4b)

_____

1c. The difference between current weight and "ideal" weight requirements: _____calories per day
You might need to modify this. (See, *Let's Talk*.)
2c. Average calories per day spent for exercise: _____
Take total calories spent per week for cardiovascular exercise, and divide that by 7. (See, *Game Plan*)

3c. Total 1c and 2c: _____ calories (modify 1c if needed)

4c. Subtract from 4a: _____ calories per day (do not consume less than 1200 calories per day)

I recommend that you vary your calories by about 100 to 200 from day to day. On the days that you exercise, consume more calories than on the days that you do not exercise. Track this in your journal.

LET'S TALK...

What do you do now? Do you plummet down to the calories required to maintain your "ideal" weight from the calories you need now to maintain your current weight? Well, if it is quite a distance, that is not a good idea. Your metabolism will become alarmed and slow down to compensate for the drop.

The safest way to lose your body fat is to spend your calories (energy) from 2 "accounts"—diet and exercise.

Let's take an example:

Say you currently weigh 160 pounds, but you are 5'3" with a small frame, so you really should weigh about 110 pounds (Table 1).

You are sedentary, so your base-line requirements to stay at your weight are approximately 1900 calories. "Wow," you say, "I'd be a house if I ate that much!" You check your thyroid function. It is very low—that is why you'd be a house if you ate that much. (Also, let's face it, if you added up every single little thing you ate during the course of the day, what do you think the number would be? Try it.)

You calculate a 20% reduction in calories to compensate for your low thyroid. That puts you at approximately 1500 calories.

You add back in 10% of that 1500 calories for "specific dynamic action of foods." That puts you at approximately 1650 calories to maintain your current weight.

Now, your base-line requirements for your "ideal" weight of 110 pounds are 1300 if you intend to remain sedentary (not a good idea) or 1400 if you have decided to move around a bit (bravo).

Compensate for your low thyroid, and you have 1100 calories.

Add back in 10% for "specific dynamic action of foods" and you have 1250 calories.

That's a difference of 400 calories per day.

So...do you just go there?

No. Drop your calories slowly. Start with spending about 200 calories per day from your diet account for the first week, then 300 calories per day for the second week, and so on if you need to. I do not want you to lose more than 2 pounds per week, so be careful. Also, we are about to factor in your exercise component. That will add to your calorie "expense" per day.

For example:

You've decided to walk for your cardiovascular "event." Okay. How frequently? How long? My recommendation to you is to start with one of two programs: Walk for an hour three times per week, or for 30 minutes five times per week at a little higher intensity (see, *Cardiovascular Conditioning*). Both programs will average out to about the same caloric expense for you at your current weight (you can even vary them)—1800 calories per week.

To average that out over the week, divide that number by 7 (days in a week) and you have approximately 250 calories per day that you are spending from your <u>exercise account</u>.

So you start by spending a total of 450 calories per day from both accounts. Multiply that by 7 (days per week) and that's approximately 3150 calories, just under one pound. Not enough? You want it to be 3500 so you can lose at least a pound a week? I recommend you spend a bit more from your <u>exercise account</u> then. It is much more effective in the long run.

(Also I want you to vary your calories daily. The best way to do that is to consume a little bit less on the days that you are sedentary.)

See how it works?

Now...go to "Your Game Plan For Fat Loss"

YOUR GAME PLAN FOR FAT LOSS

One pound of fat supplies 3500 calories (of energy). In order to lose 2 pounds of fat per week, <u>you must burn (spend) 7000 calories.</u>

Your daily caloric (energy) requirement for maintaining your current weight is approximately_____ calories (4a).

Your daily caloric requirement for maintaining your "ideal" weight is approximately _____ calories (4b).

That is a difference of_____calories per day (1c). You will modify that to start

(See, *Let's Talk*).

You want to lose a total of _____ pounds of fat to be your "ideal" weight of_____pounds

(Based on Table 1). What is the most efficient way to do that?

(Please understand that if you are also strength-training—and it is seriously recommended that you do—that the scale may not reflect the drop in body fat as dramatically as you would think. This is because muscle weighs more than fat, and you will be adding to your lean muscle mass. This is extremely desirable for the fol-

lowing reasons: Increased muscle increases your metabolism, and you will burn more fat because of that—muscle takes up less space than fat, so by all means you want to displace the fat on your body with muscle—and muscle is the only tissue you can shape, so you will be able to sculpt a more pleasing physique. Please do not obsess over the scale! It is preferable that you calculate appropriate weight by body-fat testing. Your follow-up body-fat tests will indicate fat loss, which is what you are concerned about. See Appendix D for Accumeasure.)

Each time you perform your cardiovascular exercise, you will be spending approximately_____calories per event (Table 2).

A. Your aerobic exercise account spends (approximately) the following:

1. Calories spent for each cardio event:_____

2. Frequency of event (per week):_____

3. Total calories spent per week:_____

4. Calories spent per week divided by 7 to average expense per day:_____

B. Your nutrition account spends (approximately) the following:

1. Calories per day —the difference between 4a and 4b (1c) modified:

_____

2. Calories spent from this account per week (multiply the above x 7):

_____

TOTAL CALORIES FROM BOTH ACCOUNTS (A3 + B2): _____

C. Approximate pounds of fat-loss per week (no more than 2 pounds please):_____
(Divide total calories from both accounts by 3500)

D. Approximate weeks to fat-loss goal: _____
   (Divide pounds you wish to lose by the number arrived at in C)

HOW FAT IS FAT?

Good question—and, one that I am asked all the time. If we are talking body fat, (and that is what we should be talking) the following guidelines for dangerously over-fat are provided by Jackson & Pollack:

<u>For women</u> 21-30 years old—30% and over, 31-40 years old—32% and over, 41-50 years old—33% and over, 51 and older—34% and over

<u>For men</u> 21-30 years old—22% and over, 31-40 years old—24% and over, 41-50 years old—27% and over, 51 and older—29% and over

BMI

One of the markers that is frequently used when body fat assessment is not available is called BMI, or Body Mass Index. It is flawed in that it does not take body fat to lean tissue ratio into account, but you'll find that it is used alot when government agencies want to offer guidelines for increased disease risk.

You use the metric system to figure out BMI. The equation is the following:

Bodyweight in kilograms divided by (**Height in meters**)^2

(remember "squared" from school a hundred years ago—it's when you multiply something by itself)

You convert pounds to kilograms by dividing them by 2.2

You convert inches to meters by multiplying them by 0.0254

Okay?

Let's take me as an example once again:

$$\frac{105 \text{ lbs divided by } 2.2 = 48\text{kg (my bodyweight in kilograms)}}{(60" \times 0.0254 = 1.5)^2 = 2.25 \quad \text{(my height in meters squared)}}$$

48kg divided by 2.25 = 21 BMI

*A BMI range of 20 to 25 is considered normal

  *21.3 - 22.1 is suggested for females

  *21.9 - 22.4 for men

  *BMI values above 27.8 for men and 27.3 for women are associated with increased incidence of several health problems, including high blood pressure and diabetes.

YOUR BLOOD TYPE RECOMMENDATIONS

If you know your blood type, you can also begin making adjustments with the foods you are eating. When building a *Live It Or Diet System* for someone, one of the first bits of information we get is an individual's blood type. Based on that information, we make certain adjustments before we have the rest of the information to complete the food plans. Just these preliminary modifications in diet according to blood type alone initiates weight loss, decreased bloating, and increased energy. The following guidelines are based on the work by Dr. Peter D'Adamo:

BLOOD TYPE O
"Gotta Do It-Gotta Have It-Gotta Be It-Now!"

If your blood type is O, the following are some characteristics that are unique to you—many of which you may not be aware of:

Your dietary type drives a body that runs best on pure protein foods. "Gotta Do Its..." do it best on meat, poultry, and fish. Yes, I am aware that most red meats are high in saturated fats, and this is something we have all been told to avoid. However, one of the best reasons to stay away from most red meats is that they have been intentionally fattened and shot with hormones to grow larger, and dosed with antibiotics and other drugs to counter the absurdly inhumane and unhealthy conditions they are forced to live in. I have told you about natural, organically grown, *free range* meat and poultry—which is a healthier way to give your protein-hungry metabolism what it desires.

Now, I have also told you that protein foods are "acid-producing," and eating large amounts of them will upset your body's delicate pH balance. We therefore recommend infusing your diet with many "alkaline" foods to balance the pH of your meals. These include most vegetables—making the foundation of "Gotta Do Its" diet <u>lean meats and vegetables.</u>

"Gotta Do Its..."*do not* do it so well on many grains, dairy products and beans. These foods may bloat you as they are not easily digested by your system—which has been designed for "higher octane" fuel. You might also discover that you have an allergy (sensitivity) to wheat. The gluten in wheat robs most "Gotta Do Its" of energy, and inhibits weight loss. Therefore, the <u>good news</u> is that if you eliminate wheat products from your diet, *you will lose weight.* The <u>bad news</u> is that the majority of the foods that you are used to eating *are made from wheat.* Most breads, pastas, etc. that Americans consume start out on a wheat field. You probably have been living on "fat free" refined and processed products that contain a list of ingredients beginning with *enriched wheat flour*—and you have also probably been wondering why you cannot lose weight! Most blood type O's are actually gluten-sensitive in general, and should consider avoiding all other grains that contain gluten, such as: Oats, rye, and barley, and integrate quinoa, buckwheat groats, brown rice, millet, and amaranth. You should also consider avoiding: Corn, chocolate, asparagus, cocoa, and sunflower seeds, along with all dairy products.

"Gotta Do Its" typically have sluggish thyroids as well. This makes staying lean very challenging. There are many nutrients that stimulate the thyroid, and there are also foods that suppress thyroid function—if yours is already weak (see, *Thyroid Hormone*).

BLOOD TYPE A
"Harvesting Health"

We have good news and bad news for your blood type. First—the good news. We can offer recommendations in your *Live It Or Diet Lifestyle System* that will help you become leaner and more energetic. The bad news is—this will not happen on a typical American diet of meat, potatoes, and refined and processed foods. Your blood type thrives on a primarily vegetarian diet—one that is as close to Divine design as possible—natural and organic. Once you eliminate red meats from your diet (along with refined and processed starches), *you will become leaner.*

Animal foods cause the "Health Harvester" to feel bloated and tired. They bog down your system, and your body has to work very hard to process them. Most meats, dairy products, and processed foods derived from wheat all promote fat gain for you, while vegetables and soy products, along with fruits such as pineapple, encourage fat loss.

"Health Harvesters" do very well with most fish, and a wide variety of beans. Beans (when combined with organic, whole grains) provide a complete protein your type flourishes on. Vegetables (fresh, raw or steamed, and organic) are your main-stay. Also, eat plenty of fruit. And discover tofu. Learn to love this and other soy products such as TVP (texturized vegetable protein—little soy granules that can be used in a variety of ways). There are so many ways to prepare this wonderful protein source (see, *Eating For Health, Healing, and Harmony*). Chicken and turkey are also okay for blood type A (try to find organic, free-range poultry), but not red meat. You may also consider avoiding: Tomatoes, eggplant, clams, mushrooms, and potatoes, along with wheat and dairy.

BLOOD TYPE B
"The Yin and The Yang"

One word best describes your dietary recommendations: Balanced. While "Gotta Do Its" and "Health Harvesters" have many limitations in their programs, yours includes a wide variety of foods. However, along with blood types O and A, "Yin-Yangs" need to stay away from refined and processed products derived from wheat. The gluten in wheat robs most individuals of energy, and inhibits weight loss. Also, it frequently is targeted as a culprit when testing for food allergies.

"Yin-Yangs" do well (and become leaner) on a diet that integrates meat, vegetables, and low-fat dairy products (in fact—yours is the only blood type that is not sabotaged by dairy). You thrive on most fish, but you can take or leave most beans. You can enjoy a vast assortment of grains and fruits. Besides wheat, consider avoiding: Most nuts and seeds (chestnuts and almonds are okay), black beans, black-eyed peas, chickpeas, corn, amaranth, barley, buckwheat, radishes, and nut and seed oil.

BLOOD TYPE AB
"Genetic Combo"

If you are a "Genetic Combo," your blood type is rare, complex, and a relatively new one. You don't really fit into any of the other types. You have some qualities that are similar to "Health Harvester" and some that are similar to "Gotta Do Its," and this combination could mean you have special problems.

Your genetic programming can be very confusing. "Genetic Combos" typically have low stomach acid, but their bodies do well on some meats (except beef, chicken, and organ meat). What this could mean is that because you might have an impaired ability to break down animal protein, you could store it as fat. Good advice would be to supplement with digestive enzymes (possibly a formula that contains HCL), and to eat small amounts of animal protein with vegetables. Also, you can add protein to your diet with tofu (and other soy products).

Wheat is not great for your type if you are looking to lose fat. Also, certain foods can cause an undesirable insulin reaction, resulting in hypoglycemic symptoms. It is best that you stay away from refined and processed foods. Also consider avoiding: Black beans, chickpeas, lima beans, black-eyed peas, pumpkin, sesame and sunflower seeds, corn, buckwheat, radishes, mangos, oranges, and oils from seeds.

HOW DOES THIS ALL WORK?

Once you know your approximate caloric intake to lose some body fat, what should the ratios of carbohydrates, protein, and fat be? When we build your *Live It Or Diet Lifestyle System*, we will be able to tell you what would be best for you. But for now, follow these guidelines:

Start with 20% protein, 60% carbohydrate, and 20% fat. (Based on averages.) Then review *Health Consideration Adjustments*.

Adjust your protein and fat based on those recommendations.

For example: If you are at risk for cardiovascular disease, or you are low thyroid (or both!) drop both your protein and fat intake to 15%. That leaves 70% from carbohydrates. <u>Make sure your carbohydrate sources come from whole grains, and fresh vegetables and fruits.</u>

It's Time to Get Physical

Okay, my friend... this is where you insert exercise.

That's right.

You've heard of your lymphatic system, right? It is the transit system in the body that moves wastes from the cells. But, unlike the circulatory system, it has no pump. So, daily exercise is necessary for the lymphatic system to detoxify itself. Lack of exercise can contribute to lymphatic overload and a build-up of toxins that aggravate your entire system.

Of course, exercise will also be the vehicle that escorts your unwanted fat outta here.

So...are you ready? Great!

Go to *CHAPTER 2: FITNESS-Under Construction*, page 11—and review the following section:

Cardiovascular Conditioning, page 28

Then figure out your target heart rate range for cardiovascular exercise with:

The Karvonen Formula, page 30

Put on your music, your sneakers, and let's go!

Follow the recommendations in *CHAPTER 2: FITNESS-Under Construction*, and commit to schedule some time each week to move your body.

(Remember to allow your body to cool itself during exercise. Review *Is It Ladylike to Sweat* on page 34.)

WEEKS TWO, THREE AND FOUR:
One Day At A Time

You must do the things you cannot do.

—Eleanor Roosevelt

Day 8: *Exercise Aerobically, Consider Strength Training*
Today, review the following sections in *CHAPTER 2: FITNESS-Under Construction*:

Pour The Foundation, page 15
Strength Training, page 35

Day 9: *Stop The Jiggling*
Remember, aerobic exercise will burn fat. It WILL NOT make you firm. If you are still not convinced that resistance exercise is an absolutely crucial component of <u>any</u> weight-management program, today revisit the following sections:

The Beauty Of Being Strong, page 35
The Negatives And Positives, page 37
Do Women Need To Train Differently From Men?, page 39

Day 10: *Some Cool Moves*
Okay. Ready to try something REALLY affective for those sagging body parts? Turn to:

A Little Behind In A Big Hurry, page 41
Exercises For The Rest Of You, page 57

Day 11: *How About Flexibility?*
Are you stretching when you exercise? Remember to first warm up, then stretch. Hold each stretch for at least a minute, breathing deeply in and out as you do. If you are not addressing your flexibility and your insertion points, turn to the following section for some encouragement:

Flexibility To Your Core, page 20

Day 12: *Food, Food, Glorious Food*
How about assessing your eating and shopping?

Return to page 288 and scan *Let's Go Shopping*.

Turn to page 348 for *Values Of Recommended Foods* for a quick reference guide to calories, carbohydrates, protein, fat, and fiber of many of the foods you might choose from on a healthy regimen.

Then go to page 350 for your *Shopping List.*

Day 13: *Are You Ready To Try Some New Recipes?*

Turn to page 269 and peruse Judith Lynne's section. It's a wonderful, lively adventure into the world of natural cooking. No time and stressed out? These fabulous recipes only take minutes!

By the way, if you are stressed, return to *What About Stress* on page 193.

Day 14: *Still Having Trouble Dropping Pounds Of Fat?*

There could be many reasons for that. Return to the section:

It's Not Fair! Our Stubborn Baby-boomer Fat Cells, page 219.

If you think you can, you can. And if you think you can't, you're right.

—Mary Kay Ash

Day 15: *Fat Fat Go Away!*

Arrrrrggg...don't you just hate the stuff? This is war! Arm yourself, and go back to this section that deals with our nemesis:

Cellulite, page 21

Then review how your body resists change in:

The Set Point Theory, page 151.

Meanwhile, continue exercising!

Day 16: *Still Confused About Proteins, Carbohydrates And Fats?*

I don't blame you. Recent publications are still reporting on the 'Diet Wars'— high protein-low carb, high carb-low fat, what's dangerous, what's not? Return to the following sections in *CHAPTER 3: FOOD—Now What Do I Eat*, to try and make sense of all this controversy:

Stop The Fatnasy!, page 74

Evaluating The "Big Three" Macronutrients, page 78

Fat Free—Fat Chance!, page 101

Day 17: Certain Foods Just Not "Agreeing With You?"

Chances are that you have a "sensitivity" (or "delayed onset" allergy) to them that is sabotaging your diet (by "diet" I mean as *Webster's* defines the word— "what you eat"—not what you <u>don't</u> eat—which is how our culture has come to define that word!). Turn to the following section and review a very common but often overlooked issue:

Food Allergies And Addictions, page 153

Day 18: *He Who Has The Most Toys When He Dies—Is Dead.*
I want to call your attention today to a very real, always hovering, deadly villain that threatens millions of baby-boomers—Heart Disease—our #1 killer. Please take a moment and review the following section. Thank you.

Eat To Live—Cardiovascular Disease, page 196

Day 19: *Are There Still Blocks To Your Success?*
There may be underlying issues present that you haven't addressed. In *CHAPTER 5: TAKING CONTROL,* there are many sections dealing with specific conditions. One (or more) may be sabotaging you. If you haven't already done so, review the following:

Hypoglycemia, page 165
Can I Give Myself Diabetes?, page 168
Candida Albicans, page 174
Thyroid Hormone, page 177

Day 20: *How Do You Feel?*
Check in. Ask your body what it needs today. On a scale of 1 to 10, how is your energy, mental clarity, emotional state, peace of mind? What does your body want to get it into gear, in sync with you and your day?

Go to *Your Food Must Become You* on page 189, and review the topics in that section.

Day 21: *What About Your Hormones?*
Are you experiencing the inevitable baby-boomer challenge, perimenopause? *CHAPTER 6: FEMININITY,* addresses many concerns and options. Review the following sections:

Osteoporosis, page 215
Hormone Replacement Therapy, page 225
What Is Aging Gracefully?, page 246

Day 22: *Old Habits Die Hard*
Sometimes, at this juncture, we have begun to fall back into some old habits. While some of us may be firmly entrenched in our healthy <u>new</u> habits by now, others may have started to slide. Let's go back and review some information that may bring back your fire. In *CHAPTER 3: FOOD—Now What Do I Eat*, I discussed some of your metabolic hormones. Return to:

Insulin And Glucagon—The Critical Balancing Act on page 96 for a jump start if you've stalled.
Glycemic Index vs. Effective Carbohydrate Content on page 106 for some

practical tips.

Just for kicks, if you are back in denial over sweets, go now to *Sweet Revenge* on page 117...

And get back on target!

Day 23: *Getting Bored?*

The great thing and the hard thing is to stick to things when you have outlived the first interest. —Janet Erskine Stuart

If you'd like a change in your exercise routine, try integrating cardio and strength training in one event. Turn to page 70 for *Circuit Training.*

Day 24: *Being Seduced?*

If you are being seduced by some "nasty" new diet, please go back to *Metabolism*, on page 147.

The Definition Of Insanity on page 138 is a another good section to return to if you want to bail out and "diet."

Remember our historical attitude, fellow baby-boomer, and do not just follow the masses. Turn to *We Interrupt This Broadcast* on page 141 for a memory jog.

Then, re-read my journey, *15 Rounds—My Championship Bout* on page 143, and... clear the confusion, along with your mind!

Day 25: *Now... Ready To Try Something Cool?*

Do you remember the chapter, *EATING FOR HEALTH, HEALING, AND HARMONY?* In that chapter I introduced to you The 5 Phase Theory. Return to it now, and try to integrate some of the principles of that awesome 5000 year old paradigm into your diet in the next four days. If you are still experiencing cravings, and if you feel like your body is missing something when you eat, you will be thrilled with how satisfied and nourished you feel when you prepare meals according to this awesome philosophy. Review the following sections:

The Self-Healing Cookbook Recommendations, page 261

The 5 Phase Theory, page 264

The 5 Phases, page 266

Day 27: *Applying New Principles*

Today, prepare a meal using The 5 Phase Theory. Turn to:

Incorporating Macrobiotics And The 5 Phase Theory, page 268

You will love how the 5 Phases makes you feel!

Day 28: *I'M PROUD OF YOU!*

I've been here before, just like you... and I wondered, "Why try this again?" I found the answer... deep inside me... where God has planted my strength and determination... and it changed my life. Look deep. It is there.

—Donna Michaels-Surface

Remember nothing's perfect, but you should congratulate yourself for getting this far! You have made the commitment, and learned a lot.

None of us likes getting older. Easing into this time of life (can you ever ease into aging???) is greatly assisted by <u>listening to your body</u>, and becoming intuitive and sensitive to its needs. None of us likes the inevitable changes that occur as we get older. But, oh, you can be so happy in your skin if you take care of what's under it!

Remember what I said at the beginning... this is <u>not</u> a "28 Day Program." It is a *program for life*. You have made adjustments and modifications that will dramatically impact your health, fitness, longevity, and quality of life!

VALUES OF RECOMMENDED FOODS

The following are just a few foods that you might be integrating into your food plan (they are not blood-type or metabolic-type specific). For the values of just about any other food (including many name-brand products) I recommend that you use *The Complete Book Of Food Counts* by Corinne Netzer as a reference.

White meat chicken—without skin—hormone free
Per Oz: *49 calories   8.5 grams protein   1.3 grams fat*

White meat turkey—without skin—hormone free
Per Oz: *45 calories   8 grams protein   1 gram fat*

97% extra lean ground beef—hormone free
Per Oz: *66 calories   5 grams protein   3 grams fat*

Venison
Per Oz: *45 calories   8.5 grams protein   1 gram fat*

Fish—snapper, cod, flounder, orange roughy, grouper, tile fish, sole, dolphin
Per Oz (approximately): *33 calories   7 grams protein   .5 grams fat*

Fish—tuna—chunk white in water
Per Oz: *35 calories   7.5 grams protein   .5 grams fat*

Fish—swordfish
Per Oz: *35 calories   6 grams protein   1 gram fat*

Tofu—firm

Per Oz: *41 calories   4.5 grams protein   1.2 grams carbohydrates   .7 grams fiber   2 grams fat*

Beans—black , adzuki, great northern, navy, kidney, pinto

Per 1/2 cup cooked (approximately): *90 calories   6 grams protein   15 grams carbohydrates   3 grams fiber   0 fat*

Lentils

Per 1/2 cup cooked: *115 calories   9 grams protein   20 grams carbohydrates   7.8 grams fiber   0 fat*

Egg whites—1

16 calories   3.35 grams protein   0 fat

Quinoa

1/4 cup dry: 170 calories   6 grams protein   31 grams carbohydrates   3 grams fiber   2.5 grams fat

Brown rice

1/4 cup dry: 150 calories   3 grams protein   33 grams carbohydrates   2 grams fiber   1 gram fat

Millet

1/4 cup dry: 150 calories   5 grams protein   32 grams carbohydrates   3 grams fiber   1.5 grams fat

Kamut

1/4 cup dry: 116 calories   5 grams protein   26 grams carbohydrates   4 grams fiber   .8 grams fat

Rye flakes

1/3 cup dry: 110 calories   4 grams protein   24 grams carbohydrates   4 grams fiber   .5 grams fat

Oat bran

1/3 cup dry: 150 calories   8 grams protein   23 grams carbohydrates   7 grams fiber   2.5 grams fat

Whole grain pastas—kamut & spelt

1/2 cup dry (approximately): 180-190 calories   8-10 grams protein   30-33 grams carbohydrates   5-6 grams fiber   1.5 grams fat

Wheat-free/high-fiber unrefined whole grain bread

Per slice (approximately): *100 calories   3 grams protein   15 grams carbohydrates   3 grams fiber   3 grams fat*

Baked potato in skin

5" x 2" (approximately): *220 calories   4.7 grams protein   51 grams carbohydrates   4.8 grams fiber*

Baked sweet potato in skin
5" x 2" (approximately): *118 calories   2 grams protein   28 grams carbohydrates   3.4 grams fiber*

Vegetables—broccoli, spinach, kale, zucchini, asparagus, green beans
Per 1/2 cup (approximately): *10-15 calories   1-2 grams protein   2-3 grams carbohydrates   1-2 grams fiber   0 fat*

Assorted berries—strawberries, raspberries, blueberries, blackberries
Per 3/4 cup (approximately): *70 calories   16 grams carbohydrates   2 grams fiber*

Apple
1—medium: *80 calories   21 grams carbohydrates   3.7 grams fiber*

Grapefruit
1/2 medium (approximately): *40 calories   11 grams carbs   1.3 grams fiber*

SHOPPING LIST

The following items are not blood type-specific. They are simply some reminders of wholesome foods to stock up on, and some brand names of products that I have used and worked with in my practice. If you cannot find some of these foods locally, call the numbers in Appendix G to order them.

PROTEINS

Meats & Poultry:
>Free-range Turkey
>Free-range Chicken
>Hormone-free 97% lean beef
>Buffalo
>Venison

Fish:
>Salmon (water-packed canned or fresh)
>Snapper
>Grouper
>Dolphin (Mahi-Mahi)
>Swordfish
>Tuna (water-packed canned or fresh)

Vegetable Protein:

> TVP (Texturized Vegetable-Soy Protein)
> *Eden, Hain*—Black, Adzuki, Black Soy, Pinto (other) Beans
> Dehydrated Black Beans
> Tofu (low-fat, extra firm)
> Tempeh
> *Boca Burgers*
> *LightLife* Lean Links Italian Soy Low-Fat Sausage (wheat and gluten-free)
> *White Wave* Baked Tofu (Teriaki, Mexican, etc.)

Protein Powders:
(Make sure there is no sugar and few carbs, and between 20 and 30 grams of protein)

> *Super Green Pro-96%* Protein Powder
> *Genisoy* 100% Soy Protein Powder
> *Wild Oats* Soy Protein Powder
> *Nature's Life Protein* 95% Soy Protein with Papain and Vanilla
> *The Ultimate Meal* Rice Protein Powder
> *Whey To Go* Whey Protein Powder
> *Designer Protein* Whey Protein Powder

Dairy (Alternative):

> *Better Than Milk* Lite Soy Powder
> *Rice Dream*
> Soy Milk
> Fat-Free *Soya Kaas* Soy Cheese
> *Rice-Slice* Pepper Jack Rice Cheese
> Soy Pepper Jack Cheese
> Rice Parmesan Cheese
> Goat cheese
> *White Wave* Soy Yogurt

CARBOHYDRATES

Grains:

> Quinoa
> Millet
> Kamut
> Brown or Wild Rice

Pastas (whole grain—at least 2 grams of fiber):

>   Spelt
>   Quinoa
>   Rice
>   Kamut Spirals

Breads:

>   Wheat Free/Gluten Free/Yeast Free High Fiber Bread
>   *Rudi's* Spelt Tortilla
>   *French Meadow* Wheat-Free Breads—Rice, Spelt & Millet
>   *Pacific Bakery Breads* (Spelt, Kamut, etc.)

Crackers:

>   Brown Rice Snaps
>   *Wasa* Rye
>   *Hol-Grain* Rice Crackers
>   *Finn Crisp*

Cereals:

>   *McCann's Irish Oatmeal* (in a tin)
>   *Arrowhead Mills* Steel Cut Oats
>   Oatbran
>   Kasha
>   *Puffins* Cereal
>   Amaranth Flakes (*Health Valley*)
>   Millet Rice Oatbran Flakes
>   Cream Of Rice
>   *Roman Meal* Cream of Rye (100% rye-5 grms fiber)
>   *Arrowhead Mills* Buckwheat Groats
>   Kasha
>   Kamut Flakes (*Arrowhead Mills*)
>   Spelt Flakes (*Arrowhead Mills*)

Vegetables:

>   Field Greens
>   Carrots
>   Spinach
>   Broccoli
>   Kale

Vegetables *(cont.)*:

    Sea Vegetables—Arami, Kombu, Wakame
    Pumpkin
    Squash: Acorn, Spaghetti, Winter, etc.
    Daikon Radish
    Burdock Root

Fruits:

    Raisons
    Prunes
    Pineapple
    Plums
    Apples
    Grapefruit
    Raspberries
    Strawberries

HIGH FAT FOODS

Oils:

    Cold Pressed Extra Virgin Olive Oil

Nuts & Seeds:

    Pumpkin Seeds (Spicy)

BEVERAGES

Juices:

    Prune
    Apple
    Cranberry

Misc. Beverages:

    Green Tea
    Ginger Tea
    Water With Lemon

OTHER

Spices:

> Ginger
> Cinnamon
> Cayenne Pepper
> Kelp Shaker
> *Gomasio*

Condiments:

> *Bragg Liquid Aminos*
> Lemon Juice
> Tamari (low sodium & wheat free)
> *Health Valley* No Salt Added Chicken Broth
> Low Sodium Vegetable Bouillon
> *Hain* Salt-Free Vegetable Broth
> Sweet Mellow White Miso Paste
> Brown Rice Vinegar
> Rice Butter
> Apple Butter
> Stevia

Desserts & Snacks:

> *Cliff Bars* (only the ones with 5 grms of fiber)
> *Genisoy* Soy Protein Bar
> *Pure Protein* Bar
> *Twin Labs* Diet Fuel Bar
> *Heaven Scent* Wheat Free/Sugar Free Cookies
> *Sweet Nothings* Frozen Soy Desert
> *It's Soy Delicious* Frozen Soy Dessert
> *Bearito's* Black Bean Dip
> Apple Sauce Apple/Peach   Apple/Apricot
> *Rice Dream*

BOOKS:

> *Nutrition Almanac, 4th Edition*
> *Corinne Netzer's Complete Book Of Food Counts*
> *Prescription For Nutritional Healing*

SUPPLEMENTS:

> Flax Seed:
>> *Arrowhead Mills* or *Nature's Life* Flax Seed Meal
>> *FibroFlax* Ground Flax Seed
>
> Digestive Enzymes (with Papain, Bromelain, HCL, etc.)
> *Beano*

SUPPLIES:

> *Misto* (mister for olive oil)

PHASE II

Phase II of your *Live It Or Diet System* will keep your momentum going. It will take how you look and feel to the next level.

For Phase II, and continued support, log on with us at *Live It Or Diet.com*. We will always be there for you, sharing the latest in health and fitness, and keeping our connection with you for your needs.

There is so much information to share with you beyond this book.

Stick with us...

But remember... you're in control!

No pessimist ever discovered the secrets of the stars, or sailed to an uncharted land, or opened a new heaven to the human spirit.

—Helen Keller

Live It Or Diet Lifestyle Systems®
HOME TESTING SOLUTION

Beyond Phase I (our 28 Day Foundational Plan) —
Phase II and your *Live It Or Diet System*

To build a **Phase II System** on your new healthier foundation (following your 28 Day Plan) we have researched and developed a scientific testing system (available at our Flagship Center in Fort Lauderdale, and at a growing number of health-care facilities across the country) that allows us to discover <u>exactly</u> what foods and nutritional supplements will support you, and, just as important, *which ones you should avoid.* This revolutionary testing also allows us to include *the specific exercise recommendations that fit <u>you</u>* as well.

But wait! What if we could put our Flagship Center right in your home?

If you do not have a *Live It Or Diet* Practitioner in your area, (call our toll-free hotline or log on to our website to find the LIOD Practitioner nearest you) the next best thing is to order our *Live It Or Diet* **Home-Test Kit.** This will allow you to perform the testing *we* need in the privacy of *your home.* Once we receive your Home-Test information, it will be evaluated by Dr. Gary at our Flagship Center in Fort Lauderdale. We will then send you *your* individualized *Live It Or Diet System* — a large, detailed package which will contain: your recommended daily calories for fat loss, the ratio of protein, carbohydrate, and fat appropriate for <u>you</u>, foods that will support you and foods that are sabotaging you, serving sizes, recipes, shopping list, exercise recommendations, a handy, laminated "Avoid Foods" card that fits in your wallet, plus much more valuable stuff. ☺

Call us on our *Live It Or Diet* toll-free hotline (**888-733-8537**) or visit our website, **www.LiveItOrDiet.com** for more information on **Phase I** and **Phase II.**

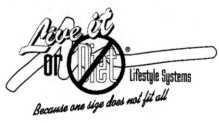

CHAPTER X

Your Live It or Diet Lifestyle System

A Holistic Approach

"Each of us is an integrated whole. We are not fragmented into separate parts each carrying a specific ailment or diagnostic category. We cannot be divided by any belief, lifestyle, relationship, or therapy without violating fundamental universal laws. Each of us is a unique individual, whole and complete, functioning as a totality in relation to the universe surrounding us. All states of health or disease must be viewed in this context. To the extent that we deviate from this perspective, we experience dis-harmony and dis-ease. Conversely, the more we live within this principle, the more we enjoy a balanced state of harmony and vitality."

—George Vithoulkas
Homeopathy: Medicine of the New Man

If we are going to deal with any individual's health and fitness issues, we must consider the <u>whole</u> person, including: Health history, family health history, genetic factors, cultural factors, social factors, relationships, experiences, perceptions, concepts and beliefs, psychological factors, spiritual factors, environment, hopes, dreams, aspirations, desires, fears, structural integrity of cells, tissues and organs, the functional efficiency of all organs and systems, diet, digestive efficiency, nutritional status, special needs, activity, etc. A lot of stuff, right? Well, you want this structure to withstand a hurricane, an earthquake, a tornado, don't you? Haven't we had enough "quick fixes" and patch jobs?

This is the "holistic" approach. George Vithoulkas in his book, *Homeopathy*, explains: "A holistic practitioner helps the 'client' to identify the various aspects of his or her life which tend to enhance the natural processes, and which aspects tend to oppose them. Thus, the primary responsibility for the recovery of his or her health is placed on the shoulders of the client. In this context, symptoms are seen as attempts by the body to heal or to signal distress, and they are respected as such—in marked contrast to the standard medical approach in which symptoms are viewed as disturbances to be suppressed." To this he adds that the "vital force" of an individual is sustained by the proper balance of nutrients, detoxification, and exercise.

Your *Live It Or Diet Lifestyle System* will be designed to amplify your <u>vital force</u>. You may not have conditions that threaten your life, but aren't they *Quality Of Life* threatening? Aren't there things you <u>don't do</u> anymore because of the way you look and feel? Haven't they been replaced by rituals that annoy or even disgust you? Haven't you had enough? You bet you have! Time for <u>your</u> "Game Plan."

THE PLAYERS IN YOUR GAME PLAN

One man's meat is another man's poison

—Lucretius
Roman philosopher (1 A.D.)

Before you get more specific about <u>your</u> plan of attack, we must first assess who <u>you</u> are, and what <u>your</u> level of health and functioning is. Remember, your plan must address many factors that contribute to the uniqueness of you. Let's review some of the key players:

- Your *Overall Health History*—recognizing and compensating for specific issues like cardiovascular disease, diabetes, hypertension, etc.
- Your *Blood Type*—which recent studies show to be a significant means of evaluating your nutrition and exercise needs
- Your *Food Allergies*—seemingly innocent but hazardous foods for you
- Your *Pancreatic Function*—identifying insulin resistance, hypoglycemia, and sugar-sensitivity
- Your *Immune Function*—and opportunistic attackers like Candida Albicans
- Your *Oxidative Rate*—the rate at which your body burns sugar
- Your *Thyroid Function*—your metabolic rate (and thus every process of the body) is affected by this gland
- Your *Glandular Balance*—the harmony necessary for wellness (homeostasis)
- Your *pH Balance*—the critical alkaline/acid condition of your body
- Your *Digestive Efficiency*—what foods you are able to assimilate without dis-<u>stress</u> to your system

•Your *Liver Function*—and your body's ability to detoxify, and metabolize fat

•Your *Gut Condition*—identifying conditions such as leaky gut & dysbiosis

•Your *Metabolic Type*—recognizing your dominant and recessive glands

Rather than giving you a "program," we will evaluate all the different players in your game plan. You will have guidelines for your players, which will increase your odds for success. For example, some people need more protein, some need more fat, and some are sabotaging themselves with excessive carbohydrate intake. Some people need to eat frequently throughout the day—and for others, this may not be a good idea at the start of his or her program. You may be eating certain foods that your body is allergic to, which sets off a whole series of undesirable metabolic consequences. You also may need serious resistance exercise with not as much emphasis on cardio, where as for others it might be just the opposite. Another group may need an activity more along the lines of yoga, while another may need to choose a more aggressive activity such as "boxer-size." Do you get the point? The fitness program that worked for your sister or your friend probably won't work for you, and chances are if it were a diet...it won't continue to work for them either. *You simply cannot randomly eliminate foods or drastically reduce calories.* It must be more specific than that, or you will set off a tailspin reaction that will result in uncontrollable craving and bingeing. We need to learn how our bodies work, and what our realistic expectations should be. We must take all of the relentlessly changing information and apply only what is appropriate to ourselves.

TRINA AND MICHELLE

I want to tell you a quick story just to illustrate the importance of diet individualization. I met Trina first. She came to me looking for what she called a "coach"...someone to guide her through the insane terrain of the diet world. She had been there several times before, and always got blown up by land mines. She didn't want to go there alone again. After Trina went through her testing and evaluation, she began a nutrition regimen designed specifically for her; one that would support her special needs and balance her body. It was filled with healthy, nutritious, organic foods that were extremely beneficial for her. Trina lost fat, gained energy, and was very excited about her new journey.

Trina moved in with her friend, Michelle, and the two roommates happily followed Trina's *Live It Or Diet Lifestyle System*. Trina cooked and shopped for both of them. They ate all of the foods that were recommended for Trina. Trina continued to lose fat, but...uh-oh...Michelle began to gain fat! How could this be? She was eating healthier than she had ever eaten. Her house was now stocked (thanks to Trina) with whole grains, organic produce, free-range poultry, and healthy snacks. What was going on?

Michelle was following <u>Trina's</u> food plan, which was designed to compensate for the foods that sabotaged <u>Trina</u>. Michelle did not know that some of the foods (and the ratios of how they should be consumed) that were great for <u>Trina</u>, were not appropriate for <u>her</u>. When she came to have her own *Live It Or Diet Lifestyle System* built, she found out that she needed <u>a different game plan</u> from Trina's. Trina was a *slow oxidizer*. Michelle's oxidative rate was extremely *fast*. Trina's blood type is A, Michelle's is O. They have some different food intolerance's. Their caloric requirements are not the same, nor are their ratios of carbohydrates to protein. Trina needed to stress cardiovascular exercise. Michelle needed more strength training. And the differences continued. Bottom line—Michelle needed <u>Michelle's</u> program.

By entering the world of Live It Or Diet, you will be embarking on an exciting and life-altering journey. Your experience will be educational, stimulating, and interactive. You will discover the appropriate program for you, and we will help you build it.

We acknowledge that our method requires your participation, while the others you have tried might have just had you lamely follow an already set plan. If that seemed to fit into your "challenged lifestyle" better than this, then why did you need another book? It didn't work, that's why!

Supplemental Support
On your *Live It Or Diet Lifestyle System*, we will determine what kind of supplemental support is needed to help your body achieve homeostasis.

Exercise
Your *Live It Or Diet Lifestyle System* will also offer you exercise recommendations—specific to <u>your</u> needs. Not everyone is drawn to the same type of exercise, and for that matter—*not everyone should do the same type of exercise*. First, you will not continue to do an activity you hate, so it makes no sense to try and force you to do it. Second, *your metabolic/oxidative type has distinct needs regarding exercise*, and they will vary in category and ratio from one to another (for example: Some people will need more strength training than cardio, and for others this will be reversed).

DIETARY TYPING

Your *Live It Or Diet Lifestyle System* will incorporate a unique way of establishing your nutritional needs. We have integrated the research and counsel from important projects involving blood type, oxidative rate, pH balance, food allergies, thyroid (metabolism) and other glandular function, hypoglycemia, dysbiosis, sugar regulation, and metabolic body type. *Certain foods will support your immune system, encourage fat loss, and increase your energy, while others may sabotage your efforts and irritate your system.* Your body reacts to irritants by trying to protect itself. One way it does this is to fill its tissues with fluid. This looks and feels and weighs like fat! When you eliminate these foods from your diet, <u>you will lose weight!</u> You will feel better! You will have more energy! This is the foundation of *Live It Or Diet Lifestyle Systems.* Remember the "tennis matches" in this book: Fat leads to fat! No, sugar leads to fat! Eat more carbs, less protein! No—more protein, less carbs! Fat free! No—more fat!

Man. And this is all from very smart folks! What's it tell you? Somewhere in the middle of this mess is the answer for <u>you</u>.

When we build your *Live It Or Diet Lifestyle System,* we will be cross-referencing the information derived from all of our researched methods of identification. We will take this information and zero-in on the overlapping recommendations. (Remember, as I worked with our system I observed exciting correlations between the above considerations.)

Your *Live It Or Diet Lifestyle System* will sort out the best foods and ratios for you to consume. We realize that simply telling you *what foods to eat,* and *what foods to stay away from* might not give you sufficient parameters in which to operate. We will therefore include guidelines for daily caloric, protein, carbohydrate, and fat requirements. These will be based on computations factoring in lean body mass, age, activity level, etc. But, remember that we do not believe in obsessing over numbers...whether it be on a scale or a food label.

If you eat the way we recommend, all of that will take care of itself. By simply adjusting your daily eating habits in the right direction...

You will become naturally leaner!

WHERE TO BEGIN

A heightened awareness of everything we eat and come in contact with is critical. Eating organically grown produce and grains, choosing hormone and drug-free animal protein, taking responsibility for as many of your daily meals as you can, drinking clean water, ingesting lots of fiber, exercising, managing stress, taking supportive nutrients—this is how to begin. Also, do you need to address some gut and liver issues? Chances are pretty good that you do (if you have picked up this book)! These are critical steps, my friend. If we do not take them, our journey will lead to <u>nowhere</u>.

For where to have a *Live It Or Diet System* built for you—turn to *Appendix C.*

See you there.

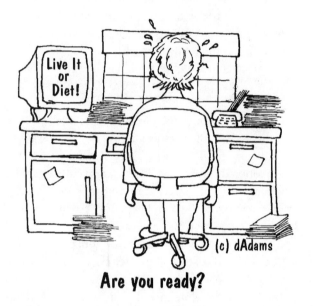

Are you ready?

"...A clear and rational approach to weight management ...offering straightforward answers to age-old questions."

—John Hinze,
Pharm. D., N.M.D.

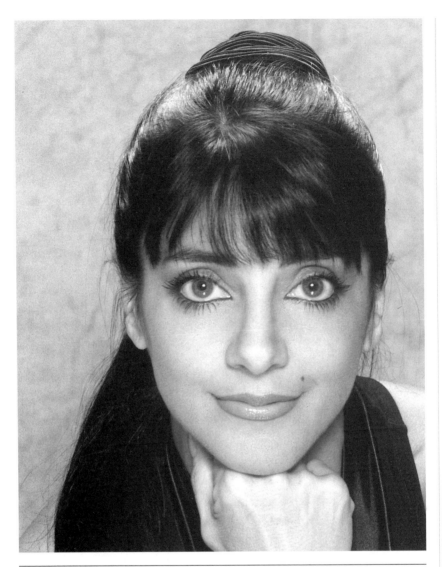

DONNA MICHAELS-SURFACE, CPTS, ACSM

Donna is certified by the American College of Sports Medicine, and an honor graduate of The Fitness Institute International (Valedictorian, class of '88). Donna's 20 years in the fitness arena have taken her from 50 pounds "over-fat"—to a nationally ranked competitive body builder. From 1997 to the present, she has been the president of Live It Or Diet, Inc. During this time she developed *Live It Or Diet Lifestyle Systems* and adapted it for health clubs, clinics, doctor's offices, and pharmacies under the direction of Dr. Gary

Snyder. She also conducted a research project studying the effects of exercise on oxidative rate.

From 1995-1997, Donna was the National Fitness Director of MET-Rx Substrates, Inc. where she: Developed programs for the modeling community, designed women's exercise protocols for METRx's "The Balance Program," lectured nationally on nutrition and exercise, and presented these at national aerobic and fitness conferences. From 1988 to 1995, Donna was the owner and president of The Fitness Team, Inc., and The US Total Fitness Team, Inc. These companies were contracted to develop, market, and pilot the fitness/weight management divisions of health clubs and corporations. Donna designed protocols, trained individuals, and developed special-needs programs for: Traumatic brain injury victims, the obese, children, the elderly, and the physically challenged. During this time Donna also created "I'm Losin' It," a nutrition program, and served as Fitness Director of US Total Fitness Health Clubs where she: Supervised the training in all clubs, hired and trained the training staff, developed and supervised the nutrition system in the clubs, developed corporate programs, and designed programs for competitive and professional athletes. Donna's fourteen years of experience as a professional actor and director enabled her to create, produce, and perform in her own fitness segments (called The Action '5' Fitness Team—which regularly aired on the NBC affiliate, WPTV in South Florida) and serve as the channel 5 health/fitness expert from 1991 to 1992. She has also written, produced and starred in a television pilot targeting "family fitness," shot on South Beach, called *The Fitness Team*.

Donna is older than 50 and younger than dirt.

GARY S. SNYDER, B.A.,B.S.,D.C.,D.N.B.H.E.

I have referred to "Dr. Gary" throughout this book. He is the person I have been working with to identify myself and my needs—and I have collaborated with him on this book and the *Live It Or Diet Lifestyle Systems*.

Dr. Snyder is the owner, founder, and director of The Clinical Nutrition Center in Ft. Lauderdale, Florida. People from all over the world come to Dr. Snyder's clinic to address their health problems with his state of the art, alternative methods of testing and treatment.

Dr. Snyder has been in practice twenty-five years, and has spent the last thirty-three years developing his own unique brand of medicine. His educational accomplishments include a bachelors in Human Biology, a doctorate in Chiropractic, and a post-graduate degree in Bio-Nutrition. He is one of only a handful of doctors that hold a specialty certification in Clinical Nutrition (proprietary drugs) and is board certified in Homeopathy. He has also logged thousands of hours studying alternative medicine around the world. Along with his clinical duties, Dr. Snyder is a consultant to several Nutritional and Homeopathic companies. He is not only involved in the development of the *"Live It Or Diet" Lifestyle System*, but he has formulated the system's natural metabolic formulas with Dr. Jack Hinze (Doctor of Pharmacy, Doctor of Naturopathic Medicine, and certified Clinical Nutritionist).

But, to me, Dr. Gary's most impressive credit is that he profoundly cares. His knowledge, generosity, tenacity, and spirit have helped and inspired me more than I could write in ten books.

KEEP THE FIRE BURNING!

Remember, your results will be proportionate to your commitment. You are in control. What else in life can you say that about? Relationships? Your job? Your kids? You can do this. Hey, you know all about me now, so you must also know that if *I* can do it, *anyone* can. But, the most difficult task I have ever undertaken is to somehow communicate to you what sparked my fire and kept it burning these past seventeen years. It is like trying to describe another realm—another *dimension*. We exist in a four dimensional world, but most of us only *live* in three dimensions. When you tap into your *innate intelligence*—the force within you—you have entered the fourth dimension. This is the dimension where all things are possible. But, we only have three dimensional words to describe an experience that exists beyond that. The best I can do with the language that we have is to tell you that *it's not just your* presented in this book is *within all of us*. Not just me.

And now, my friend, I leave you to it...with these words:

When one exercises in a way that increases range of motion,
one necessarily opens up areas of the body
which have become closed over time.
With this opening,
pathways of energy are freed
that were locked up
holding incomplete experience.
"Incomplete" meaning...not fully experienced,
or, not learned from and released.
An experience of this type stays lodged in the body
until:
One learns from it...
realizes why one brought it on himself...
understands the teaching it is in his life...
forgives himself and everyone else for the pain involved...
then lets it go...
thus releasing any hold the experience had on his life.

This is the true meaning of fitness,
where one cleanses oneself
of both the physiological and psychological blocks
to full range of motion and expression.

Many people these days exercise
to avoid a lifetime of incomplete experiences,
never breaking up the patterns of resistance,
and thus not letting go of what about them
is stuck and blocked.
Hence, they look fit,
But are not free.

The popular concept of fitness has been narrowed

to mean a particular look, a performance level.
It is not seen as a complete
mental, emotional and physical relationship.
One can feel refreshed after a workout
through simple physiological exertion.
This is quite different
from working within oneself
to remove resistance to full range of motion,
to re-establish patterns of smooth effortless strength,
and let go of memories and experiences lodged in the body
which hold one back from fuller self expression.
When one begins to see fitness
as a mental, emotional, physical, spiritual interrelationship
which has its purpose,
not distance, time, number of reps, or an appearance,
but rather a broadening, deepening and freeing
of the self within,
then one can exercise
in a truly creative and regenerating way.

—Author Unknown

RESOURCES

NUTRITION
Essentials of Nutrition, Edward Dratz, Ph.D. D.
University of California at Berkeley Wellness Letter, 1995
Modern Nutrition In Health And Disease, Lea & Febiger
Coaches Guide to Nutrition & Weight Control, Human Kinetics Publishers
Understanding Nutrition, Whitney & Hamilton
International Journal of Sport Nutrition, Priscilla M. Clarkson, Ph.D.
The Zone and Mastering The Zone, Barry Sears, Ph.D.
Protein Power, Michael R. Eades, M.D. & Mary Dan Eades, M.D.
New Diet Revolution, Robert C. Atkins, M.D.
Healing With Whole Foods, Paul Pitchford
The Vegetarian Way, Virginia Messina, M.P.H., R.D. & Mark Messina, Ph.D.
Eat Right For Your Type, Peter J.D'Adamo, N.D.
Outsmarting The Female Fat Cell, Debra Waterhouse, M.P.H., R.D.
Outsmarting The Midlife Fat Cell, Debra Waterhouse, M.P.H., R.D.
The Complete Book Of Food Counts, Corinne T. Netzer
The Nutrition Almanac, Gayla and John Kirschmann/Fourth Edition
Eating Alive, Jonn Matsen, N.D.
Physiology—Little, Brown Text Book, Charles H. Tadlock
Leaky Gut Syndrome, Elizabeth Lipski, M.S., C.C.N.
Prescription For Nutritional Healing, James Balch, M.D.
The MSM Miracle, Earl Mindell, R.Ph., Ph.D.
Earl Mindell's Vitamin Bible, Earl Mindell, R. Ph., Ph.D.
Food Is A Wonder Medicine, Neal Barnard, M.D.
Foods That Can Cause You To Lose Weight, Neal Barnard, M.D.
Nutrition For Fitness And Sport, Melvin H. Williams
The Self-Healing Cookbook, Kristina Turner
The Natural Gourmet, Annemarie Colbin
The Carbohydrate Addict's Diet, Richard F. Heller, Ph.D. &
Rachael F. Heller, Ph.D.
Sugar Busters!, H. Leighton Steward, Morrison C. Bethea, M.D.,
Sam S. Andrews, M.D., Luis A. Balart, M.D.

BODY FAT
Anti-Fat Nutrients, Dallas Clouatre, Ph.D.
The McDougall Program For Maximum Weight Loss, John A. McDougall, M.D.
Eat More, Weigh Less, Dean Ornish, M.D.
The Pritikin Weight Loss Breakthrough, Robert Pritikin

The Cellulite Solution, Elizabeth Dancey, M.D.
Outsmarting The Female Fat Cell, Debra Waterhouse, M.P.H., R.D.
Outsmarting The Midlife Fat Cell, Debra Waterhouse, M.P.H., R.D.

EXERCISE

Medicine and Science in Sports and Exercise, G.A. Brooks
Medicine and Science in Sports and Exercise, G.L. Dohm
It's Better To Believe, Kenneth H. Cooper, M.D.
Fitness Motivation, W. Jack Rejeski, Ph.D & Elizabeth A. Kenney, MA
Designing Resistance Training Programs, Steven Fleck, Ph.D.&
William Kraemer, Ph.D.
Exercise, Fitness, And Health: A Consensus Of Current Knowledge,
Human Kinetics
Guidelines For Exercise Testing And Prescription, A.C.S.M.
Exercise Metabolism, Mark Hargreaves, Ph.D.
The Body You Love, Phil Kaplan

AGING

What Every Woman Should Know...Staying Healthy After 40, Lila Nachtigall,
M.D.
On Women Turning 50, Cathleen Rountree
The Youth Corridor, Gerald Imber, M.D.
The Bodywise Woman, The Melpomene Institute for Women's Health Research
How And Why We Age, Leonard Hayflick, Ph.D.

HORMONE REPLACEMENT THERAPY

Women's Bodies, Women's Wisdom, Christiane Northrup, M.D.
Growth Hormone Synergism-DMC Health Sciences, Douglas M. Crist
The New England Journal of Medicine, July 5,1990, Effects of Human Growth
Hormone
Journal of Endocrinology, J.M. Tanner & R.H. Whitehouse
DHEA Reference Supplement to Health and Healing, Dr. Julian Whitaker
DHEA A Practical Guide, Ray Sahelian, M.D.
What Your Doctor May Not Tell You About Menopause, John R. Lee, M.D.
What Your Doctor May Not Tell You About Premenopause, John R. Lee, M.D.
The Superhormone Promise, William Regelson, M.D. & Carol Colman
The Miracle of Natural Hormones, David Brownstein, M.D.
Natural Hormone Replacement, Jonathan V. Wright, M.D. & John
Morgenthaler
The Living Soy Superfood, Tonita d'Raye

FOOD ALLERGIES AND ADDICTIONS
Food Addiction...The Body Knows, Kay Sheppard
Food Allergy And Nutrition Revolution, James Braly, M.D.
Winning The War Against Asthma & Allergies, Ellen W. Cutler, D.C.
Say Goodbye To Illness, Devi S. Nambudripad, D.C., R.N., Ph.D.
Your Hidden Food Allergies Are Making You Fat, Rudy Rivera, M.D. & Roger D. Deutsch

HYPOGLYCEMIA
The Do's And Don'ts Of Low Blood Sugar, Roberta Ruggiero

SUGAR-SENSITIVITY AND SEROTONIN
Potatoes Not Prozac, Kathleen DesMaisons, Ph. D.
5-HTP Boosts Serotonin Levels The Natural Way, Michael T. Murray, N.D.

CANDIDA ALBICANS
The Missing Diagnosis, C. Orian Truss, M.D.
The Yeast Connection: A Medical Breakthrough, William G. Crook, M.D.

ACID-ALKALINE BALANCE AND TOXIC WASTES
Alkalize Or Die, Theodore A. Baroody, N.D.,D.C.,Ph.D.
Reverse Aging, Sang Whang
Detoxification & Healing, Sidney MacDonald Baker, M.D.
The 20-Day Rejuvenation Diet Program, Jeffrey Bland, Ph.D.
Your Health...Your Choice, Dr. M. Ted Morter, Jr., M.A.
Homeopathy—Medicine Of The New Man, George Vithoulkas

OXIDATIVE RATE
Nutrition And Your Mind, George Watson, Ph.D.
The Balance, Oz Garcia

METABOLIC TYPING
Your Body Knows, Ann Louise Gittleman, M.S.
Different Bodies—Different Diets, Carolyn L. Mein, D.C.
The Body Code, Jay Cooper, M.S.
Medicine's Missing Link, Tom and Carole Valentine
Personalized Metabolic Nutrition Practictioners Manual, Harold J. Kristal, D.D.S

THYROID FUNCTION
Hypothyroidism: The Unsuspected Illness, Broda O. Barnes, M.D.

CANCER
The Breast Cancer Prevention Diet, Bob Arnot, M.D.
Prostate Health In 90 Days, Larry Clapp, Ph.D.

HEART DISEASE
Dr. Dean Ornish's Program For Reversing Heart Disease, Dr. Dean Ornish
Is Heart Surgery Necessary?, Julian Whitaker, M.D.

BALANCE
Between Heaven And Earth, Harriet Beinfield L.Ac. & Efrem Korngold, L.Ac., O.M.D.
Your Body's Many Cries For Water, F. Batmanghelidj, M.D.

MEDICINE
Ask The Doctor, Derrick M. DeSilva Jr., M.D.

CHIROPRACTIC
The Neurobiologic Mechanisms In Manipulative Therapy, Irvin M. Korr
Chiropractic Speaks Out, Chester A. Wilk, D.C.
The Chiropractor's Adjustor, D.D. Palmer

PHASE I: STARTING THE PROCESS
Acidophilus and Colon Health, David Webster
An Analytical System of Clinical Nutrition, Guy R. Schenker, D.C.
The Homeopathic Review, Institute of Quantum and Molecular Medicine

APPENDIX

APPENDIX A: AMERICAN COLLEGE OF SPORTS MEDICINE RISK FACTOR CHECKLIST

Individuals at higher risk are those with at least one major coronary risk factor, and/or symptoms suggestive of cardiopulmonary or metabolic disease. An exercise test prior to beginning a vigorous exercise program is desirable for high risk individuals of any age.

Major Coronary Risk Factors:
Age: 45 + years
History of high blood pressure (above 140/90)
Sedentary lifestyle
Current cigarette smoking
High cholesterol (above 180)
Diabetes
Heart attack, coronary bypass, or other cardiac surgery
Chest discomfort—especially with exertion
Extra, skipped, or rapid heart beats/palpitations
Heart murmurs, clicks, or unusual cardiac findings
Rheumatic fever
Ankle swelling
Peripheral vascular disease
Phlebitis
Unusual shortness of breath
Lightheadedness or fainting
Pulmonary disease including asthma, emphysema, and bronchitis
Abnormal blood lipids
Stroke
Family history
Coronary disease, sudden death, congenital heart disease—prior to age 50

Other Considerations:
Emotional disorders
Medications of all types
Recent illness, hospitalization or surgical procedure
Drug allergies
Orthopedic problems, arthritis
Habits

Caffeine, including cola drinks
Alcohol
Unusual habits of dieting

APPENDIX B: GLYCEMIC INDEX OF FOODS

The higher the number, the faster the absorption rate into the bloodstream, the more rapid the secretion of insulin.

Quickly Absorbed

Tofu frozen dessert 155
Glucose 138
Rice cakes 133
Puffed rice 132
Puffed wheat 132
French bread 131
Honey 126
Instant white rice 12I
Corn Flakes 121
Instant potato 120
Peeled potato 117
Rice Crispies 112
40% Bran Flakes 104
Crackers, plain, no fiber 100
White bread 100
Corn chips 100

"Whole wheat" bread 100
Grape-Nuts 100
Carrots 92
Rolled oats 90
Brown rice 82
Corn 82
Banana 82
Most cookies 80
White Potato 80
All-Bran 74
Kidney beans 74
Canned baked beans 70

Moderately Absorbed

Couscous 66
Bulgur 65
Orange juice 65
Pasta 64
Raisins 64
Beets 64
Chickpeas 60
Yams 52
Peas 50
Butter beans 46
Rye kernels 46
Grapes 45

Apple juice 45
Whole grain rye bread 42
Navy beans 40
Pinto beans 40
Oranges 40

More Slowly Absorbed

Apple 39	Lentils 30
Fat-free yogurt 39	Peaches 29
Yogurt 36	Grapefruit 26
Lima beans 36	Plums 25
Ice cream 36	Cherries 23
Pears 34	Soybeans 20
Black-eyed peas 33	Peanuts 13

CONTACT US AT LIVE IT OR DIET

For Products, Services, Support, And Information

    Live It Or Diet Information Hotline: 888-733-8537

    Our Virtual Live It Or Diet Center: www.liveitordiet.com

APPENDIX C: LIVE IT OR DIET LIFESTYLE SYSTEM LOCATIONS

Visit our website or call our hotline to locate a *Live It Or Diet* practitioner in your area.

APPENDIX D: TOOLS AND TOYS

PowerBlock 800-466-3215

For additional product information, visit our website or call our hotline.

APPENDIX E: TESTING

Live It Or Diet Home Testing & Starter Kit

Food Allergy Testing

Hormone Testing

For product information, visit our website or call our hotline. (See above)

APPENDIX F: LIVE IT OR DIET PRODUCTS AND INFORMATION

Phase I Protocol-*Let's Get Started*

Donna Michaels Audio and Video Tapes

Daily Food Journal

For product information, visit our website or call our hotline. (See above)

APPENDIX G: ADDITIONAL PRODUCTS AND INFORMATION

Dr. John Lee's Medical Letter 800-528-0559

Paul Perlow Design 212-758-4398

Paul Greco Studio 305-893-0433

Minnie Pauz www.minniepauz.com

Magni Publishing Company www.magnico.com

APPENDIX H: DOCTORS, CLINICS, AND PROGRAMS

Live It Or Diet Flagship Center in Fort Lauderdale 888-733-8537

Dr. Gary S. Snyder

   Clinical Nutrition Center 954-486-4000

Radiant Recovery 888-579-3970 www.radiantrecovery.com

The Fitness Institute International 954-786-1442

Lee-Benner Institute 800-968-8418

Dr. Helene Friedberg   The Skin Care Center 954-202-7388

Daniel G. Clark, M.D.

   Bio Active Nutritional   800-288-9525

James Braly, M.D.

   www.drbralyallergyrelief.com

Sidney MacDonald Baker, M.D.

   www.sbakermd.com

APPENDIX I: INTERNATIONAL LIVE IT OR DIET INFORMATION

For Products And Services In The United Kingdom:

   01442 266244 (phone number to be used within the U.K.)

AFTERWORD

Dear Friend...

There is something I'd like to share with you before I close. It took me six years to write this book—partly because of the research—but mostly because I became confused about the message I wanted to deliver to you. Then, mercifully, I came out of the fog and saw clearly what I needed to say.

You see, for most of my life I behaved very irresponsibly. And, I figured, it was pretty much a write-off. You know—no sense in changing now—the damage is done. Then, at a place called Calvary Chapel Fort Lauderdale, God showed me that I could start all over again—just like a brand new child—any time I was ready to. And, when I did, my entire life changed.

You can start over too—any time at all. With each moment comes a fresh new opportunity to keep a promise to yourself—renew a commitment—begin again. That's the awesome thing about Living In The Moment...each moment comes with a clean slate. You don't have to beat yourself up over failure. Don't look back, and you can give this to yourself.

But, always remember, my friend...it's the contents, not the container, that is the gift. Honor that...and you will succeed.

God bless you, and your journey home

Donna

Stay in touch with Donna & Dr. Gary

At

LiveItOrDiet.com

Visit us at our exciting virtual center, where we will be keeping you up-to-date on the ever-changing world of health & fitness. When you enter our center, you will be able to explore this fascinating world without leaving the comfort of your home or office! Feel free to drop in often. There will always be something new to share with you.

Donna

SO MUCH TO LOOK FORWARD TO

- Your <u>own</u> Virtual Live It Or Diet System…built on line for <u>you</u>!
- Directions to your nearest Live It Or Diet Center to have <u>your</u> system built ONE ON ONE
- Links to other incredible web-sites to widen your world of knowledge
- Browse in our <u>Free</u> area and have <u>fun</u> while you access cutting-edge information
- Order new Live It Or Diet products as they become available
- Subscribe to our Live It Or Diet newsletter
- Learn when and where Donna and Dr. Gary will be speaking in your area
- Receive <u>Free</u> updates on late-breaking research and discoveries

And much, much more!

Live It Or Diet™
The Health/Fitness Solution For The New Millennium

Fort Lauderdale, Florida
888-733-8537
www.liveitordiet.com

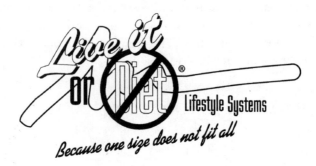

Donna Michaels-Surface

President

Live It Or Diet Lifestyle Systems®

**1400 East Oakland Park Blvd.
Suite 100
Fort Lauderdale, Fl. 33334**

954-564-5053 / 888-733-8537

www.LiveItOrDiet.com

livefit@aol.com